Late Onset Schizophrenia

Late Onset Schizophrenia

Edited by

ROBERT HOWARD

Senior Lecturer and Consultant in Old Age Psychiatry,
Institute of Psychiatry and Maudsley Hospital, London, UK

PETER V. RABINS

Professor of Psychiatry, Johns Hopkins University School of Medicine,
Baltimore, Maryland, USA

DAVID J. CASTLE

Clinical Director, Directorate of Mental Health Services,
Fremantle Hospital and Health Services, Western Australia

WRIGHTSON BIOMEDICAL PUBLISHING LTD
Petersfield, UK and Philadelphia, USA

The cover illustration is Daphne Reynolds' *The Watchers*.
© Crown Copyright: UK Government Art Collection.
Harold Wilson (British Prime Minister 1964–70 and 1974–76) hung this picture in his study at
10 Downing Street. Obsessed with the clandestine activities of the security services, Wilson
would tell visitors that the light socket above a portrait of Gladstone was really a secret
bugging device and on the day he became premier in 1974 he remarked to an aide, 'There
are only three people listening – you, me and MI5'. George Bush as head of the CIA had to
fly to London to reassure Wilson that the agency had not infiltrated his office. Painted as *The
Watcher*, Reynolds' intention that the foreground figure was observing the distant figures
took on a more persecutory interpretation with a change in the picture's name during
Wilson's tenure.

Editorial Office:

Wrightson Biomedical Publishing Ltd
Ash Barn House, Winchester Road, Stroud,
Petersfield, Hampshire GU32 3PN, UK
Telephone: 44 (0)1730 265647
Fax: 44 (0)1730 260368

British Library Cataloguing in Publication Data
Late onset schizophrenia
   1. Schizophrenia in old age
   I. Howard, Robert, 1961– II. Rabins, Peter V. III. Castle,
   David J.
   618.9'768982

Library of Congress Cataloging in Publication Data
Late onset schizophrenia / edited by Robert Howard, Peter V. Rabins,
   David J. Castle.
      p. cm.
   Includes bibliographical references and index.
   ISBN 1-871816-39-4 (hard cover)
   1. Schizophrenia in old age. Cross-cultural studies.
   2. Psychiatry, Transcultural. I. Howard, Robert, 1961– .
   II. Rabins, Peter V. III. Castle, David J.
   [DNLM: 1. Schizophrenia. 2. Cross-Cultural Comparison. 3. In Old
   Age.   WM 203 L351 1999]
   RC514.L35 1999
   616.89'82--dc21
   DNLM/DLC   99-22797
   for Library of Congress   CIP

ISBN 1 871816 39 4

Composition by Scribe Design, Gillingham, Kent
Printed in Great Britain by Biddles Ltd, Guildford

Contents

Contributors

Kirsten Abelskov, *Psychogeriatic Department, Psychiatric Hospital, 8240 Risskov, Denmark*

Luis Agüera-Ortiz, *Psychiatry Department, University Hospital 12 de Octubre, Madrid, Spain*

Osvaldo P. Almeida, *Department of Psychiatry and Behavioural Science, Queen Elisabeth II Medical Centre, Nedlands, Perth, Western Australia 6009*

Nancy C. Andreasen, *Mental Health Clinical Research Center, Department of Psychiatry, The University of Iowa Hospitals and Clinics, 200 Hawkins Drive, Iowa City, Iowa 52242-1057, USA*

David J. Castle, *Directorate of Mental Health Services, Fremantle Hospital and Health Service, Alma Street Centre, Fremantle, Western Australia 6160*

Jean-Pierre Clément, *Psychiatric Service of the University Hospital, Esquirol Hospital Centre, 15 rue du Dr Marcland, 87025 Limoges, France*

P. Fitzgerald, *The Centre for Addictions and Mental Health, Clarke Division, Department of Psychiatry, 250 College Street, Toronto, Ontario M56 1R8, Canada*

Heinz Häfner, *University Psychiatric Outpatient Department, Petersgraben 4, CH-4031, Basel, Switzerland*

Robert Howard, *Section of Old Age Psychiatry, Institute of Psychiatry, De Crespigny Park, London SE5 8AF, UK*

Dilip V. Jeste, *Department of Psychiatry and Neurosciences, Geriatric Psychiatry Intervention Center, University of California, San Diego, California 92161, USA*

Shitij Kapur, *Department of Psychiatry, University of Toronto, 250 College Street, Toronto, Ontario M56 1R8, Canada*

David W.K. Kay, *Visiting Professor in the Department of Psychiatry, University of Newcastle, 1–4 Claremont Terrace, Newcastle upon Tyne NE2 4AE, UK*

Sudhir Khandelwal, *Department of Psychiatry, B.P. Koirala Institute of Health Sciences, Dharan, Nepal*

Fauzia Simjee McClure, *Department of Psychiatry, Geriatric Psychiatry Intervention Center, University of California, San Diego, California 92161, USA*

Pøvl Munk-Jørgensen, *University Psychiatric Outpatient Department, Petersgraben 4, CH-4031 Basel, Switzerland*

Godfrey D. Pearlson, *Johns Hopkins University School of Medicine, 600 N. Wolfe Street, Baltimore, Maryland 21287-7279, USA*

Peter V. Rabins, *Johns Hopkins University School of Medicine, 600 N. Wolfe Street, Baltimore, Maryland 21287-7279, USA*

Blanca Reneses-Prieto, *Regional Ministry of Health and Social Services, Madrid, Spain*

Anita Riecher-Rössler, *University Psychiatric Outpatient Department, Petersgraben 4, CH-4031, Basel, Switzerland*

Mary V. Seeman, *The Centre for Addictions and Mental Health, Clarke Division, Department of Psychiatry, 250 College Street, Toronto, Ontario M56 1R8, Canada*

Phillip Seeman, *Departments of Psychiatry and Psychopharmacology, University of Toronto, 250 College Street, Toronto, Ontario M56 1R8, Canada*

Noriyoshi Takei, *Department of Psychiatry and Neurology, Hamamatsu University School of Medicine, 3600 Handa-cho, Hamamatsu 431-3192, Japan*

Preface

Few areas within psychiatry are subject to as much debate and controversy as schizophrenia-like states that have their first onset in middle or old age. Many colleagues who work with younger patients are either ignorant or sceptical about the concept of an illness that has anything in common with schizophrenia, yet has such a delayed onset. Add to such healthy scepticism a perverse insistence among late onset workers to adopt different cut off ages, diagnostic criteria and nomenclature and it is not difficult to see why late onset schizophrenia failed to find a place in DSM-IV or ICD-10. This book is the product of a two-day meeting at Leeds Castle, England in July 1998 to which representative late onset schizophrenia workers from around the world and a couple of 'mainstream' schizophrenia researchers were invited by Peter Rabins and Robert Howard. The meeting had some modest aims: to review the current state of knowledge concerning late onset schizophrenia, to debate the case for heterogeneity based on onset age and to reach consensus on diagnosis, terminology and future research directions. The meeting was seen as an opportunity for clinicians and researchers interested in late onset schizophrenia to get their house in order, determine if agreement existed on the international stage and to forge cooperation between individuals and centres with common research agendas. In suitably historic surroundings we found we agreed on more than we disagreed, and the resulting Consensus Statement is included as the final chapter. As the contributions to this volume show, late onset schizophrenia represents more than an eccentric interest confined to old age psychiatry. Consideration and study of these cases informs issues of heterogeneity, gender, brain maturation and ageing, putative structural or functional cerebral substrates for psychosis and receptor psychopharmacology in schizophrenia as a whole. Anita Riecher-Rössler reminds us at the beginning of her chapter that Kraepelin himself considered late onset psychoses represented the 'darkest area of psychiatry'. We hope that the material covered by our contributors sheds some light, not only upon late onset psychosis, but more widely into schizophrenia. This is a good place to express our thanks to the staff of Janssen, Gardiner–Caldwell and Leeds Castle who supported our meeting, and to our authors and Judy Wrightson for painless book production.

ROBERT HOWARD, PETER RABINS, DAVID CASTLE
January 1999

I

Historical Development

Late Onset Schizophrenia
Edited by Robert Howard, Peter V. Rabins, David J. Castle
© 1999 Wrightson Biomedical Publishing Ltd

1

Late Onset Schizophrenia: The German Concept and Literature

ANITA RIECHER-RÖSSLER

University Psychiatric Outpatient Department, Basel, Switzerland

INTRODUCTION

'Man kann sich kaum mit den spätschizophrenen Krankheitsbildern abgeben, ohne immer wieder daran erinnert zu werden, wie sehr Kraepelin recht hatte, wenn er die Lehre von den Psychosen des höheren Lebensalters als "das dunkelste Gebiet der Psychiatrie" bezeichnete. In der Tat scheint einem heute wie früher der Boden unter den Füssen zu schwanken, und unsere grundlegenden psychiatrischen Begriffe scheinen ihren Sinn zu verlieren, wenn man um Erkenntnisse über die Spätschizophrenien ringen will' (M. Bleuler 1943, S. 259).

'One can hardly deal with late onset schizophrenic pictures without being reminded again and again how right Kraepelin was when he called the science of psychoses of old age "the darkest area of psychiatry". Indeed, today as in earlier times the ground seems to shake under our feet, and our basic psychiatric terms seem to lose their meaning, when one grapples with late onset schizophrenias' (M. Bleuler, 1943, p. 259).

Hardly any psychiatric disorder exists that is described so inconsistently, defined in such an imprecise manner and about which we still have so little sound empirical knowledge as late onset schizophrenia. The reasons for this are manifold. First, there is still a 'dearth of published data' on late onset schizophrenia, as was stated by Jeste (1993). Furthermore, the few studies conducted so far are mainly older studies, which suffer from severe method-ological limitations (Riecher-Rössler, 1994; Riecher-Rössler *et al.*, 1997; Riecher-Rössler *et al.*, see this volume, Chapter 4). Finally most studies on this disease group have so far been done in German speaking countries and have only been published in German language. Their results have either not been received at all in Anglo-American psychiatry or have often been misin-terpreted. This has led to an unfortunate international confusion in terms

and concepts. The term 'late onset schizophrenia' is now used for two different entities. In the classic Bleulerian tradition, late onset schizophrenia is
diagnosed when a patient first manifests specific schizophrenic symptoms
after age 40. Schizophrenia beginning after age 60 is included but it is considered very rare. Other, mainly British and American, psychiatrists often use
the term 'late onset schizophrenia' interchangeably with late paraphrenia or
as a generic term for both these diseases, even though the concept of late
paraphrenia is quite different from that of late onset schizophrenia — late
paraphrenia being a British concept that includes all schizophrenia-like but
also all delusional disorders after age 60. One of the causes for this confusion, which has so far seriously impeded research, is the misunderstanding of
Kraepelin's concept of 'paraphrenia'.

The aim of this article therefore is

– to give a brief overview of the studies on classic late onset schizophrenia
  (i.e. according to the original definition by Manfred Bleuler, 1943)
  conducted in German speaking countries and so far only published in
  German. Studies from other European countries — except Great Britain
  — are also mentioned, as far as they refer to the same concept and were
  published in German or English;
– briefly to describe the development of the original term and concept of
  'paraphrenia' as introduced by Emil Kraepelin (1909–15);
– to discuss the international confusion of terms and concepts regarding late
  onset schizophrenia and late paraphrenia and its unfortunate impact on
  research.

In Chapter 4 of this volume, the results of these studies are summarized and
critically discussed, taking into consideration their methodological short-
comings. Chapter 4 also gives a tabular overview of the studies mentioned
here.

HISTORICAL DEVELOPMENT IN GERMAN-SPEAKING
PSYCHIATRY BEFORE 1943

Kraepelin (1893) chose the term 'dementia praecox' to describe the endogenous psychoses whose progression has a distinct process resulting in dementia. In 1905 Kraepelin wrote: 'I chose the term dementia praecox because of
the terrible outcome as well as the fact that the suffering develops in early
age. At the time, these two characteristics seemed to apply to this group of
newly described patients' (p. 557). However, he quickly realised that dementia praecox did not always begin in youth. In his textbooks he sketched a
diagram showing that two-thirds of the cases began between ages 15 and 30.

The number of first onset cases then dwindled as age progressed, although in a small number of cases the illness developed in the fourth, fifth, and even the sixth decade of life. Even so, Kraepelin found that only 0.2% of the 1,054 patients he studied experienced their first symptoms after age 60 (Kraepelin, 1909–15, cf. Riecher-Rössler *et al.*, this volume, Chapter 4, Table 1).

Kraepelin also realised early on that not all patients suffering from dementia praecox had the same symptoms. So he tried to identify specific subgroups. For example, he tried to isolate a group with paraphrenia ('Paraphrenie'). He characterised this group as having a minimal disturbance of affect and will, and no progression to dementia. Patients had a very insidious development of an ever-worsening paranoia with ideas of grandiosity in the later stages, but personality was preserved (Kraepelin, 1909–15, p. 974). Hallucinations were also observed. The symptoms were described as beginning mainly between ages 30 and 50. Mayer (1921) followed up on the 78 cases that Kraepelin had diagnosed as having paraphrenia and found that 50 of them had developed a clear diagnosis of 'dementia praecox' in the meantime. This is why Kraepelin himself later abandoned the distinction between paraphrenia and schizophrenia.

Paraphrenia, then, was never a diagnostic entity based on age but on phenomenology (Kraepelin, 1919, 1971). Kraepelin never tried to delineate a specific symptomatology of dementia praecox in elderly patients, even when his work was presented in Anglo-Saxon literature in such a way as to justify the term 'late paraphrenia' for elderly patients experiencing schizophrenia-like symptomatology.

Gaupp (1905) was one of the first to try to distinguish specific cases of late onset from dementia praecox. He described a rare illness in women, characterised by a depressive climacteric agitation resulting in mental weakness. The beginning of this disease was observed between ages 45 and 60. Stransky (1906) also made an effort to differentiate between dementia praecox and similar illnesses that occur in old age. He named the latter group 'dementia tardiva'. Typical symptoms were 'a prephase of depression, the contrast between the absurdity and incoherence of delusions as well as the clearness of hallucinations on the one hand as compared to the well-preserved affectivity' (quoted in Bleuler, 1943, p. 263). Bleuler (1943) believed that Stransky had described the main characteristics of late onset schizophrenia, which many authors after him have confirmed. Stransky considered dementia tardiva to be a subtype of dementia praecox.

Berger (1913) unsuccessfully attempted to delineate 'paranoia chronica' as an independent mental illness of later life separate from schizophrenia. What he obviously described was the clinical picture of paranoid schizophrenia.

Kleist (1913) coined the term 'involutional paranoia' ('Involutionsparanoia') for an illness that supposedly affected mostly women aged 40–50. It was regarded as an exacerbation of 'hyperparanoic' pre-psychotic personality characteristics into pathological symptomatology. This illness was supposedly caused by 'innersecretory change'. Unlike in dementia praecox, in involutional paranoia delusions and their accompanying affect would remain in a clear relationship and the disease would never result in 'imbecility'.

Albrecht (1914) studied 138 patients with a 'late-life psychosis not explained by brain pathology'. Among these cases he could identify 24 with a so-called 'presenile paraphrenia' ('präsenile paraphrenie'), the symptoms of which were similar to those of Kleist's involutional paranoia. Another 19 cases were characterized by a 'depressive madness resulting in imbecility', which according to Bleuler (1943) could be regarded as late onset schizophrenia. Later, Serko (1919) coined the term 'involutional paraphrenia' ('Involutionsparaphrenie') and Medow (1922) came up with the term 'stiffening involutional psychosis' ('erstarrende Rückbildungspsychose'). In both clinical pictures late onset schizophrenia according to M. Bleuler can at least be suspected. Kolle (1931) took up the term 'paraphrenia' ('Paraphrenie') or 'schizophrenia of paraphrenic type' for schizophrenia occurring in middle and old age, mainly between ages 40 and 50. He examined 142 late onset cases of Carl Schneider and 33 of his own cases (cf. Riecher-Rössler et al., this volume, Chapter 4, Table 1). He described his late onset patients as usually showing a pyknic structure of the body, a cyclothymic character and having a favourable prognosis.

However, most German psychiatrists, among them Leonhard (1957), used the term 'paraphrenia' as Kraepelin had originally intended, that is, for a specific category of paranoid schizophrenia patients with characteristic psychopathology and independent of age.

MANFRED BLEULER AND THE CONCEPT OF 'LATE ONSET SCHIZOPHRENIA'

As early as 1908 E. Bleuler, medical director of the 'Burghölzli', the University Psychiatric Hospital of Zurich, had suggested the term 'schizophrenia' (Schizophrenie) instead of the Kraepelian 'dementia praecox', as according to his observations the disconnection or splitting of mental functioning was an outstanding symptom of this group of diseases. In 1943, his son, Manfred Bleuler, then director of the same institute, coined the term 'late onset schizophrenia' ('Spätschizophrenie'). He defined late onset schizophrenia as a group of psychoses fulfilling the following criteria:

1. The psychosis must begin after the 40th year of life.
2. Symptomatology does not differ fundamentally from that of schizophrenia in early life.

3. There is neither an amnestic syndrome nor accompanying physical findings unequivocally indicating that symptoms could be due to brain disease (M. Bleuler, 1943, p. 269).

M. Bleuler had examined 130 late onset cases, an unsystematic selection of patients, 'who became known to me'. He personally examined the patients — and partly also their relatives — from different hospitals and countries. M. Bleuler does not give many details about his investigations, but obviously part of his studies were based on hospital records only, as some of the patients, as he reports, had already died at the time of investigation. According to M. Bleuler's results, 15% of all schizophrenic disorders begin between ages 40 and 60, and onset after age 60 is negligible. Half the patients with late onset schizophrenia that he investigated did not differ in symptomatology from early onset schizophrenia patients, the other half, however, did:

'In somewhat more than half of late onset schizophrenics we see a symptom colouring as it has been described as somehow characteristic and especially frequent: paraphrenia-like states on the one hand, depressive–anxious–catatonic on the other hand, and additionally a small group of confused agitations which can be easily mistaken for amentia. In the second, smaller half of the late onset schizophrenics, symptomatology does not show anything differing from early-onset schizophrenics' (translated from M. Bleuler, 1943, p. 283).

The course of late onset schizophrenia he found to be more favourable than that of early onset patients (cf. Riecher-Rössler et al., this volume, Chapter 4).

THE ERA AFTER MANFRED BLEULER

Over the years, many German-speaking researchers have continued to use M. Bleuler's criteria for diagnosing late onset schizophrenia (Klages, 1961; Siegel and Rollberg, 1970; Berner et al., 1973; Huber et al., 1975, 1979; Gabriel, 1978). Some authors have used other diagnostic labels such as 'paranoid-hallucinatory psychosis in involutional age' ('paranoid-halluzinatorische Psychose im Umbildungsalter'), 'paranoid involutional psychosis with schizophrenic colouring' ('paranoide Rückbildungspsychose mit schizophrener Färbung') and 'paranoid climacteric psychosis' ('paranoide klimakterische Psychose'). Knoll (1952) studied 114 patients who had developed paranoid illnesses for the first time after age 40 and found their symptoms to be so close to schizophrenia that he saw no need to create an independent diagnostic group for them.

Janzarik (1957) was one of the few German psychiatrists interested in patients whose first signs of illness occurred after age 60. He used the term

'Altersschizophrenie' (old-age schizophrenia) for this patient group. According to his observations, these cases were comparatively rare. Although he screened all patients of the Psychiatric University Hospital of Heidelberg during 5 years and did not limit his study to first-admitted or non-organic patients, he could identify only six patients whose schizophrenia had begun after age 60. In fact, among these six and another 44 patients from other institutions, he noted relevant organic findings in a large number of cases. These cases would certainly be excluded from a diagnosis of schizophrenia according to modern diagnostic criteria. Janzarik wrote: 'When schizophrenic, cyclothymic, and organic symptomatology are mixed, and when reactive and endogenous symptoms are intertwined, then the dubiosity of the term schizophrenia becomes obvious' (1957, p. 541). These results underline the rarity of schizophrenia onset after age 60.

Müller (1959) examined 30 inpatients aged over 65 years who had experienced their first psychotic symptoms after age 40. Only nine of them in the meantime had not developed an organic brain syndrome. Klages (1961) was one of the authors who used the term and concept of late onset schizophrenia according to M. Bleuler's criteria but his schizophrenia diagnosis was already based on Kurt Schneider (1957) with a more restrictive and exact definition. As to the onset of the disease he even set a clear upper age limit at age 60 as, according to his studies, in patients after this age 'presenile and senile components' cannot safely be excluded. Klages examined all 53 late onset cases who were hospitalised at the Tübingen University Hospital over 4 years. Patients with suspected organic brain disorder were excluded. He found the symptomatology of these patients not distinctly different from that of early onset patients, although he observed their paranoid ideas to be more concrete, more systematic and 'ich-nah' (close to the self). Quite often he also observed 'physical malsensations'. He stated that age without doubt has a symptom-colouring, pathoplastic influence on psychosis. However, like most other authors, he had not directly examined a control group of early onset patients and his comparisons were mainly based on literature.

Schimmelpenning (1965) published a study on 117 patients with a schizophrenic or paranoid psychosis who had been admitted to the Münster University Psychiatric Hospital during a time period of 5 years. Of 82 patients who could be examined directly, only 15 were diagnosed with late onset schizophrenia. The other 67 patients he labelled as 'schizophreniforme Psychose', as he could not observe a typical course but rather an organic disease as potentially underlying the disorder. In the few cases of real late onset schizophrenia he described a 'Verbalhalluzinose' (verbal hallucinosis) as characteristic symptomatology.

Siegel and Rollberg (1970) conducted a similar study. Over a period of 10 years they examined all 60 inpatients of the Erfurt University Hospital with late onset schizophrenia. They found no clear differences in symptomatology as compared with early onset patients. Their comparisons, however, were also based on literature only. Angst *et al.* (1973) in a study on 291 consecutive admissions in seven hospitals in five countries did not aim at late onset schizophrenia. But they have contributed to the topic by showing that illness onset of the paranoid subgroup of schizophrenia is later than in schizoaffective and especially later than in catatonic psychoses. This would be in accordance with the observations of other authors who found more paranoid symptoms in late onset schizophrenia. Berner *et al.* (1973) and also Gabriel (1974a,b, 1978) did a catamnestic investigation of the late onset patients of the Lausanne study (Ciompi and Müller, 1976). They re-examined all former patients of the Lausanne University Hospital originally first admitted between ages 40 and 65, who could still be contacted after an average period of over 20 years. Only one-fifth of the original population could be re-examined. From these patients, who in the meantime had an average age of 77 years, only 13% were assessed to be 'healthy', one-third of them were hospitalized at the time of assessment — most of them since a long time. Although they had investigated a very selected population only, Gabriel concluded from this that the course of late onset schizophrenia patients was worse than that of early onset patients (for further results see Riecher-Rössler, this volume, Chapter 4).

One of the first authors to examine also a control group of early onset patients and to compare them directly with the late onset cases was Hinterhuber (1973). At the same time he was one of the first who restricted his investigations to *first* admitted. All first admissions of the University Hospital of Innsbruck over a time period of 5 years were re-examined after a medium catamnestic period of 30–40 years. Diagnoses were made based on case records according to Bleuler, onset of illness was defined by the occurrence of the first psychotic symptom or, if that was not possible, by first admission. He also found the course of late onset patients to be comparably less favourable than in early onset patients (for further results see Riecher-Rössler *et al.*, this volume, Chapter 4).

Huber *et al.* (1979) used the concept of late onset schizophrenia in the same way as M. Bleuler did but, like Klages, based on the schizophrenia criteria of K. Schneider (1957). Huber *et al.* were the first researchers after Hinterhuber (1973) to compare a group of late onset patients empirically with early onset cases. They examined all admissions of the Bonn University Hospital over a period of 4 years. The retrospective investigation covered a medium illness duration of 17.8 years. Patients with suspected organic brain disease were excluded. Of 502 patients, 70 had their illness onset after age 40. At 'illness onset' they found more paranoid and paranoid-hallucinatory symptoms in late onset as compared with early onset patients. Nevertheless, their general conclusion from their empirical comparison was that late onset cases do not substantially differ from early onset cases as regards symptomatology. As to the course of these patients Huber *et al.* (1979) found this to be milder in late onset than in early onset patients (see Riecher-Rössler *et al.*, this volume, Chapter 4).

Marneros and Deister (1984) analysed the case-notes of 1208 schizophrenia patients (diagnosed according to K. Schneider's criteria). They only found 170 late onset cases. However, as opposed to almost all other German speaking authors, their age boundary was not age 40 but age 50. Also in contrast to most other authors since M. Bleuler, they did not definitely exclude patients with suspected organic brain syndrome, or at least did not mention this criterion.

Marneros *et al.* (1992) used diagnostic criteria similar to DSM-III (American Psychiatric Association, 1980). But they considered schizophrenia with onset after age 45, which DSM-III did not regard as schizophrenia, as late onset schizophrenia. With this age cut-off, which is slightly later than that of other German authors, they found the proportion of late onset cases to be lower, i.e., 8% of all those with schizophrenia. However, like most authors, they did not give an exact definition of 'onset'.

Mayer *et al.* (1993) have for the first time analysed patients directly at first admission, however based on clinical routine documentation only. They compared extreme groups: patients first admitted between ages 18 and 23 with patients first admitted between ages 40 and 63. They found only marginal differences, with more vegetative symptoms in the late onset group.

Recently, we have for the first time conducted a direct study on a representative sample of 43 *first admitted* late onset patients in direct comparison to a control group of 224 early onset patients (Riecher-Rössler, 1994; Riecher-Rössler *et al.*, 1997; for details and results see Riecher-Rössler *et al.*, this volume, Chapter 4).

RUSSIAN LITERATURE

The concept of late onset schizophrenia is also known in Russian literature. These authors however do not use clear criteria for the schizophrenia diagnosis itself, rather the schizophrenia concept of Russian tradition seems to be quite broad. To define 'late onset' Sternberg (1972) and also Rokhlina (1975) used age 50 years as the age boundary. They did not exclude organic brain disorder.

SCANDINAVIAN LITERATURE

Sjögren (1964) used the term 'paraphrenic state' for psychoses of the 'presenile–senile period of life'. But he did not give an exact definition of his concept apart from stating that he was influenced by M. Bleuler (1943) and Kay and Roth (1961). As characteristic symptoms he described a well-organized, persisting and not correctable system of fixed paranoid delusions with frequent halluzinations. Funding (1963) divided the paranoid psychoses of old age into schizophrenic and paraphrenic forms, not giving an exact definition of either.

Jørgensen and Munk-Jørgensen (1985) in a case-register study analysed 108 patients first admitted after age 60 years for a schizophrenic or paranoid disorder according to ICD-8 or DSM-III. Among these patients they could identify 50 cases with paranoid psychoses, 39 cases with reactive psychoses, 10 cases with other psychoses and only seven cases of schizophrenia.

CONCLUSIONS AND DISCUSSION

As has been shown, late onset schizophrenia is a term and concept invented by early German speaking psychiatrists. It was originally used to describe the relatively small subgroup of schizophrenic patients whose illness started after age 40. The reasons to delineate these patients from the majority with an earlier illness onset were not only this unusual age of onset but also the fact that these patients were mainly women and that many of them seemed to be different from earlier onset schizophrenia patients as regards symptomatology and course of their disease.

German speaking psychiatrists have used this term and concept ever since and have repeatedly stated to have found differences between late and early onset patients. However, this has never been proven on an empirically sound basis. In fact, studies so far have suffered from serious methodological problems. Thus, for example, there was never a control group of early onset patients which was directly compared with the late onset patients on a sound empirical basis. Further methodological problems will be discussed in Riecher-Rössler et al., this volume, Chapter 4. The result is a serious deficit in empirically sound knowledge in this area.

A further reason for our scarce knowledge is the conceptual and terminological confusion which has occurred internationally regarding this illness group. British and American psychiatrists often use the term late onset schizophrenia interchangeably with late paraphrenia or as a generic term for both these diseases. Even so, the concept of late paraphrenia is quite different from that of late onset schizophrenia.

This concept of late paraphrenia derives from British psychiatry and includes patients with the onset of not only schizophrenic but also delusional disorders after age 60. The diagnosis is 'a peculiarly British [one] and has no international counterpart' (Howard, 1992, p. 63). Even so, this concept had some impact on the International Classification of Diseases (ICD, World

Health Organization 1967, 1978, 1993) as well as on international research and literature. Thus, authors do not unequivocally distinguish between late onset schizophrenia and late paraphrenia (e.g. Grahame, 1984; Stoudemire and Riether, 1987; Gurland, 1988; Flint *et al.*, 1991; Yassa, 1991; Hasset *et al.*, 1992; Howard *et al.*, 1993; Yassa and Suranyi-Cadotte, 1993). Reviews of late onset schizophrenia do not adhere to stringent definition of this disease, and they mix findings on late onset schizophrenia with those on late paraphrenia (e.g. Castle and Howard, 1992). The same is true for reviews of late paraphrenia (e.g. Bridge and Wyatt, 1980a,b).

One of the causes of confusion is the above described evolution of the term 'paraphrenia'. Kraepelin (1919, 1971) originally defined this disease phenomenologically and did not set age boundaries. Since then the term has undergone an unorthodox change in definition to include only patients with late onset. Roth (1955), who coined the term 'late paraphrenia', originally used it to describe elderly patients with paraphrenia-like symptoms, e.g. 'patients ... with a well organized system of paranoid delusions with or without hallucinations existing in the setting of a well-preserved personality and affective response' (Roth, 1955, p. 283). From two studies (Roth and Morrissey, 1952; Roth, 1955) he concluded that most patients with this clinical picture experience their first symptoms after age 60. However, this conclusion seems precarious, because he only investigated patients over 60 years old. As early as 1960, Fish criticised the term 'late paraphrenia'. First, the studies conducted in Germany showed that the diagnosis of paraphrenia merges into that of paranoid schizophrenia. Secondly, he wrote 'late paraphrenia can also be confused with Bleuler's late onset schizophrenia. Thus, it would appear that Roth's choice is unfortunate' (Fish, 1960, p. 940).

The described confusion in terminology and concept has recently grown even more in importance because in the past years it has become clear that one can encounter many diseases under the umbrella of a late paraphrenia diagnosis. These diseases not only include late onset schizophrenia and other delusional disorders, but also those that are of clear organic origin (Naguib, 1991). Up to now, however, it is not known how many late paraphrenia patients in fact have late onset schizophrenia, i.e. how often 'true' schizophrenia occurs after age 60. According to the pertinent literature, which is mainly German, the number of patients with very late onset schizophrenia is minimal.

In summary, these problems of terminology and nosology have until now seriously limited the international comparability of studies and thereby contribute to our scarce knowledge in this area. When researchers report on the same sort of patients using different terms (and vice versa) it is not possible to arrive at a reliable and valid description of late onset schizophrenia. In my opinion, it is therefore important to (re)establish clear boundaries between schizophrenia and other delusional disorders with onset in old age, especially those disguised as late paraphrenia that are partly of organic origin. In practical terms, this means that, first, the term 'late paraphrenia' should be abandoned to avoid further confusion. There is now enough evidence that this is not a valid entity, but an umbrella diagnosis for a heterogeneous group of diseases, including many cases of organic aetiology. Secondly, we have to question the validity of 'late onset schizophrenia'. Are there really decisive differences between late and early onset patients which justify the use of an extra diagnostic label for this illness group? If we really look at late onset schizophrenia only and not at a mixed group of diagnoses and (the few) methodologically sound studies, do we then really find significant differences between late and early onset patients concerning risk factors, symptomatology and course of the disease, as to regard late onset schizophrenia as a valid entity? An attempt to answer this question is made in Chapter 4 of this volume by Riecher-Rössler *et al.*

REFERENCES

Albrecht, H. (1914). Die funktionellen Psychosen des Rückbildungsalters. *Z Neurol Psychiatr* **22**, 306–344.

American Psychiatric Association (1980). *Diagnostic and Statistical Manual of Mental Disorders, 3rd edn* (DSM-111). American Psychiatric Association, Washington, DC.

Angst, J., Baastrup, P., Grof, P. *et al.* (1973). Statistische Aspekte des Beginns und Verlaufs schizophrener Psychosen. In: Huber, G. (Ed.), *Verlauf und Ausgang schizophrener Erkrankungen*. Schattauer, Stuttgart, New York, pp. 67-78.

Berger, H. (1913). Klinische Beiträge zur Paranoiafrage. *Mschr Psychiatr* **34**, 181–229.

Berner, P., Gabriel, E. and Naske, R. (1973). Verlaufstypologie und Prognose bei sogenannten Spätschizophrenien. In: Huber, G. (Ed.), *Verlauf und Ausgang schizophrener Erkrankungen*. Schattauer, Stuttgart, New York, pp. 85–95.

Bleuler, E. (1908). Die Prognose der Dementia praecox (Schizophreniegruppe). *Allg Z Psychiatr* **65**, 436–464.

Bleuler, M. (1943). Die spätschizophrenen Krankheitsbilder. *Fortschr Neurol Psychiatr* **15**, 259–290.

Bridge, P.T. and Wyatt, R.J. (1980a). Paraphrenia: paranoid states of life life. I. European research. *J Am Geriatr Soc* **28**, 193–200.

Bridge, P.T. and Wyatt, R.J. (1980b). Paraphrenia: paranoid states of late life. II. American research. *J Am Geriatr Soc* **28**, 201–205.

Castle, D.J. and Howard, R. (1992). What do we know about the aetiology of late-onset schizophrenia? *Eur Psychiatry* **7**, 99–108.

Ciompi, L. and Müller, C. (1976). *Lebensweg und Alter der Schizophrenen*. Springer, Berlin, Heidelberg, New York.

Fish, F. (1960). Senile schizophrenia. *J Mental Sci* **106**, 938–946.

Flint, A.J., Rifat, S.L. and Eastwood, M.R. (1991). Late-onset paranoia: distinct from paraphrenia? *Int J Geriatr Psychiatry* **6**, 103–109.

Funding, T. (1963). Paranoid psychoses in later life. *Acta Psychiatr Scand* **39** (suppl 169), 356–361.

Gabriel, E. (1974a). Der langfristige Verlauf schizophrener Späterkrankungen im Vergleich mit Schizophrenien aller Lebensalter. *Psychiatrica Clinica* **7**, 172–180.

Gabriel, E. (1974b). Über den Einfluss psychoorganischer Beeinträchtigungen im Alter auf den Verlauf sogenannter Spätschizophrenien. *Psychiatrica Clinica* **7**, 358–364.

Gabriel, E. (1978). *Die langfristige Entwicklung der Spätschizophrenien*, Karger, Basel.

Gaupp, R. (1905). Depression des höheren Lebensalters. *Münchner Medizinische Wochenschrift* **52**, 1531–1537.

Grahame, P.S. (1984). Schizophrenia in old age (late paraphrenia). *Br J Psychiatry* **145**, 493–495.

Gurland, B.J. (1988). Schizophrenia in the elderly. In: Tsuang, M.T. and Simpson, J.C. (Eds), *Handbook of Schizophrenia: Nosology, Epidemiology and Genetics*. Elsevier, Amsterdam, New York, Oslo, pp. 288–317.

Hasset, A.M., Keks, N.A., Jackson, H.J. and Copolov, D.L. (1992). The diagnostic validity of paraphrenia. *Austr NZ J Psychiatry* **26**, 18–29.

Hinterhuber, H. (1973). Zur Katamnese der Schizophrenien. *Fortschr Neurol Psychiatr* **41**, 527–558.

Howard, R. (1992). Late paraphrenia: an update. *J Roy Soc Med* **3**, 63–65.

Howard, R.J., Almeida, O. and Levy, R. (1993). Phenomenology of late-onset schizophrenia. *Schizophr Res* **9**, 100.

Huber, G., Gross, G. and Schüttler, R. (1975). Spätzschizophrenie. *Arch Psychiatr Nervenkr* **221**, 53–66.

Huber, G., Gross, G. and Schüttler, R. (1979). *Schizophrenie: Verlaufs- und sozialpsychiatrische Langzeituntersuchung an den 1949–1959 in Bonn hospitalisierten schizophrenen Kranken*. Springer, Berlin.

Janzarik, W. (1957). Zur Problematik schizophrener Psychosen im höheren Lebensalter. *Nervenarzt* **28**, 535–542.

Jeste, D.V. (1993). Late-life schizophrenia: Editor's introduction. *Schizophr Bull* **19**, 687–689.

Jørgensen, P. and Munk-Jørgensen, P. (1985). Paranoid psychosis in the elderly. *Acta Psychiatr Scand* **62**, 358–363.

Kay, D.W.K. and Roth, M. (1961). Environmental and hereditary factors in the schizophrenia of old age ('late paraphrenia') and their bearing on the general problem of causation in schizophrenia. *J Mental Sci* **107**, 649–686.

Klages, W. (1961). *Die Spätschizophrenie*. Enke, Stuttgart.

Kleist, K. (1913). Die Involutionsparanoia. *Allg Z Psychiatr* **70**, 1–134.

Knoll, H. (1952). Wahnbildende Psychosen der Zeit des Klimakteriums und der Involution in klinischer und genealogischer Betrachtung. *Arch Psychiatr Z Neurol* **189**, 59–92.

Kolle, K. (1931). *Die primäre Verrücktheit: psychopathologische, klinische und genealogische Untersuchungen*. Thieme, Leipzig.

Kraepelin, E. (1893). *Psychiatrie, ein Lehrbuch für Studierende und Ärzte, Vol. 4*. Barth, Leipzig.

Kraepelin, E. (1905). Fragestellungen der klinischen Psychiatrie. *Zentralblatt Nervenheilkunde Psychiatrie* **28**, 573–590.

Kraepelin, E. (1909–15). *Psychiatrie, ein Lehrbuch für Studierende und Ärzte, Vol. 8*. Barth, Leipzig.

Kraepelin, E. (1919). *Dementia praecox und Paraphrenie*. Krieger, New York (reprint in English, 1971).

Kraepelin, E. (1971). *Dementia praecox and Paraphrenia (1919)*. [Translated by R.M. Barclay.] Robert E. Krieger, New York.

Leonhard, K. (1957). *Aufteilung der endogenen Psychosen*. Akademie, Berlin.

Marneros, A. and Deister, A. (1984). The psychopathology of 'late schizophrenia'. *Psychopathology* **17**, 264–274.

Marneros, A., Deister, A. and Rohde, A. (1992). Schizophrenic, schizoaffective and affective disorders in the elderly: a comparison. In: Katona, C. and Levy, R. (Eds). *Delusions and Hallucinations in Old Age*. Gaskell, London, pp. 136–152.

Mayer, C., Kelterborn, G. and Naber, D. (1993). Age of onset in schizoprenia: relations to psychopathology and gender. *Br J Psychiatry* **162**, 665–671.

Mayer, W. (1921). Über paraphrene psychosen. *Z Gesamte Neurol Psychiatr* **71**, 187–206.

Medow, (1922). Eine Gruppe depressiver Psychosen des Rückbildungsalters mit ungünstiger Prognose. *Arch Psychiatr* **64**, 480–506.

Müller, (1959). *Über das Senium der Schizophrenen*. Karger, Basel, New York.

Naguib, M. (1991). Paraphrenia revisited. *Br J Hosp Med* **46**, 371–375.

Riecher-Rössler, A. (1994). *Die Spätschizophrenie — eine valide Entität? Eine empirische Studie zu Risikofaktoren, Krankheitsbild und Verlaug*. Habilitationsschrift. Medizinische Fakultät der Universität Heidelberg.

Riecher-Rössler, A., Löffler, W. and Munk-Jørgensen, P. (1997). What do we really know about late-onset schizophrenia? *Eur Arch Psychiatry Clin Neurosci* **247**, 195–208.

Rokhlina, M.L. (1975). A comparative clinico-genetic study of attack like schizophrenia with late and early manifestations with regard to age (in Russian). *Zh Nevrograt Psikhiatr* **75**, 417–424.

Roth, M. (1955). The natural history of mental disorders in old age. *J Mental Sci* **101**, 281–301.

Roth, M. and Morrissey, J.D. (1952). Problems in the diagnosis and classification of mental disorder in old age; with a study of case material. *J Mental Sci* **98**, 66–80.

Schimmelpenning, G.W. (1965). *Die paranoiden Psychosen der zweiten Lebenshälfte*. Karger, Basel.

Schneider, K. (1957). Primäre und sekundäre Symptome bei Schizophrenie. *Fortschr Neurol Psychiatr* **25**, 487.

Serko, A. (1919). Die Involutionsparaphrenie. *Mschr Psychiatr* **45**, 245–286.

Siegel, E. and Rollberg, I. (1970). Über Spätschizophrenien. *Wien Z Nervenheilk Grenzg* **28**, 145–151.

Sjögren, H. (1964). Paraphrenic, melancholic and psychoneurotic states in the presenile–senile period of life. *Acta Psychiatr Scand* **40** (suppl 176), 1–63.

Sternberg, E. (1972). Neuere Forschungsergebnisse bei spätschizophrenen Psychosen. *Fortschr Neurol Psychiatr* **40**, 631–646.

Stoudemire, A. and Riether, A.M. (1987). Evaluation and treatment of paranoid syndromes in the elderly: a review. *Gen Hosp Psych* **9**, 267–274.

Stransky, E. (1906). Dementia tardiva. *Mschr Psychiatr* **18**, 1–38.

World Health Organization (1967). *International Classification of Diseases, ICD, 8th revision*. World Health Organization, Geneva.

World Health Organization (1978). *Mental Disorders: Glossary and Guide to their Classification in Accordance with the Ninth Revision of the International Classification of Diseases*. World Health Organization, Geneva.

World Health Organization (1993). *Tenth Revision of the International Classification of Diseases. Chapter V (F): Mental and Behavioural Disorders (Including Disorders of Psychological Development). Clinical Description and Diagnostic Guidelines*. World Health Organization, Geneva.

Yassa, R. (1991). Late-onset schizophrenia. In: Walker, E.F. (Ed.), *Schizophrenia.* Academic Press, New York, Boston, London, pp. 243–255.
Yassa, R. and Suranyi-Cadotte, B. (1993). Clinical characteristics of late-onset schizophrenia and delusional disorder. *Schizophr Bull* **19**, 701–707.

Late Onset Schizophrenia
Edited by Robert Howard, Peter V. Rabins, David J. Castle
© 1999 Wrightson Biomedical Publishing Ltd

2

The English Language Literature on Late Paraphrenia from the 1950s

DAVID W.K. KAY

Newcastle Project for Health in Later Life, Department of Psychiatry, University of Newcastle, Newcastle upon Tyne, UK

EARLY OBSERVATIONS

Until the 1950s there was little in the English literature about schizophrenia-like illnesses in old age. Most of what was known derived from the German literature, known to British readers mainly through translation by Fish and others. The German psychiatrists' interest in schizophrenia in later life was for the most part an extension of their interest in schizophrenia in general. But in the United Kingdom Lewis (1946) had noted that the clinical psychiatry of old age was a neglected field and these conditions became prominent in the course of the development of psychogeriatrics (Roth and Morrissey, 1952; Post, 1965). However, Fish's study of senile schizophrenia seems to have been a response to the studies of Roth (Fish, 1960).

In the course of their enquiries Roth and Morrissey (1952) undertook a study of patients aged over 60 admitted to Graylingwell, a county mental hospital in England. Their main interest was in affective disorders and suicide, and they noted that paranoid delusions often occurred in depressive illness. However, in 12 of 150 patients admitted during one year with illnesses commencing after the age of 60, the delusions were paraphrenic in character, often primary, and were usually associated with passivity feelings or other volitional disturbances and hallucinations in clear consciousness, a clinical picture virtually pathognomonic of schizophrenia. These observations were extended over a period of 4 years and showed that there was a well-defined group of 10% of patients with an organized system of paranoid delusions, and frequently hallucinations, in the setting of well-preserved intellect, personality and affective response (Roth, 1955). The term late paraphrenia was chosen because of the late onset (age 60 or over) and the clinical resemblance to the illness described by Kraepelin. Roth's (1955) hypothesis that it was distinct from the organic psychoses required that the illness took a different course, and this was shown to be true by significant differences in mortality at 6 months and 2 years. Overlap between these groups was small; only one late paraphrenic patient had begun to show signs of dementia at follow-up, and a review of the histories of patients with organic psychoses had not shown any that had commenced with a well-integrated system of paranoid delusions. Roth (1955) concluded that the combination of late paraphrenia and organic dementia was rare.

Fish (1960) based his conclusions on a study of all elderly patients (N=264) admitted to psychiatric institutions including nursing homes in the City of Edinburgh during 1957. He found 16% with illnesses with marked paranoid symptoms but only 2.7% with schizophrenia beginning after the age of 60 years; the remaining paranoid cases were schizophrenias of earlier onset (3.4%), paranoid depressions (2.3%), organic psychoses (6.1%) or psychogenic reactions (1.1%). Earlier Robertson and Mason-Browne (1953) had reviewed all female patients admitted to a section of the Royal Edinburgh Hospital over a 6 year period, and found schizophrenic or paraphrenic states beginning after age 60 in only 1.5%. Differing views of the frequency of the types of paranoid disorders in the elderly have persisted till today.

Kay and Roth (1961) drew their cases from two sources: 42 patients with a mean age of 71 and onset over 55 admitted to Graylingwell Hospital, over a 5 year period, most of whom were followed up for at least 5 years; and 57 patients identified from the case records of the Psychiatric Hospital, Stockholm, during 1931–1940, whose mean age was 68 and age of onset over 60, and followed retrospectively through the system of parish registers till death or 1956 (Kay, 1962). The Graylingwell patients were all interviewed, but in Stockholm the information was derived from records and only one patient had survived long enough to be interviewed. After noting that the relationship between paraphrenic, paranoid and schizophrenic illness had long been disputed, Kay and Roth (1961) used late paraphrenia as a suitable descriptive term, without prejudice as to aetiology, for cases with a paranoid symptom complex in which signs of organic dementia or sustained confusion were absent, and in which the condition was judged from the content of the delusional and hallucinatory symptoms not to be due to a primary affective disorder. In this and accompanying studies late paraphrenia was found to be associated with a number of characteristics in its demography (sex, civil state and fertility), family history (Kay, 1959), premorbid personality, social circumstances, and sensory functions – Houston and Royse (1954) had already noted an association between deafness and paranoid schizophrenia – which distinguished it from affective disorders, and with an absence of gross cognitive impairment and progressive cerebral organic disease, which distinguished it from the dementia disorders. General physical health seemed to be compatible with patients' age (Kay and Roth, 1955). These findings were based on hospital cases and a small field study yielded little information about late paraphrenia outside hospital (Kay et al., 1964), except that it was probably rare.

Symptomatology

Kay and Roth (1961) were impressed by the uniformity of the clinical picture (except in a subgroup described below), the bizarreness of the delusions, and the vivid, often multi-modal, hallucinations, which tended to be worse at night. Persecution, often by the neighbours, was the most common delusion and might lead to assault and complaints to police, but erotic, hypochondriacal and grandiose delusions also occurred. Ideas of mental or physical influence were found in 28% (being drugged, hypnotized, sexually molested). Auditory hallucinations were found in 75%, and visual, olfactory and tactile hallucinations were rather frequent. Insight was totally lacking. Gross formal thought disorder, incoherent speech, inappropriate affect and catatonic symptoms were rare or absent, though in long-lasting cases, some emotional blunting, mild incongruity or euphoria might occur. (The duration of illness varied from a few weeks to many years.) These differences in symptomatology from that in younger schizophrenic patients were attributed to the pathoplastic effects of ageing. It was concluded that, employing an operational definition based on symptoms, the main group of cases of late paraphrenia had to be regarded as schizophrenic, though the aetiology (risk factors) might differ in certain respects. Study of these differences and the factors that had postponed onset to late life would be relevant for schizophrenia as a whole (Kay and Roth, 1961).

In a minority (about 20%) of the patients, hallucinations were absent, the delusions were almost confined to ideas of theft or poisoning by those in everyday contact, and personality and illness seemed to merge into one another (Kay and Roth, 1961). Relatives tended to regard the illness as a caricature of the premorbid personality. However, since there were many features in common with the majority of patients (sensory impairment, social isolation), and no firm line could be drawn clinically between this group and the remaining patients, who resembled paranoid schizophrenia, its nosological standing remained uncertain.

Demographic features, social isolation

Kay and Roth (1961) made a number of observations and interpretations. Both groups had a very marked excess of females, who were usually unmarried, and even in ever-married females fertility was low; hearing impairment was more common than in elderly patients with affective disorders; paranoid or schizoid personality traits were present in over 40% of patients, and others were described as explosive, sensitive or eccentric; 38% of Graylingwell patients had experienced social isolation, operationally defined, before the onset of overt illness. This raised the question: had the isolation contributed independently to the development of the psychosis, or was the isolation itself a result of personal difficulties in forming relationships, due to the personality traits, which might themselves be a prodromal form of the illness? When, for instance, the isolation seemed to have been a consequence of being unmarried or childless, or was associated with domestic quarrels and estrangement from relatives, it could have been related to the traits of personality. Some degree of hereditary predisposition, probably multifactorial, was suggested by the estimated risk of 3.6–5.6% for schizophrenia among sibs and children of patients (minimal/maximal values, with risk period age 20–50), compared with an estimated risk of 1.6% in the general population (Kay, 1959). However, circumstances sometimes existed for which qualities in the patient could not have been responsible, such as being the youngest in the family, loss of sibs through death, or progressive deafness, when the isolation seemed to be only partly explained by the existence of inherent personality traits. This suggested the possibility of intervention through social action. Finally, solitariness, eccentricity or aggressive independence might have been a defensive response, successful earlier but leading in old age to further isolation and breakdown (Kay and Roth, 1961). Multiple factors appeared to be involved and their relative importance could not be determined. A somewhat similar situation existed in schizophrenia (Faris and Dunham, 1939).

Cerebral disease

The role of cerebral disease was examined at the onset of illness, during follow up, and at death. It was known that psychoses associated with organic brain disease or dysfunction, as in amphetamine psychosis, alcoholism, or temporal lobe epilepsy, could closely simulate schizophrenic illness, and that in old age the role accorded to cerebral disease in the aetiology of mental disorder was ubiquitous (Kay and Roth, 1961). To exclude these cases, who constituted a separate group, patients with signs of clinical dementia, intoxication or active neurological disease at the onset of psychosis were carefully excluded. Psychometric tests (Progressive Matrices, vocabulary subtest from the Wechsler Bellevue Scale, and an information and orientation test) were found to discriminate sharply between late paraphrenia and dementia but not between late paraphrenia and affective disorder (Hopkins and Roth, 1953; Roth and Hopkins, 1953). Follow up (Kay and Roth, 1961; Kay,1962) and neuropathological studies (Corsellis, 1962) also showed that cerebral changes of the kind found in the organic dementias were unlikely to be a major factor in late paraphrenia, as did the finding that the certified causes of death were similar to those in the general population of similar age and differed from those of demented patients (Kay, 1962). A hypothetical role for focal cerebral disease could be postulated in the 8% of patients who had a history of focal cerebral damage or disease usually originating many years previously, including congenital conditions and childhood hemiplegia, and which though apparently inactive and completely unconnected with the psychosis, might have increased susceptibility in predisposed persons. Greater relevance was attached to the 5% of patients in whom signs of cerebrovascular disease or seizures arose later but the time relations suggested that the disease could have been present at the onset of psychosis. As regards senile degeneration, evidence of dementia eventually appeared in one patient at Graylingwell (2.4%) and so far as could be judged from records, in seven patients (12.4%) in Stockholm, where the follow-up was longer, often after many years of illness. Since the average life expectation in the Stockholm patients was almost normal, the incidence of organic changes was thought to be within the normal range; in fact 50% were still living after 10 years. It was not possible, however, to reach a definite conclusion as to the role of organic factors in late paraphrenia, including normal cerebral ageing, on the basis of the data available.

LATER DEVELOPMENTS

In this chapter, the aim is to determine to what extent these early observations and ideas have been supported or need to be modified or discarded in the light of more recent studies. In addition to the topics just mentioned, new data on epidemiology (Castle and Murray, 1993), response to neuroleptic drugs, brain imaging and neuropathology (Blessed, 1989) will be summarized. The main sources, limited to those describing at least 20 patients with late paraphrenia or LOS, are identified in Tables 1 and 2; the final columns cite studies of subsets selected for detailed investigation, including brain imaging. The data on late paraphrenia are based mainly on patient series assembled by Sjögren (1964), Herbert and Jacobson (1967), Grahame (1984), Holden (1987), Naguib and Levy (1987), Flint et al. (1991), Castle and Murray (1993), Howard et al. (1994a) and Almeida et al. (1995a). Data on LOS are derived from studies by Marneros and Deister (1984) and Häfner et al. (1992) in Europe and by Craig and Bregman (1988), Rabins et al. (1984, 1987), Pearlson et al. (1989, 1993) and Jeste et al. (1988, 1995) in the USA. Some authors have used non-committal terms such as paranoid ideation (Christenson and Blazer, 1984), late-life psychosis (Miller and Lesser, 1988) or persistent persecutory states (Post, 1966) to describe similar but not

Table 1. European studies ($N > 20$) showing size and source of samples and diagnostic criteria.

Authors describing sample	Source of data[a]	Years sample collected[b]	Sample size/age onset	Diagnosis	Comments and references to related papers[c]
Roth (1955)	IP, Graylingwell Hospital, UK	1934, 1936 1948–1949 records	46/>59	Late paraphrenia	2 year social follow-up, Hopkins and Roth (1953)
Fish (1960)	Institutions, Edinburgh	1957 interview	256/>60	With marked paranoid delusions	2.7% LOS, onset >60
Kay (1962)	IP, Psychiatric Hospital, Stockholm	1931–1940 records	57/>60	Late paraphrenia, Roth's criteria	Retrospective follow-up till 1956 or death, Kay (1959)
Kay and Roth (1961)	IP, Stockholm and Graylingwell Hospitals	1931–1940, 1951–1955 records + interview	ST 57, GW 42/>59	Late paraphrenia, Roth's criteria	Stockholm + new Graylingwell patients
Sjögren (1964)	IP, Lillhagen Hospital, Gothenburg	1964, not stated	202/not stated	Late paraphrenia, Roth's criteria	14% of geriatric first admissions
Post (1966)	IP, Bethlem Hospital, London	1954–1961, interview	93/not stated	Persistent persecutory states	17% organic aetiology, 1–3 year follow-up
Herbert and Jacobson (1967)	IP, St Francis Hospital, UK	1958–1964, not stated	45/ >middle age	Late paraphrenia, Roth's criteria	Restrospective follow-up
Marneros and Deister (1984)	IP, Cologne University Psychiatric Hospital	1950–1979, records	170/>50	Schneider's criteria for schizophrenia	Comparison of first hospitalized patients age >50 and <50

Study	Setting	Period/method	N/age	Diagnostic criteria	Comments
Grahame (1984)	Psychiatric services, City/East London	1981–1982, clinical	25/>60	Late paraphrenia, Roth's criteria	GMS to study Schneider first rank symptoms
Holden (1987)	Camberwell, London, cumulative psychiatric register	1971–1975, records+interview	37/>59	Late paraphrenia, Roth's criteria	10 year follow-up survivors and relatives interviewed
Naguib and Levy (1987)	IP, OP and DP, Bethlem/Maudsley, London	Not stated, GMS interview	43/>59	Late paraphrenia, Roth's criteria	Psychometric tests, CT scans. Burns et al. (1989); Hymas et al. (1989); Howard et al. (1992b)
Castle and Murray (1993)	Camberwell, London, cumulative psychiatric register	1965–1984 records OPCRIT	343/<45 134/>44 57/>64	ICD-9: schizophrenia, schizophrenia/affective, paraphrenic, other non-organic	Rates peaked at 16–25 and >65. Castle et al. (1997); Howard et al. (1993a)
Howard et al. (1994a)	IP, OP, DP, community and hospital services, London	1991–1992, records and PSE	101/>60	Late paraphrenia, Roth's criteria	CAMCOG, NART. Howard et al. (1992a), 1993b, 1994b, 1995a,b)
Almeida et al. (1995a)	As above. Normal controls from local clubs	1990–1992 interview	47/>54	Late paraphrenia, Roth's criteria	PSE, SAPS, HEN. Normal controls matched for age/sex/education/IQ. Almeida et al., 1995b,c,d, 1996
Häfner et al. (1992)	(1) 10 Mental hospitals, Germany	(1) 1987–1989 interview	76/35–59	ICD-9 schizophrenia, paranoid, psychogenic psychosis	PSE, IRAOS. Comparisons with younger patients. Riecher-Rössler et al. (1997); Häfner et al. (1998)

[a]IP, Inpatient; OP, outpatient; DP, day patient.
[b]GMS, Geriatric mental status examination; OPCRIT, operational criteria checklist for psychotic illness; PSE, present state examination (Wing et al., 1973).
[c]GMS, Geriatric mental status examination; NART, national adult reading test; SAPS, scale for assessment of positive symptoms; HEN, High Royds evaluation of negativity scale; IRAOS, instrument retrospective assessment of onset of schizophrenia (Häfner et al., 1992).

Table 2. North American studies (N>20) showing size and source of samples and diagnostic criteria.

Authors describing sample	Source of data[a]	Years sample collected[b]	Sample size/age onset	Diagnosis	Comments and references to related papers[c]
Christenson and Blazer (1984)	Community living persons, USA	1972, questionnaire by interview	40/>65	General persecutory ideation	4% prevalence. Diagnosis by Mini-Mult paranoid scale
Craig and Bregman (1988)	IP, Rockland Psychiatric Center	1972–1976, chart review	32 LOS/>45	DSM-III schizophrenia (except age)	Affective symptoms in 20%, organic deterioration in 41%
Miller and Lesser (1988)	IP, OP, Harbor-UCLA Medical Center	1986–1992, interview	24/27 total/>45	DSM-IIIR schizophrenia, delusional disorder, psychosis NOS	SPECT. Lesser et al. (1992); Miller et al. (1986,1989,1991,1992)
Flint et al. (1991)	IP, Clark Psychiatric Institute, Canada	1972–1987, chart review	21 LOS, 12 delusional disorder/>59	ICD-8,9 schizophrenia, paraphrenia, delusional disorder	CT scans (n=16) and drug response (n=33) in LOS and delusional disorder compared

Study	Setting	Period/method	N/age	Diagnostic criteria	Comments
Rabins et al. (1984)	IP, OP, Henry Phipps Clinic	1984–1987, chart review+ interview	35 LOS/>45	DSM-III schizophrenia (except age)	Comparison with 35 patients with major depression onset >45
Rabins et al. (1987)	As above	1983–1986	29 LOS/>45	DSM-III schizophrenia (except age)	VBR studies. Comparisons with AD and normal controls
Pearlson et al. (1989)	As above	1982–1986, chart review	54 LOS/>45	DSM-IIIR schizophrenia	Comparison of LOS versus 22 EOS-E, 54 EOS-Y. Pearlson et al. (1993)
Jeste et al. (1988)	Four centres, USA	1983–1987	37 LOS, >44	DSM-IIIR schizophrenia	Comparisons across four centres
Jeste et al. (1995)	San Diego VA and UCSD Medical Center and County Unit	Not stated. Over 3 year period	25 LOS/>45	DSM-IIIR schizophrenia	Study of LOS versus 39 EOS and 35 normal controls. Jeste et al. (1993); Corey-Bloom et al. (1995) (MRI)
Yassa and Suranyi-Cadotte (1993)	IP, Douglas Hospital, Quebec	1984–1990, interview	40 total/>45	DSM-IIIR LOS, ICD-9 delusional disorder	Comparison of LOS, paraphrenia and delusional disorder

[a]IP, Inpatient; OP, outpatient; DP, day patient.
[b]AD, Alzheimer's disease. EOS, Early onset schizophrenia < age 45; EOS-E, grown old; EOS-Y, young; LOS, late onset schizophrenia > age 45. MRI, magnetic resonance imaging. SPECT, Single photon emission computerized tomography. VBR, Ventricle/brain ratio.

necessarily identical groups. Studies by Breitner *et al.* (1990), Leuchter and Spar (1985), Krull *et al.* (1991) and Marneros *et al.* (1992) contained too few late onset patients for inclusion in the tables.

Symptomatology

Controversy exists as to whether the differences in symptomatology between schizophrenia in general and late paraphrenia (or LOS) are compatible or not with the latter being the manifestation of schizophrenia in later life. Riecher-Rössler *et al.* (1997) listed the clinical and epidemiological studies of LOS and concluded that differences between early and late onset illness (mostly with onset after 40 or 45 years) were only marginal both cross-sectionally and longitudinally. Interest has focused on symptoms regarded as typically schizophrenic, such as formal thought disorder, inappropriate affect, and first rank symptoms of Schneider (FRS). The main findings are that FRS of some kind occur in about one-third of patients with late paraphrenia but that thought insertion and withdrawal are uncommon (Post, 1966; Grahame, 1984; Howard *et al.*, 1993a,b, 1994a); that the incidence of FRS in LOS (onset > 45 years) does not differ significantly from that in early onset schizophrenia (Pearlson *et al.*, 1989), although some individual FRS are relatively common (Howard *et al.*, 1993a); and that formal thought disorder, inappropriate affect and other negative symptoms are rare in LOS and late paraphrenia (Almeida *et al.*, 1995a; Marneros and Deister, 1984) and much less common than in young people with schizophrenia or in people with schizophrenia who have grown old. Pearlson *et al.* (1989) found an inverse relation between age at onset and thought disorder, and between age at onset and marked affective flattening. In contrast, Riecher-Rössler *et al.* (1997) did not find significant differences on the SANS scale of negative symptoms between schizophrenic patients first admitted aged 40–59 and younger patients.

As regards positive symptoms, mainly delusions and hallucinations, delusions of persecution have been found to be more common in LOS than EOS (Howard *et al.*, 1993a) but their prevalence was also related to current age (Pearlson *et al.*, 1989). Marneros and Deister (1984) emphasized the richness of the psychotic productions in late schizophrenia. In contrast Riecher-Rössler *et al.* (1997), did not find significant differences in the PSE (Wing *et al.*, 1973) total score or subscore for delusions and hallucinations, or in FRS. However, Häfner *et al.* (1998) reported linear increases in paranoid symptoms and systematic delusions from adolescence to the age group 75 years and over (incoherent thought and ego disturbances displayed a linear decrease). Mayer *et al.* (1993) compared two groups of patients with onset aged 18–23 and with onset 40–63, both with ICD-9 diagnoses of schizophrenia or paranoid disorders; the paranoid subtype and paranoid disorders were much more common in the older onset group. In late paraphrenia, delusions of persecution, reference, misinterpretation and misidentification were the most common types, followed by alien control, and primary, hypochrondriacal and sexual delusions, while delusions of jealousy were much less common (Howard *et al.*, 1994a; Almeida *et al.*, 1995a). So-called partition delusions are characteristic both of late paraphrenia (Herbert and Jacobson, 1967; Howard *et al.*, 1992a) and LOS (Pearlson *et al.*, 1989); they may represent the mode in which older people experience boundary disturbances between self and non-self (Howard *et al.*, 1994a). A variant of the delusion of 'phantom boarders' may occur (Rowan, 1984). Hallucinations of any kind were more common in elderly than in younger patients; visual, tactile, olfactory and multimodal hallucinations were characteristic of patients with LOS (Pearlson *et al.*, 1989), while in late paraphrenia olfactory, visual, non-verbal and third person auditory hallucinations occurred, in that order, in from 30 to 70% (Howard *et al.*, 1994a).

Subtypes

About one-third of patients fulfil ICD-10 or DSM-IV criteria for delusional disorder (Howard *et al.*, 1994a; Almeida *et al.*, 1995a); nearly all the remainder can be diagnosed as paranoid schizophrenia. Principal components factor analysis generated five factors and three clusters which, however, did not closely correspond with the clinical ICD-10 diagnoses (Howard *et al.*, 1994a). Häfner *et al.* (1998) found that the symptoms of elderly patients fulfilling ICD-9 criteria for paranoid disorder differed from those of patients with schizophrenia quantitatively but not qualitatively, the largest differences being in tangential speech and disorders of self; FRS were present in both disorders.

In conclusion, while there is substantial agreement about the similarities and differences that exist in the symptomatology of patients with EOS and LOS, interpretations differ. Riecher-Rössler *et al.* (1997) conclude that LOS, strictly defined, with age at onset 40–59, is the same condition as schizophrenia at any age, differences being due to the pathoplastic effects of ageing, but Howard *et al.* (1993a) using broader criteria and including onsets over 60 consider that the early and late onset syndromes cannot be regarded as phenotypically homogeneous. The existence of a distinct group or subgroup akin to delusional disorder has received some support.

Response to treatment

Post (1966) was one of the first to report the striking immediate response to neuroleptics in a proportion of patients, and a good short term response has generally been confirmed (Raskind *et al.*, 1979; Rabins *et al.*, 1984; Pearlson *et al.*, 1989). Elderly patients are susceptible to side effects including tardive dyskinesia and Parkinsonism (Jeste *et al.*, 1993; Raskind and Risse, 1986) and are usually prescribed low doses, but despite this the short term response to treatment appears not to differ much from that of younger people with schizophrenia; this could be a consequence of the higher plasma concentrations. About 30% do not respond to the usual regimes. Soni (1988) noted that treatment of a physical condition may help to relieve psychotic symptoms. In the longer term, response is largely dependent on compliance and for this reason depot medication is advised (Howard and Levy, 1992). Non-compliance may result from lack of insight, which is related to the severity of positive symptoms, which in turn are the symptoms most likely to respond to neuroleptics (Almeida *et al.*, 1996). In a 5–15 year follow up of patients with paranoid psychoses in Denmark (9% DSM-III schizophrenia, 59% paranoid states and 31% reactive or other type), 91% received neuroleptic drugs; 27% had fully remitted and only 9% remained continuously psychotic (Jørgensen and Munk-Jørgensen, 1985).

Demography

The excess of females in late paraphrenia has been repeatedly observed (Post, 1966; Herbert and Jacobson, 1967; Naguib and Levy, 1987; Holden, 1987; Howard *et al.*, 1994a) and has also been found in most studies of LOS, based on DSM-IIIR criteria for schizophrenia (Rabins *et al.*, 1984; Pearlson *et al.* 1989). As regards civil status, being single or divorced is more common (31%) than in the general population or in affective disorders (Post, 1966) but not to the extent described by Kay and Roth (1961). Though a high proportion (37–51%) of females are childless (Herbert and Jacobson, 1967; Rabins *et al.*, 1984; Howard *et al.*, 1994a), fertility overall is not greatly reduced (Pearlson *et al.*, 1989; Almeida *et al.*, 1995a). In conclusion, an excess of females is one of the best attested facts in late paraphrenia, and is also found in most studies of LOS with onset after 45 but the cause is unclear. It appears to be a continuation of the increasing female preponderance that begins in schizophrenia in the fourth decade (Castle and Murray, 1993) for which endocrine changes (oestrogen deficit) have been thought responsible (Häfner *et al.*, 1991). Childlessness is often cited as a contributory cause of social isolation later in life but the possible effects of accidental factors such as being the youngest in the family, with a loss of older siblings, do not seem to have been evaluated.

Sensory impairment. (1) Hearing

Post (1966) found 30% of his paranoid patients to have impaired hearing compared with 11% of elderly depressives. Cooper *et al.* (1974) used the criteria of Wilkins (1948) to measure social deafness and calculated that deafness was about three times more common in elderly paranoid patients in England and Wales, whereas patients with affective disorder resembled the general elderly population (Wilkins, 1948). Forty-one per cent of the paranoid but only 17% of the depressed patients possessed hearing aids. These authors also employed pure tone audiometry to compare hearing loss in these groups: the paranoid patients had significantly more severe hearing loss in the better ear and, after controlling for age, the difference was also significant between patients who were first admissions. Otological examination of an enlarged sample showed that though sensorineural deafness was the most common type in both groups, significantly more paranoid than affective patients had deafness of conductive or mixed type, due to chronic middle-ear disease or otosclerosis, which was usually severe and bilateral, and had begun on average over 30 years before the onset of psychosis (Cooper and Curry, 1976). Patients with late paraphrenia have also been found to be more often socially deaf than psychiatrically normal age-matched controls (Naguib and Levy, 1987; Almeida et al., 1995b), and patients with LOS had significantly worse hearing than schizophrenic patients of similar age who had grown old (Pearlson et al., 1989).

The contribution of deafness among other factors to the aetiology of paranoid disorders was investigated by discriminate function analysis, which showed that social deafness present at onset of psychosis was one of four variables that independently differentiated between the paranoid and affective patient groups (Kay et al., 1976). Premorbid personality, number of surviving children, and family loading with affective disorder were the other variables. The finding that the patients with long-standing deafness had fewer abnormal personality traits than the remainder suggested that the deafness might have played a determining role in this subgroup (Cooper et al., 1976) (a similar observation in respect of visual impairment was made by Castle et al., 1997).

Not all studies have agreed with these findings. Sjögren (1964) found no difference between elderly paranoid and melancholic patients. Watt (1985) did not find significant differences in pure tone audiograms of paranoid patients whose illnesses began before the age of 60, and those of age-, sex- and social class-matched depressed patients or population controls. Moore (1981) found that hearing impairment was apparently rare in patients with affective disorders, which would suggest that these patients were not a valid control group; however, poor inter-observer reliability and other factors may have influenced the results in this study (Moore, 1981). In fact, major depression was the most frequent psychiatric diagnosis among patients attending hearing clinics (Mahapatra, 1974; Kalayam et al. 1991).

The specificity of hearing loss in late paraphrenia has been questioned. In a hospital study Stein and Thienhaus (1993) found that non-demented psychotic patients (mean age 66) had significantly worse unilateral poor tone averages and significantly poorer speech discrimination than controls, but patients whose delusions were paranoid were less impaired in both respects than non-paranoid subjects. Prager and Jeste (1993) carried out a controlled study of patients with LOS, EOS and mood disorders, and normal controls. The psychiatric patients as a group were significantly more impaired than the normal controls on a self-report hearing handicap inventory but they did not differ significantly on pure tone audiometry, and the patient groups did not differ between themselves on either measure. The authors noted that fewer schizophrenic patients wore hearing aids than the other groups although their uncorrected hearing loss was equally severe, suggesting that suboptimal correction of deficits might account for some of the findings in the literature. The pathology of the hearing impairment was not examined. The finding of Cooper and Curry (1976), that hearing loss in paranoid psychosis was largely due to long-standing middle-ear disease, has not been replicated; in their study sensorineural deafness was actually more common in depressed patients, though its presence in some paranoid patients might have been obscured by conductive defects.

In conclusion, the nature and role of the hearing deficits frequently reported in late paraphrenia remain incompletely elucidated. Various factors may contribute to this, including the exponential decline in auditory threshold with age, the only moderate correlation between pure tone audiometry and social deafness (Working Group on Speech Understanding and Aging, 1988), ambiguity in the diagnosis of social deafness (Cooper et al., 1976; Eastwood et al., 1985), and the likelihood that the prevalence of the potentially treatable conductive defects described in late paraphrenia varies by time and place. However, the reported disappearance of hallucinations after fitting a hearing aid (Eastwood et al., 1981) and the occurrence of unilateral hallucinations associated with unilateral conductive deafness (Khan et al., 1988) suggest that ear disease may play a part in the genesis of hallucinations in some patients.

Sensory impairment. (2) Vision

Herbert and Jacobson (1967) found visual loss in one or both eyes in 47% of their patients, and bilateral defects in 27%. However, most studies have not found visual impairments to be significantly increased in late paraphrenia (Sjögren, 1964; Naguib and Levy, 1987; Pearlson et al., 1989; Prager and Jeste, 1993; Almeida et al., 1995a). Cooper and Porter (1976) studied visual acuity and ocular pathology in the two groups of patients described by Cooper and Curry (1976) and found that vision was not significantly associated with diagnosis in either eye but when vision was optimized by spectacles, if they were worn, it was significantly worse in the less good eyes of paranoid patients. Prager and Jeste (1993) also found that their patient groups did not differ significantly from normal controls in uncorrected visual acuity in either eye but when vision was corrected by spectacles, all patient groups performed worse than controls. A possible explanation was that psychiatric patients in general (not LOS in particular) tend to have their eyesight inadequately corrected (Prager and Jeste, 1993). Visual impairment appears to have a closer connection with visual hallucinations (Berrios and Brook, 1984) than hearing impairment with auditory hallucinations. Some parallels have been drawn (Roth and Cooper, 1992; Howard and Levy, 1994) between the hallucinations of late paraphrenia and the syndromes of musical hallucinosis (Fuchs and Lauter, 1992) and of Charles Bonnet (Damas-Mora et al., 1982).

Premorbid personality

Post (1966) drawing on clinical impressions and relatives' reports considered that 40% of his patients had been paranoid, sensitive, quarrelsome or odd, while 30% had been anxious or depressive and 30% seemed to have been normal. Sjögren (1964) found paranoid patients tended to have been socially and economically insecure; 7% were isolated. Herbert and Jacobson (1967) also found many of their patients' premorbid personalities were paranoid or schizoid; only 9% were normally sociable. Howard and Levy (1993) administered the preliminary ICD-10 version of a personality assessment schedule to 25 consecutively referred patients with late paraphrenia and 10 controls. Ten (40%) of the index cases had a diagnosable ICD-10 personality disorder, all of which were of paranoid type, compared with two (20%) of the controls (none of paranoid type). Relatives judged seven of 13 (54%) to have paranoid personality disorder and one also to be dissocial. In addition, 10 index cases had one or more personality difficulties not amounting to diagnosable disorders (schizoid eight, paranoid six, dissocial two) compared with four of the controls (four anxious, two dependent). Twenty per cent of patients had no recognizable personality difficulty. The time of origin of the disorders or difficulties, and their relationship to living alone and family circumstances, such as position in the family and the number of surviving sibs or children, or to the presence of sensory deficits or psychiatric symptomatology, were not described. However, in a community study of elderly people Gurland and Wilder (1987) found a significant association between suspiciousness and having never been married, and between suspiciousness and hearing impairment.

Pearlson et al. (1989) recorded the presence or absence of 12 premorbid traits derived from earlier studies. Sixty-three per cent of LOS patients showed schizoid traits compared with 50% of elderly patients with EOS and 28% of young schizophrenics. A principal components factor analysis of the premorbid traits of LOS index cases produced two factors, one including

items such as outgoing and energetic, the other items like reclusive, intro-
verted, holding peculiar religious beliefs, which together accounted for 45%
of the variance. Jeste *et al.* (1995) noted that patients with LOS sometimes
showed schizoid or paranoid traits but did not meet DSM-IIIR criteria for
personality disorders; LOS and EOS patients both differed significantly from
normal subjects on psychosocial history (childhood and psychosexual
subscales of a premorbid social adjustment scale) and on the interpersonal
relations item of an outcome and prognostic scale. EOS patients differed
from controls on some items on which LOS patients showed non-significant
differences in the same direction. The authors considered that the similarities between LOS and EOS supported the diagnosis of schizophrenia in the
late onset group (Jeste *et al.*, 1995).

In conclusion, the earlier observations that the majority of patients with
late paraphrenia have personality disturbances, mainly of paranoid or
schizoid type, have been confirmed. Their relationship to the psychosis and
the existence of a minority of patients whose personality seems to have been
within normal limits are topics for further study.

Social isolation and living alone

Of late paraphrenia patients, 40–80% are reported to have experienced social
isolation (Herbert and Jacobson, 1967; Holden, 1987; Almeida *et al.*, 1995a),
the proportion depending in part on how it is measured but in any case much
more frequently than controls. Herbert and Jacobson (1967) found that lack
of social contact due to being single or widowed, bereavement or moving
house were common, and had probably intensified existent personality
defects, with a contribution from sensory loss. Almeida *et al.* (1995b) found
that 70% of patients with late paraphrenia were living alone compared with
18% of age- and sex-matched normal controls and that only 13% were in
sheltered accommodation compared with 64% of controls; they were less
involved than controls in regular leisure activities ($p < 0.001$) and 78% were
judged to be socially isolated, at the time of assessment, compared with 18%
of controls ($p < 0.001$). There was a non-significant excess of never-married
among controls (presumably related to recruitment from clubs) but more of
the patients were divorced or widowed (66% versus 33%). The number of
children born to ever-married persons did not differ significantly between the
groups. The results suggested that social isolation was due to the current state
rather than to premorbid factors (Almeida *et al.*, 1995b). In the USA, studies
of patients with DSM-IIIR LOS found that 34–50% were living alone,
compared with 26% of elderly patients with major depression ($p > 0.05$), and
with none of elderly schizophrenics with early onset (who presumably were
living in institutions) (Rabins *et al.*, 1984; Pearlson *et al.*, 1989). More LOS
patients were childless compared with controls but not to a significant extent.

In conclusion, there has been little systematic investigation of the mode of development and causes of social isolation in late paraphrenia, and its relationship to the prodromal stages of the psychosis remains unclear. Psychoses could sometimes be the result of defensive reactions by vulnerable personalities to the adverse cirumstances that affect many old people (Cordeiro, 1992). However, Gurland and Wilder (1987) found no association between social isolation and hearing loss or between social isolation and suspiciousness among elderly subjects living in the community. Gurian et al. (1992) proposed that early trauma and failure to have children among a group of patients who were war refugees contributed to their social isolation and eventual psychosis, and Fuchs (1994) found that nearly half of patients with late onset paranoid psychosis had been war refugees. Careful reconstruction of the sequence of events leading to social isolation is required.

Family history

Funding (1962) and Watt et al. (1980) found no increase in risk of schizophrenia among relatives of patients with paranoid psychoses. Pearlson et al. (1989) found 17% with family history of schizophrenia among LOS patients, compared with 32% in elderly EOS and 18% in young EOS patients ($p > 0.5$). Kay (1959) had found no increase in risk of affective disorder in first-degree relatives of late paraphrenics but Howard et al. (1997) reported no excess of schizophrenia but a significant excess of depressive states in the relatives of patients compared with relatives of controls, a new finding requiring confirmation. The advanced age and psychosis of probands and the estrangement of many of them from their families make reliable family histories difficult to obtain.

Epidemiology

Statistics based on first admissions to hospital (Kay, 1972; Riecher-Rössler et al., 1997) or first contact with a case-register (Holden, 1987; Castle and Murray, 1993) have shown age-specific rates for late onset schizophrenia including paranoid states of 10–26 per 100,000 per year. Castle and Murray (1993) found onset to be after age 64 in 12% of patients with diagnosis of schizophrenia but Riecher-Rössler et al. (1997) estimated that only 3–4% of first admissions to hospital occurred after age 60. Van Os et al. (1995) reported an increase in age-specific admission rates aged 60 and over with non-affective non-organic psychoses in the Netherlands and regions of England and Wales in both sexes, and Castle et al. (1993) observed a peak after 65 which was much more pronounced in women. Castle et al. (1993) and Riecher-Rössler et al. (1997) also observed a small peak in incidence in mid-life, which was confined to women and compatible with the oestrogen hypothesis, while the later peak suggested an effect of brain degeneration.

The hope that the mode of development of late paraphrenia would be illuminated by field studies has not yet been realized, chiefly because of the low yield. Most prevalence estimates of schizophrenia of late onset in the general elderly population vary from 0.1 to 1.0% (review by Henderson and Kay, 1997), but Skoog (1993) found a higher rate and an association of schizophrenic but not delusional syndromes with Alzheimer's disease. Generalized persecutory ideation was found in 4% of an elderly community-living population, based on self-report utilizing the Duke–OARS Multidimensional Functional Assessment Questionnaire, and was associated with cognitive impairment and sensory deficit (Christenson and Blazer, 1984).

Cognition and cerebral changes

As regards cognitive functioning, Naguib and Levy (1987) found that patients with late paraphrenia performed significantly less well than independently living, healthy controls on two of the three psychological tests administered but observed that the lack of correlation of cognitive performance either with duration of illness (range 3 to 240 months) or the VBR (ventricle/brain ratio) suggested that there was not a simple relationship between cognitive deficit, psychotic illness and brain degeneration. Howard and Almeida (1994) compared the performance of patients and controls on the CAMCOG subsections (Roth et al., 1988) and found lower scores in attention, retrieval of remote information and expressive language, the pattern differing from that in Alzheimer's disease. More elaborate testing including computerized tests for frontal lobe dysfunction (executive functions) were carried out on patients with late paraphrenia (onset over age 55) and normal controls by Almeida et al. (1995c,d). A clear pattern of impairment could not be distinguished overall but two subgroups of patients could be discerned: one manifested a wide range of psychotic symptoms but cognitive deficits were restricted to executive functions, while in the other the psychotic symptoms were less complex but cognitive impairment was generalized and there were neurological soft signs, compatible with the existence of an organic basis (Almeida et al.,1995c,d). In LOS patients (onset after age 45) the neuropsychological deficits resembled those reported in young people with schizophrenia but differed from those of patients with Alzheimer's disease (Cullum et al., 1988), and in another study they were found to differ from normal controls but to resemble the deficits in patients with EOS who had become old (Jeste et al., 1995).

Is cognitive impairment progressive? Holden (1987) identified new cases of functional paranoid psychoses retrospectively from a case-register and after excluding those with low scores on a routine cognitive test, followed them up for 10 years or till death, using records and interviewing survivors and next of kin. Ten of these patients were considered after follow-up and review to be suffering from depression or from secondary symptomatic psychoses, and were excluded. Of the remaining 37, 13 (35%) had become demented within 3 years, and it was observed that the initial mean test scores of these patients had been significantly lower than the remainder; they seemed to form a separate organic subgroup. The findings in this study pointed to the presence of cerebral change in a proportion of cases diagnosable as late paraphrenia but the criterion of absence of dementia at onset of illness, required by Kay and Roth (1961), may not have been fulfilled.

In the patients studied by Naguib and Levy (1987), cognitive performance had deteriorated after a mean period of 3.7 years to a greater extent in surviving patients with late paraphrenia than in controls, but only 6.5% of patients and 5.9% of controls showed a global deterioration suggestive of dementia (Hymas *et al.*, 1989). Follow-up performance was not related to initial ventricular size, duration of symptoms, or medication. Longer follow-up has also been reported. In the Danish study of paranoid psychoses already referred to, the diagnosis changed to dementia in only 8% after 5–15 years (Jørgensen and Munk-Jørgensen, 1985). Gabriel (1992) found no significant difference in the frequency of signs of organic brain syndrome in patients with delusions with onset in mid-life (aged 40–64) who had survived, compared with the whole group of schizophrenics; the mean duration of follow-up was 26 years, when the mean age was 75, but there was no information about those who had died.

Examination of the overlap between late paraphrenia and organic cerebral disease has been hampered by the fact that patients with neurological disease are usually excluded by the diagnostic criteria. Post (1966), who did not exclude them, found 17% with clinically suspected or confirmed progressive cerebral disease; he noted that the psychotic symptoms of these patients were indistinguishable from those of patients with intact brains. More recently clinico-pathological correlations have been studied by cerebral imaging. A series of papers from the Harbor-UCLA Medical Center (Miller *et al.*, 1986, 1989; Lesser *et al.*, 1992) reported clinically silent lesions, revealed only by CT, including subcortical infarctions and white matter abnormalities, in up to 60% of patients with late-life psychosis (DSM-IIIR schizophrenia, delusional disorder or psychosis not otherwise specified). However, the structural lesions were not significantly correlated with neuropsychological test performance, which resembled that described in schizophrenia (Miller *et al.*, 1991). Utilizing single brain photon emission computerized tomography (SPECT), Miller *et al.* (1992) compared the regional cerebral blood flow of patients with late onset psychosis and of patients with late onset psychotic depression with elderly controls. Both patient groups differed significantly from controls in extent of temporal or frontal hypoperfusion. Somewhat similar observations were made by Breitner *et al.* (1990) but Corey-Bloom *et al.* (1995) and Krull *et al.* (1991), using MRI, found no difference in white matter abnormalities between patients with DSM-IIIR LOS and controls, though the LOS patients had larger ventricles.

Brain imaging studies were also conducted by the Johns Hopkins group. Rabins *et al.* (1987) found the mean ventricle/brain ratio (VBR) was significantly higher in patients with LOS than in age-matched healthy controls but significantly lower than in patients with Alzheimer's disease (AD) who also had hallucinations or delusions; they considered the increased VBR was unlikely to be a manifestation of early progressive dementia (Rabins *et al.*, 1987). Pearlson *et al.* (1993) found that patients with AD had significantly larger lateral VBR, third ventricle volumes and more total CSF than controls but detected no significant differences between LOS and EOS patients.

CT studies carried out on patients with late paraphrenia at the Institute of Psychiatry and Maudsley Hospital, London, revealed dilatation of the lateral ventricle (Naguib and Levy, 1987); since this was not accompanied by the sulcal widening present in the age-matched normal controls, it was suggesting that the dilatation was not merely age-related (Burns *et al.*, 1989). Howard *et al.* (1992b) re-examined the same patients and found that those exhibiting first rank symptoms of Schneider (FRS) had less cortical atrophy than those who did not, and was similar to that seen in age-matched normal controls. In a new cohort of patients, using MRI, Howard *et al.* (1994b) found significantly greater lateral and third ventricle volumes than in controls, but the differences were limited to a subgroup of patients who fulfilled criteria for ICD-10 delusional disorder. An inverse relation between auditory hallucinations and VBR in schizophrenia (Owens *et al.*, 1985) and between cortical atrophy and paranoid delusions in senile dementia (Jacoby and Levy, 1980) had suggested that a relatively intact brain was necessary for the occurrence of complex psychotic symptoms (Forstl *et al.*, 1992). Howard *et al.* (1995a) also made quantitative volumetric measurements of the superior temporal and parahippocampal gyri, the hippocampal, frontal and temporal lobes, and the basal ganglia structures, and again found differences between controls and the delusional disorder subgroup which were not present between controls and the remaining patients. The delusional disorder patients also had more right–left temporal lobe asymmetry. These findings are compatible with the view that late paraphrenia includes a subgroup of patients with neurodegenerative changes, which are not present or only doubtfully present in the remaining patients, who are suffering from paranoid schizophrenia. The VBR did not correlate either with the cognitive performance of patients or with duration of illness (range 3–240 months), suggesting that the ventricular enlargement may have preceded the onset of overt symptoms; however, its unimodal distribution pointed to late paraphrenia being a unitary condition (Naguib and Levy, 1987). In a further study, Howard *et al.* (1995b) looked for white matter signal hyperintensities (WMI) and found these were very common in both patients and controls, were associated with blood pressure, and were not significantly different in patients with late paraphrenia and community-living controls; none of the patients had MRI evidence of cerebral infarction. Symonds *et al.* (1997) made similar observations. This conclusion does not agree with the findings of Miller *et al.* (1992) or Breitner *et al.* (1990) but accords with other studies (Krull *et al.*, 1991; Pearlson *et al.*, 1993; Corey-Bloom *et al.*, 1995), and is compatible with the report of Flint *et al.* (1991) that silent areas of cerebral infarction are more common in paranoia (chronic delusional disorder) than in late paraphrenia.

Neuropathological studies of late paraphrenia are few in number. Blessed (1989) referred to nine patients with paranoid illness of late onset with mean plaque counts and neurofibrillary tangle density within the range found in patients with multi-infarct dementia, acute confusion, affective disorder or physical illness, and much less than in patients with senile dementia; the volume of infarction was not increased.

In conclusion, apart from a putative subgroup diagnosable as delusional disorder, the evidence for cerebral changes in the main group, identified as paranoid schizophrenia with late onset, has been inconsistent; any changes that may exist are subtle and may be related to non-specific atrophy or hypoplasia associated with schizophrenias of any age rather than to age-related, progressive neurodegeneration.

GENERAL CONCLUSIONS

The existence of non-affective, non-organic psychoses occurring for the first time late in life is now well established. The relationship of these psychoses to schizophrenia is still debated but it is widely accepted that at least a proportion are manifestations of schizophrenia, as acknowledged by the revision of DSM-III in 1987 (American Psychiatric Association, 1987). The occurrence of schizophrenia-like psychoses in the presence of neurological disease is also well established, though the frequency with which these phenocopies occur requires further study. The brain changes and psychological impairments most consistently reported in the late-life psychoses without overt neurological disease are compatible with the advances that have taken place in schizophrenia, and are different from those occurring in the dementia disorders.

Of the features earlier thought to be characteristic of late paraphrenia, female predominance and deviant premorbid personality have been strongly supported, while data on family history, marital status, fertility and the role of sensory impairment have been less consistent, and the causes and significance of social isolation remain unresolved. The relative importance of innate and accidental factors is an open question.

As regards nomenclature, there is some doubt whether the schizophrenias of very late onset (i.e. after the age of 60 or 65) can be regarded as identical, aside from pathoplastic effects of greater age, with the traditional disorder. Here the term late paraphrenia, which has been criticized as being ill-defined and overinclusive, appears to be serving a useful purpose by embracing conditions whose boundaries are as yet unclear and whose relationship to schizophrenia is conjectural. In contrast, narrow definitions pre-empt these issues by excluding just those residual and atypical disorders whose affinity to schizophrenia calls for elucidation. Late paraphrenia, or an equivalent non-committal term, will be superfluous when schizophrenia has been biologically defined and the full range of its phenomenology becomes apparent.

REFERENCES

Almeida, O., Howard, R.J., Levy, R. and David, A.S. (1995a). Psychotic states arising in late life. Psychopathology and nosology. *Br J Psychiatry* **166**, 205–214.

Almeida, O., Howard, R.J., Levy, R. and David, A.S. (1995b). Psychotic states arising in late life. The role of risk factors. *Br J Psychiatry* **166**, 215–228.

Almeida, O.P., Howard, R.J., Levy, R., David, A.S., Morris, R.G. and Sahakian, B.J. (1995c). Cognitive features of psychotic states arising in late life (late paraphrenia). *Psychol Med* **25**, 685–698.

Almeida, O.P., Howard, R.J., Levy, R., David, A.S., Morris, R.G. and Sahakian, B.J. (1995d). Clinical and cognitive diversity of psychotic states arising in late life (late paraphrenia). *Psychol Med* **25**, 699–714.

Almeida, O.P., Levy, R., Howard, R. and David, A.S. (1996). Insight and paranoid disorders in late life (late paraphrenia). *Int J Geriatr Psychiatry* **11**, 653–658.

American Psychiatric Association (1987). *Diagnostic and Statistical Manual of Mental Disorders, 3rd edn revised* (DSM-IIIR). APA, Washington, DC.

Berrios, G.E. and Brook, P. (1984). Visual hallucinations and sensory delusions in the elderly. *Br J Psychiatry* **144**, 662–664.

Blessed, G. (1989). Clinicopathological studies in mental disorder in old age. The Newcastle studies 1963–1977. In: Davison, K. and Kerr, A. (Eds), *Contemporary Themes in Psychiatry*. Gaskell, London, pp. 14–321.

Breitner, J.C.S., Husain, M.M., Figiel, G.S., Ranga, K., Krishman, R. and Boyko, O.B. (1990). Cerebral white matter disease in late-onset paranoid psychosis. *Biol Psychiatry* **28**, 266–274.

Burns, A., Carrick, J., Ames, D., Naguib,M. and Levy, R. (1989). The cerebral cortical appearance in late paraphrenia. *Int J Geriatr Psychiatry* **4**, 31–34.

Castle, D.J. and Murray, R.M. (1993). The epidemiology of late-onset schizophrenia. *Schizophr Bull* **19**, 691–700.

Castle, D.J., Wessely, S. and Murray, R.M. (1993). Sex and schizophrenia: effects of diagnostic stringency, and associations with premorbid variables. *Br J Psychiatry* **162**, 658–664.

Castle, D.J., Wessely, S., Howard, R. and Murray, R.M. (1997). Schizophrenia with onset at the extremes of adult life. *Int J Geriatr Psychiatry* **12**, 712–717.

Christenson, R. and Blazer, D. (1984). Epidemiology of persecutory ideation in an elderly population in the community. *Am J Psychiatry* **141**, 1088–1091.

Cooper, A.F. and Curry, A.R. (1976). The pathology of deafness in the paranoid and affective psychoses of later life. *J Psychosomatic Res* **20**, 97–105.

Cooper, A.F. and Porter, R. (1976). Visual acuity and ocular pathology in the paranoid and affective psychoses of later life. *J Psychosomatic Res* **20**, 107–114.

Cooper, A., Kay, D., Curry, A., Garside, R. and Roth, M. (1974). Hearing loss in the paranoid and affective psychoses of later life. *Lancet* **ii**, 851–854.

Cooper, A.F., Garside, R.F. and Kay, D.W.K. (1976). A comparison of deaf and non-deaf patients with paranoid and affective psychoses. *Br J Psychiatry* **129**, 532–538.

Cordeiro, J.D. (1992). Late chronic delusions – psychopathology and nosography. In: Katona, C. and Levy, R. (Eds). *Delusions and Hallucinations in Old Age*. Gaskell, London, pp. 177–186.

Corey-Bloom, J., Jernigan, T., Archibald, S., Harris, M.J. and Jeste, D.V. (1995). Quantitative magnetic resonance imaging of the brain in late-life schizophrenia. *Am J Psychiatry* **152**, 447–449.

Corsellis, J.A.N. (1962). *Mental Illness and the Ageing Brain*. Maudsley Monograph No. 9. Oxford University Press, London.

Craig, T.J. and Bregman, Z. (1988). Late onset schizophrenia-like illness. *J Am Geriatr Soc* **36**, 104–107.

Cullum, C.M., Heaton, R.K. and Nemiroff, B. (1988). Neuropsychology of late-life psychoses. *Psychiatric Clin North Am* **11**, 47–59.

Damas-Mora, J., Skelton-Robinson, M. and Jenner, F. (1982). The Charles Bonnet syndrome in perspective. *Psychol Med* **12**, 251–261.

Eastwood, M.R., Corbin, S. and Reed, M. (1981). Hearing impairment and paraphrenia. *J Otolaryngology* **10**, 306–308.

Eastwood, M.R., Corbin, S.L., Reed, M., Nobbs, H. and Kedward, H.B. (1985). Acquired hearing loss and psychiatric illness: an estimate of prevalence and co-morbidity in a geriatric setting. *Br J Psychiatry* **147**, 552–556.

Faris, R.E.L. and Dunham, H.W. (1939). *Mental Disorders in Urban Areas*. University of Chicago Press, Chicago.

Fish, F. (1960). Senile schizophrenia. *J Mental Sci* **106**, 938–946.

Flint, A.J., Rifat, S.L. and Eastwood, M.R. (1991). Late-onset paranoia: distinct from paraphrenia? *Int J Geriatr Psychiatry* **6**, 103–109.

Forstl, H., Howard, R., Almeida, O. and Stadtmuller, G. (1992). Psychotic symptoms and the paraphrenic brain. In: Katona, C. and Levy, R. (Eds). *Delusions and Hallucinations in Old Age*. Gaskell, London, pp. 153–170.

Fuchs, T. (1994). Uprooting and late-life psychosis. *Eur Arch Psychiatry Clin Neurosci* **244**, 126–130.

Fuchs, T. and Lauter, H. (1992). Charles Bonnet syndrome and musical hallucinations in the elderly. In: Katona, C. and Levy, R. (Eds) *Delusions and Hallucinations in Old Age*. Gaskell, London, pp. 187–198.

Funding, T. (1962). Genetics of paranoid psychoses in later life. *Acta Psychiatr Scand* **37**, 267–282.

Gabriel, E. (1992). Delusional disorders (of earlier onset) in old age. In: Katona, C. and Levy, R. (Eds). *Delusions and Hallucinations in Old Age*. Gaskell, London, pp. 173–176.

Grahame, P.S. (1984). Schizophrenia in old age (late paraphrenia). *Br J Psychiatry* **145**, 493–495.

Gurian, B.S., Wexler, D. and Baker, E.H. (1992). Late-life paranoia: possible association with early trauma and infertility. *Int J Geriatr Psychiatry* **7**, 277–284.

Gurland, B.J. and Wilder, C. (1987). Deafness as a precursor to paraphrenia. In: Miller, N.E. and Cohen, G.D. (Eds). *Schizophrenia and Aging: Schizophrenia,*

Paranoia, and Schizophreniform Disorders in Later Life. Guilford Press, New York, pp. 239–245.

Häfner, H., Behrens, S., de Vry, J. and Gattaz, W.F. (1991). Oestradiol enhances the vulnerability threshold for schizophrenia in women by an early effect on dopaminergic neurotransmission. *Eur Arch Psychiatry Clin Neurosci* **24**, 65–68.

Häfner, H., Riecher-Rössler, A., Hambrecht, M. *et al.* (1992). IRAOS: an instrument for the retrospective assessment of onset and early course of schizophrenia. *Schizophr Res* **6**, 209–223.

Häfner, H., Hambrecht, M., Löffler, W., Munk-Jørgensen, P. and Riecher-Rössler, A. (1998). Is schizophrenia a disorder of all ages? A comparison of first episodes and early course across the life-cycle. *Psychol Med* **28**, 315–365.

Henderson, A.S. and Kay, D.W.K. (1997). The epidemiology of functional psychoses of late onset. *Eur Arch Psychiatry Clin Neurosci* **247**, 176–189.

Herbert, M.E. and Jacobson, S. (1967). Late paraphrenia. *Br J Psychiatry* **113**, 461–469.

Holden, N.L (1987). Late paraphrenia or the paraphrenias? A descriptive study with a 10-year follow-up. *Br J Psychiatry* **150**, 635–639.

Hopkins, B. and Roth, M. (1953). Psychological test performance in patients over sixty. II. Paraphrenia, arteriosclerotic psychosis and acute confusion. *J Mental Sci* **99**, 451–463.

Houston, F. and Royse, A.B. (1954). Relationship between deafness and psychotic illness. *J Mental Sci* **100**, 990–993.

Howard, R. and Almeida, O.P. (1994). Cognitive changes in late paraphrenia. In: Burns, A. and Levy, R. (Eds). *Dementia.* Chapman & Hall, London, pp. 710–716.

Howard, R. and Levy, R. (1992). Which factors affect treatment response in late paraphrenia? *Int J Geriatr Psychiatry* **7**, 667–672.

Howard, R. and Levy, R. (1993). Personality structure in the paranoid psychoses of later life. *Eur Psychiatry* **8**, 59–66.

Howard, R. and Levy, R. (1994). Charles Bonnet syndrome plus: complex visual hallucinations of Charles Bonnet type in late paraphrenia. *Int J Geriatr Psychiatry* **9**, 399–404.

Howard, R., Castle, D., O'Brien, J., Almeida, O. and Levy, R. (1992a). Permeable walls, floors, ceilings and doors. Partition delusions in late paraphrenia. *Int J Geriatr Psychiatry* **7**, 719–724.

Howard, R.J., Forstl, H., Naguib, M., Burns, A. and Levy, R. (1992b). First-rank symptoms of Schneider in late paraphrenia: cortical structural correlates. *Br J Psychiatry* **160**, 108–109.

Howard, R., Castle, D., Wessely, S. and Murray, R. (1993a). A comparative study of 470 cases of early-onset and late-onset schizophrenia. *Br J Psychiatry* **163**, 352–357.

Howard, R., Almeida, O. and Levy, R. (1993b). Schizophrenic symptoms in late paraphrenia. *Psychopathology* **26**, 95–101.

Howard, R.J., Almeida, O. and Levy, R. (1994a). Phenomenology, demography and diagnosis in late paraphrenia. *Psychol Med* **24**, 397–410.

Howard, R.J., Almeida, O., Levy, R., Graves, P. and Graves, M. (1994b). Quantitative magnetic resonance imaging volumetry distinguishes delusional disorder from late-onset schizophrenia. *Br J Psychiatry* **165**, 474–480.

Howard, R.J., Mellers, J., Petty, R. *et al.* (1995a). Magnetic resonance imaging volumetric measurements of the superior temporal gyrus, hippocampus, parahippocampal gyrus, frontal and temporal lobes in late paraphrenia. *Psychol Med* **25**, 495–503.

Howard, R., Cox, T., Almeida, O., Mullen, R., Graves, P., Reveley, A. and Levy, R.

(1995b). White matter signal hyperintensities in the brains of patients with late paraphrenia and the normal community-living elderly. *Biol Psychiatry* **38**, 86–91.

Howard, R.J., Graham, C., Sham, P. *et al.* (1997). A controlled family study of late-onset non-affective psychosis (late paraphrenia). *Br J Psychiatry* **170**, 511–514.

Hymas, N., Naguib, M. and Levy, R. (1989). Late paraphrenia. A follow-up study. *Int J Geriatr Psychiatry* **4**, 23–29.

Jacoby, R.J. and Levy, R. (1980). Computerised tomography in the elderly. 2. Senile dementia: diagnosis and functional impairment. *Br J Psychiatry* **136**, 256–269.

Jeste, D.V., Lacro, J.P., Gilbert, P.L., Kline, J. and Kline, N. (1993). Treatment of late-life schizophrenia with neuroleptics. *Schizophr Bull* **19**, 817–830.

Jeste, D.V., Harris, M.J., Pearlson, G.D. *et al.* (1988). Late-onset schizophrenia. Studying clinical validity. *Psychiatric Clin North Am* **11**, 1–13.

Jeste, D.V., Harris, M.J., Krull, A., Kuck, J., McAdams, L.A. and Heaton, R. (1995). Clinical and neuropsychological characteristics of patients with late-onset schizophrenia. *Am J Psychiatry* **152**, 722–730.

Jørgensen, P. and Munk-Jørgensen, P. (1985). Paranoid psychosis in the elderly. A follow-up study. *Acta Psychiatr Scand* **62**, 358–363.

Kalayam, B., Alexopoulos, G.S., Merrell, H.B., Young, R.C. and Shindledecker, R. (1991). Patterns of hearing loss and psychiatric morbidity in elderly patients attending a hearing clinic. *Int J Geriatr Psychiatry* **6**, 31–136.

Kay, D. (1959). Observations on the natural history and genetics of old age psychoses: a Stockholm material, 1931–1937. *Proc Roy Soc Med* **52**, 791–794.

Kay, D.W.K. (1962). Outcome and cause of death in mental disorders of old age: a long-term follow-up of functional and organic psychoses. *Acta Psychiatr Scand* **38**, 249–276.

Kay, D.W.K. (1972). Schizophrenia and schizophrenia-like states in the elderly. *Br J Hosp Med* October, 369–376.

Kay, D.W.K. and Roth, M. (1955). Physical accompaniments of mental disorder in old age. *Lancet* **259**, 740–745.

Kay, D.W.K. and Roth, M. (1961). Environmental and hereditary factors in the schizophrenia of old age ('late paraphrenia') and their bearing on the general problem of causation in schizophrenia. *J Mental Sci* **107**, 649–686.

Kay, D.W.K., Beamish, P. and Roth, M. (1964). Old age mental disorders in Newcastle upon Tyne. Part 1: a study of prevalence. *Br J Psychiatry* **110**, 146–158.

Kay, D.W.K., Cooper, A.F., Garside, R.F. and Roth, M. (1976). The differentiation of paranoid from affective psychoses by patients' premorbid characteristics. *Br J Psychiatry* **129**, 207–215.

Khan, A.M., Clark, T. and Oyebode, F. (1988). Unilateral auditory hallucinations (letter). *Br J Psychiatry* **152**, 297–298.

Krull, A.J., Press, G., Dupont, R., Harris, M.J. and Jeste, D.V. (1991). Brain imaging in late-onset schizophrenia and related psychoses. *Int J Geriatr Psychiatry* **6**, 651–658.

Lesser, I.M., Jeste, D.V., Boone, K.B. *et al.* (1992). Late-onset psychotic disorder, not otherwise specified: clinical and neuroimaging findings. *Biol Psychiatry* **31**, 419–423.

Leuchter, A.F. and Spar, J.E. (1985). The late-onset psychoses. Clinical and diagnostic features. *J Nervous Mental Dis* **173**, 488–493.

Lewis, A.J. (1946). Ageing and senility: a major problem of psychiatry. *J Mental Sci* **12**, 150–170.

Mahapatra, S.B. (1974). Deafness and mental health: psychiatric and psychosomatic illness in the deaf. *Acta Psychiatr Scand* **50**, 596–611.

Marneros, A. and Deister, A. (1984). The psychopathology of 'late schizophrenia'. *Psychopathology* **17**, 264–274.

Marneros, A., Deister, A. and Rohde, A. (1992). Schizophrenic, schizoaffective and affective disorders in the elderly: a comparison. In: Katona, C. and Levy, R. (Eds). *Delusions and Hallucinations in Old Age.* Gaskell, London, pp. 136–152.

Mayer, C., Kelterborn, G. and Naber, D. (1993). Age of onset in schizophrenia: relations to psychopathology and gender. *Br J Psychiatry* **162**, 665–671.

Miller, B.L. and Lesser, I.M. (1988). Late-life psychosis and modern neuroimaging. *Psychiatric Clin North Am* **11**, 33–45.

Miller, B.L., Benson, F., Cummings, J.J. and Neshkes, R. (1986). Late-life paraphrenia: an organic delusional syndrome. *J Clin Psychiatry* **47**, 204–207.

Miller, B.L, Lesser, I.M, Boone, K. *et al.* (1989). Brain white-matter lesions and psychosis. *Br J Psychiatry* **155**, 73–78.

Miller, B.L., Lesser, I.M., Boone, K., Hill, E., Mehringer, M.C. and Wong, K. (1991). Brain lesions and cognitive functions in late-life psychosis. *Br J Psychiatry* **158**, 76–82.

Miller, B.L., Lesser, I.M., Mena, I. *et al.* (1992). Regional cerebral blood flow in late-life-onset psychosis. *Neuropsychiatr Neuropsychol Behav Neurol* **5**, 132–137.

Moore, N.C. (1981). Is paranoid illness associated with sensory deficits in the elderly? *J Psychosomatic Res* **25**, 69–74.

Naguib, M. and Levy, R. (1987). Late paraphrenia. *Int J Geriatr Psychiatry* **2**, 83–90.

Owens, D.G.C., Johnstone, E.C., Crow, T.J. *et al.* (1985). Lateral ventricular size in schizophrenia: relationship to the disease process and its clinical manifestations. *Psychol Med* **15**, 27–41.

Pearlson, G.D., Kreger, L., Rabins, P.V. *et al.* (1989). Late life onset schizophrenia: a chart review study. *Am J Psychiatry* **146**, 1568–1574.

Pearlson, G.D., Tune, L.E., Wong, D.F. *et al.* (1993). Quantitative D_2 dopamine receptor PET and structural MRI changes in late-onset schizophrenia. *Schizophr Bull* **19**, 783–795.

Post, F. (1965). *The Clinical Psychiatry of Late Life.* Pergamon Press, Oxford.

Post, F. (1966). *Persistent Persecutory States of the Elderly.* Pergamon Press, Oxford.

Prager, S. and Jeste, D.V. (1993). Sensory impairment in late-life schizophrenia. *Schizophr Bull* **19**, 755–772.

Rabins, P., Pauker, S. and Thomas, J. (1984). Can schizophrenia begin after age 44? *Compr Psychiatry* **25**, 290–293.

Rabins, P., Pearlson, G.D., Jayaram, G., Steele, C. and Tune, L. (1987a). Increased ventricle-to-brain ratio in late-onset schizophrenia. *Am J Psychiatry* **144**, 1216–1218.

Raskind, M.A. and Risse, S.C. (1986). Antipsychotic drugs and the elderly. *J Clin Psychiatry* **46**, 17–22.

Raskind, M.A., Alvarez, C. and Herlin, S. (1979). Fluphenazine enanthate in the outpatient treatment of late paraphrenia. *J Am Geriatr Soc* **27**, 459–463.

Riecher-Rössler, A., Löffler, W. and Munk-Jørgensen, P. (1997). What do we really know about late-onset schizophrenia? *Eur Arch Psychiatry Clin Neurosci* **247**, 195–208.

Robertson, E.E. and Mason-Browne, N.L. (1953). Review of mental illness in the old age group. *Br Med J* **ii**, 1076–1079.

Roth, M. (1955). The natural history of mental disorders in old age. *J Mental Sci* **101**, 281–301.

Roth, M. and Cooper, A.F. (1992). A review of late paraphrenia and what is known of its aetiological basis. In: Katona, C. and Levy, R. (Eds). *Delusions and*

Hallucinations in Old Age. Gaskell, London, pp. 25–42.

Roth, M. and Hopkins, B. (1953). Psychological test performance in patients over sixty. I. Senile psychosis and the affective disorders of old age. *J Mental Sci* **99**, 439–450.

Roth, M. and Morrissey, J.D (1952). Problems in the diagnosis and classification of mental disorders in old age. *J Mental Sci* **98**, 66–80.

Roth, M., Huppert, F.A., Tym, E. and Mountjoy, C.Q. (1988). *CAMDEX; The Cambridge Examination for Mental Disorders in the Elderly*. Cambridge University Press, Cambridge.

Rowan, E.L. (1984). Phantom boarders as a symptom of late paraphrenia. *Am J Psychiatry* **141**, 580–582.

Sjögren, H. (1964). Paraphrenic, melancholic and psychoneurotic states in the prese-nile–senile period of life. *Acta Psychiatr Scand* **40** (suppl 176), 7–63.

Skoog, I. (1993). The prevalence of psychotic, depressive and anxiety syndromes in demented and non-demented 85-year-olds. *Int J Geriatr Psychiatry* **8**, 247–253.

Soni, S.D. (1988). Relationship between peripheral sensory disturbance and onset of symptoms in elderly paraphrenics. *Int J Geriatr Psychiatry* **3**, 275–279.

Stein, L.M. and Thienhaus, O.J. (1993). Hearing impairment and psychosis. *Int Psychogeriatrics* **5**, 49–56.

Symonds, L.L., Olichney, J.M., Jernigan, T.L. *et al.* (1997). Lack of clinically signifi-cant gross structural abnormalities in MRIs of older patients with schizophrenia and related psychoses. *J Neuropsychiatry Clin Neurosci* **9**, 251–258.

van Os, J., Howard, R., Takei, N. and Murray, R. (1995). Increasing age is a risk factor for psychosis in the elderly. *Social Psychiatry Psychiatric Epidemiology* **30**, 161–164.

Watt, J.A.G. (1985). Hearing and premorbid personality in paranoid states. *Am J Psychiatry* **142**, 1453–1455.

Watt, J.A.G., Hall, D.J., Olley, P.C., Hunter, D. and Gardiner, A.Q. (1980). Paranoid states of middle life. Familial occurrence and relationship to schizophrenia. *Acta Psychiatr Scand* **61**, 413–426.

Wilkins, L.T. (1948). *The Prevalence of Deafness in the Population of England, Scotland and Wales*. Central Office of Information, London.

Wing, J.K., Cooper, J.E. and Sartorius, N. (1973). *Present State Examination (PSE)*. Cambridge University Press, Cambridge.

Working Group on Speech Understanding and Aging (1988). Speech understanding and aging. *J Acoustics Soc Am* **83**, 859–890.

World Health Organization (1993). *The ICD-10 Classification of Mental and Behavioural Disorders. Diagnostic Criteria for Research*. WHO, Geneva.

Yassa, R. and Suranyi-Cadotte, B. (1993). Clinical characteristics of late-onset schizophrenia and delusional disorder. *Schizophr Bull* **19**, 701–707.

II

An International Perspective

Late Onset Schizophrenia
Edited by Robert Howard, Peter V. Rabins, David J. Castle
© 1999 Wrightson Biomedical Publishing Ltd

3

Schizophrenia Beginning in Late Life: An American View

PETER V. RABINS

Johns Hopkins University School of Medicine, Baltimore, Maryland, USA

The American concept of schizophrenia has differed from the European view for much of the twentieth century. Emil Kraepelin (1915) chose the name 'dementia praecox' 100 years ago to identify a condition that had an early life (that is, 'precocious') onset and followed a course of social dilapidation (by which he meant 'dementia'). This choice of name and Kraepelin's concept reflected his emphasis on course of illness as a defining feature. Eugen Bleuler (1950) shifted to an emphasis on symptomatology or phenomenology and chose the name 'schizophrenia' to highlight the split from reality and fracture of mental processing (cognition) that occurs.

For the first third of the twentieth century, the most influential view in the United States was that of the Swiss-born psychiatrist Adolph Meyer (Lief, 1948). Meyer was trained as a neuropathologist and recognized the importance of brain disease in generating psychiatric symptoms. However, he was greatly influenced by the inability to find a neuropathology associated with schizophrenia or the major mood disorders. During his tenure at Johns Hopkins (1912–1940), he promoted a view of psychiatry that downplayed diagnostic categories, emphasized the interplay between biology, environment and inner psychological forces, and conceptualized most psychiatric disorders as being 'reactive' to external events. He was an early promoter of prevention as well. Not surprisingly, Meyer rejected the Kraepelinian concept of dementia praecox because of its implication that schizophrenia was primarily a brain disease and yet had no neuropathology, and because he rejected categorical approaches to mental illness.

In the middle third of the twentieth century, psychoanalysis became the predominant theme in American psychiatry. The emigration of many psychoanalysts from Europe had a prominent influence on this development as did the lack of progress resulting from Meyer's conceptualization. The promise that psychoanalysis would explain and treat all mental disorders also influenced the widespread acceptance of the explanatory model proposed by Freud in the United States.

Both the Meyerian and psychoanalytic traditions undervalued diagnosis. One result was a marked broadening of the concept of schizophrenia in the USA. In the 1940s, concepts such as 'pseudoneurotic schizophrenia' (Hoch and Polatin, 1949) were developed, and by the 1950s the diagnosis of schizophrenia was being given to any patient with unusual or severe symptoms.

By the 1960s these differences were obvious. The recognition that American psychiatrists were diagnosing schizophrenia much more frequently than British psychiatrists led to the establishment of the US–UK Study (Kramer, 1963), which compared the symptomatology of patients in America and England. Its results clearly demonstrated that the higher prevalence of schizophrenia in the USA was due to differences in diagnostic practices rather than differences in symptom presentations or population prevalence. These results began being published about the time that lithium carbonate was established as an effective treatment for bipolar disorder. Since many of the patients diagnosed in the United States as suffering from schizophrenia were diagnosed in England as having bipolar disorder, the efficacy of lithium carbonate validated the British rather than the American practice.

One result of the US–UK study was a renewed interest in the USA in the standardization of criteria for psychiatric diagnosis. This furthered the work of those psychiatric research centres in the USA that had an existing emphasis on the importance of diagnosis. For example, psychiatrists at Washington University, St Louis, under the direction of Eli Robins, devised the Research Diagnostic Criteria (Feighner *et al.*, 1972). These developments led to the operationalized criteria of the 3rd edition of the *Diagnostic and Statistical Manual* of the American Psychiatric Association (DSM-III) (American Psychiatric Association, 1980). The DSM-III sought to develop criteria that would be used by clinicians and researchers. The criteria were developed by reaching consensus among those writing and devising them rather than being based on validity data because there were no data on the reliability and validity of any set of criteria.

The DSM-III diagnosis of schizophrenia fully embraced the Kraepelinian concept. It required that symptoms be present for 6 months or more and that an impairment in social functioning be present. The Bleulerian emphasis on thought disorder, hallucinations and delusions was also embraced.

DSM-III also included a criterion that required onset of schizophrenia before age 45. No data were presented to support this requirement. This criterion reflected the 'praecox' view of Kraepelin, that is, the belief that schizophrenia usually begins in adolescence or early adulthood. It was likely added to narrow the definition of schizophrenia and avoid the 'excesses' of the 1940s–1960s. It also reflected the lack of contact among schizophrenia researchers in the USA with older outpatients.

In retrospect, it is understandable (using historical methods) that onset of schizophrenia after age 44 was thought to be unlikely by American psychiatrists and was included in DSM-III as a criterion. There was little interest in geriatric psychiatry in the USA in the middle of the twentieth century, and those centres that did promote the study of the elderly did not focus on the major mental illnesses. The predominant view was that most late onset mental illness was 'organic' or structural in aetiology and therefore of no interest to psychiatrists.

The first papers suggesting that schizophrenia might begin in mid- and later life published in an American journal were review articles by Bridge (who was British trained) and Wyatt (1980). The rapid, widespread acceptance of DSM-III (APA, 1980) by the American mental health community after its publication in 1980 exposed these criteria to a scrutiny that its predecessors, DSM-I and DSM-II, had not had. Thus, a revised edition, DSM-IIIR (APA, 1987), was published within 7 years and its developers sought input from a broader spectrum of advisors. Based on the published literature supporting onset after 44, the criterion requiring onset of schizophrenia before age 45 was dropped and a sub-categorization that indicated 'late onset' was created.

Interest in old age or geriatric psychiatry began crystallizing in the USA in the mid-1970s. Psychiatrists such as Alvin Goldfarb, Jack Weinberg and Ewald Busse had been writing on late-life issues relevant to psychiatrists in the 1950s and 1960s but sections or divisions of geriatric psychiatry did not become widespread within academic departments in the USA until the 1970s and 1980s. As a result, most psychiatrists trained in the USA had little exposure to elderly individuals until the mid-1980s. This was especially true of individuals in the research community who focused on the study of patients with schizophrenia. Therefore, even though the DSM-IIIR dropped the criterion requiring onset of schizophrenia before age 45, many researchers and clinicians remained (and still remain) skeptical that schizophrenia could develop in mid- and late life because they had 'never seen it'.

Appropriate debates about the essential elements of schizophrenia continue in the USA and the rest of the world. The findings that thought disorder and affective blunting are very uncommon in mid-life and late onset cases (Harris *et al.*, 1988; Jeste, 1988; Pearlson *et al.*, 1989) are offered as evidence, by those who believe that these are essential features of schizophrenia, that the mid-life and late onset cases have 'a different disorder' than early onset cases. Cross-sectional studies showing that patients with mid- and late onset schizophrenia-like illnesses have hallucinations and delusions similar to young patients in both prevalence and phenomenology (Jeste, 1988; Pearlson *et al.*, 1989) are unconvincing to many. The central question has become an issue of validity: what is the gold standard by which schizophrenia should be diagnosed? Since psychiatry as a whole has not been able to come to agreement on how to validate the diagnosis, many American psychiatrists are likely to remain skeptical about schizophrenia developing in mid- and late life.

WHERE DO WE GO FROM HERE?

What then might it take to convince skeptics? This is an important question because it returns to the question of validity. The most obvious answer is the development of a valid biological marker to identify schizophrenia. However, it seems likely that schizophrenia is not one illness but rather a syndrome with many different aetiologies (a point made by Bleuler). Thus, while it is possible that there is a final common pathway or common mechanism that leads to the symptoms of schizophrenia no matter what the initiating event, the discovery of a single biomarker is unlikely because of the heterogeneity of the illness. It is more likely that multiple biomarkers will be identified, each linked to a specific aetiology.

Attempts to prove the hypothesis that mid- and late onset cases are similar to young onset cases have utilized convergent validity. That is, multiple sources and types of data are collected and point to a single conclusion. Attempts have been made to identify consistent abnormalities in young individuals and determine if similar abnormalities exist in older individuals. Cross-sectional comparisons of symptoms (e.g. Pearlson et al., 1989; Jeste, 1988), neuropsychological variables and ADL functioning (Heaton et al., 1994; Jeste et al., 1995), and treatment response (Rabins et al., 1984) support similarities between early and later onset cases except for lower rates of thought disorder and affective blunting in the later onset cases.

Neuroimaging offers the best hope, at present, for determining whether patients with schizophrenia-like symptoms beginning in mid- and later life have the same illness as patients whose symptoms develop between ages 15 and 30 (Rabins et al., 1987; Lesser et al., 1992; Pearlson et al., 1993; Andreasen et al., 1994; Gur, 1997). Unfortunately, no consensus has been reached about which neuroimaging changes are characteristic of young onset schizophrenia except for the non-specific ventricular dilatation that was first demonstrated on pneumoencephalography (Moore and Nathan, 1933) and prior to that by post-mortem ventricular volume studies. This issue is discussed by Pearlson in Chapter 15 of this volume. If the research community can develop a set of imaging markers that both identifies schizophrenia and distinguishes it from other diseases (such as affective disorder and Alzheimer's disease), important clues to pathogenesis should become evident. These could become biomarkers and provide the answer to the validity question.

SPECULATION

Psychiatrists studying mid- and late onset schizophrenia in the USA are in agreement that a disorder with schizophrenia-like features can begin in the fourth, fifth and sixth decades and that the study of this condition might illuminate the genesis and treatment of schizophrenia beginning before age 30. There is agreement that thought disorder is almost non-existent in mid-life and late onset cases and that affective blunting is infrequent. There is also agreement that neuropsychological changes and neuroimaging changes are similar across the age span, although specific neuroimaging abnormalities are yet to be identified.

Where can such research go and what role should 'outliers', in this instance cases of late onset schizophrenia, play in future research? Science makes advances in starts and stops and there is no single best strategy for advancing knowledge. A strong case can be made that very typical cases (and perhaps the most severe and clear cases) should be studied before unusual, variant or atypical cases, because the inclusion of atypical cases sometimes dilutes potential findings and results in type 2 or false negative error. (That is, abnormalities which are truly present are not identified because they are diluted out by the inclusion of atypical cases or because an inadequate number of cases are studied.)

An equally strong argument can be made that the study of atypical cases is sometimes very illuminating. In medicine this has been found to be true for genetic forms of diseases not commonly genetic such as Parkinson's disease and amyotrophic lateral sclerosis (ALS). In physics, the study of black body radiation, a seemingly insignificant anomaly, led the physicist Niels Bohr to develop quantum mechanics. Thus, the study of mid-life and late onset schizophrenia might well identify important leads that will be informative about schizophrenia-like illnesses that begin in early life and adolescence.

How might the lack of thought disorder and affective/social blunting in later onset cases be explained? If we assume that the same site of injury occurs in early and late onset cases (not a necessary assumption since different injuries could lead to those symptoms that are shared), then we must seek lesions that cause some symptoms to be the same in early and late onset schizophrenia and some symptoms to differ.

The brain structures underlying language develop sequentially during the first decade of life. Before age 8 or 10, damage to the left hemisphere from brain injury or left hemispherectomy does not grossly impair the development of language in most individuals. Apparently, other brain regions, perhaps in the other hemisphere, are able to 'take over' and express language. Injury after 12 years of age, however, results in aphasia (Benson, 1973). Since late onset schizophrenia is not associated with aphasia, a direct insult to the language areas of the frontal and temporal lobes is unlikely in late onset cases.

Likewise, an injury before development is completed is unlikely in late onset cases because of the lack of thought disorder (Benson, 1973). Thus, the lack of thought disorder in mid-life and late onset cases would be best explained by an injury that occurs *outside* the language areas but that involves structures and/or pathways that connect to the frontal and temporal language areas. If the same lesion is present in early onset cases, then it is likely that it occurs before the development of the language is completed, thus explaining the development of thought disorder in young onset cases only.

One useful model for explaining the similarities and differences between early and late onset cases is the concept of neural plasticity. Stevens (1982) has suggested that this might be a useful model to explain the positive symptoms of schizophrenia and it has been hypothesized elsewhere (Rabins, 1994, 1995) that the positive symptoms in schizophrenia (hallucinations, delusions, and thought disorder) might result from aberrant (plastic) connections that develop in response to injury. If the positive and negative symptoms of schizophrenia arise from the same primary lesion(s), then that injury could directly cause the negative symptoms (affective blunting, social dilapidation and cognitive dysfunction). This mirrors the Kraepelinian view that negative symptoms are the 'essence' of schizophrenia (because they are the direct result of the pathological abnormality) and that the positive symptoms are 'secondary' (since they result from the brain's attempt to repair the primary damage).

This hypothesis suggests that: aberrant connections develop via plasticity mechanisms and cause hallucinations by abnormal connections to the auditory cortices in cases of any age of onset; delusions by aberrant connections to and within the 'meaning centre' in the left temporal cortex (Gazzaniga, 1985) at any age of onset; and thought disorder by aberrant frontal and temporal lobe connections in early onset cases only.

Lower rates of affective blunting and social dilapidation in late onset cases could be explained by a similar mechanism. A direct injury to the frontal lobes is unlikely because of the lack of personality and initiative change. Rather, a remote injury that prevents normal myelination or causes aberrant myelination in early onset cases is more plausible. Again, the lesion would be outside the frontal lobes but involve structures that send afferents to and/or receive efferents from them. This would result in negative symptoms only if the injury precedes myelination of the frontal lobes and therefore be manifest only in early onset cases.

This proposal parallels the developmental hypothesis of schizophrenia (Weinberger, 1989) by suggesting that the negative symptoms of schizophrenia and thought disorder result from an interruption of usual development. It differs from the developmental hypothesis by explaining hallucinations, delusions and thought disorder as resulting from plasticity. The thalamus (Andreasen, 1997), nucleus accumbens (Stevens, 1982) and putamen (R. Powers, pers. comm.) are plausible sites of the primary injury.

If aberrant connectivity due to plasticity is present, functional imaging paradigms that can identify usual and abnormal connectivity could test the hypothesis proposed here. The hypothesis presented here predicts a shared site of initial injury in early and later onset cases. A test of the hypothesis depends on finding an inability to stimulate certain structures because of a primary injury, a linkage between this inability and the presence of negative symptoms, and the demonstration of aberrant pathways that can be linked to positive symptoms. Paradigms such as that tested by Andreasen *et al.* (1997) could test this proposal. While the ultimate demonstration of pathology in schizophrenia is likely to rely on morphometric and neurochemical methods, these studies could point researchers to the correct brain areas to be examined.

CONCLUSION

Geriatric psychiatrists in the United States see patients with a disorder beginning after age 40 or 45 which has many similarities to schizophrenia. Further research is needed to convince those who are skeptical that this condition is indeed a form of schizophrenia. More importantly, research into the pathobiology of the late onset condition has the potential to teach us about the underlying structural and functional abnormalities associated with schizophrenia-like illnesses regardless of age of onset and may lead to crucial insights that unravel the mysteries of this devastating illness. Whatever the ultimate answer to the questions that remain, research is the best way to answer them.

REFERENCES

American Psychiatric Association (1980). *Diagnostic and Statistical Manual of Mental Disorders, 3rd edn* (DSM-III). American Psychiatric Association, Washington, DC.

American Psychiatric Association (1987). *Diagnostic and Statistical Manual of Mental Disorders, 3rd edn revised* (DSM-IIIR). American Psychiatric Association, Washington, DC.

Andreasen, N.C., Arndt, S., Swayze, V. *et al.* (1994). Thalamic abnormalities in schizophrenia visualized through magnetic resonance image averaging. *Science* **266**, 294–298.

Andreasen, N.C., O'Leary, S.D., Flaum, M. *et al.* (1997). Hypofrontality in schizophrenia: distributed dysfunctional circuits in neuroleptic-naive patients. *Lancet* **349**, 1730–1734.

Benson, D.F. (1973). Psychiatric aspects of aphasia. *Br J Psychiatry* **123**, 555–566.

Bleuler, E. (1950). *Dementia praecox; or, the Group of Schizophrenia* (translated by J. Zinkin). International Universities Press, New York.

Bridge, T.P. and Wyatt, R.J. (1980). Paraphrenia: paranoid state of life. II. American research. *J Am Geriatr Soc* **28**, 201–205.

Feighner, J.P., Robins, E. and Guze, S.B. (1972). Diagnostic criteria for use in psychiatric research. *Arch Gen Psychiatry* **26**, 57–63.

Gazzaniga, M.S. (1985). *The Social Brain: Discovering the Networks of the Mind.* Basic Books, New York.

Gur, R. (1997). Data presented at the International Psychogeriatrics Association Meeting, Jerusalem, Israel.

Harris, M.J., Cullum, C.M. and Jeste, D.V. (1988). Clinical presentation of late-onset schizophrenia. *J Clin Psychiatry* **49**, 356–360.

Heaton, R., Paulsen, J.S., McAdams, L.A. *et al.* (1994). Neuropsychological deficits in schizophrenics. *Arch Gen Psychiatry* **51**, 469–476.

Hoch, P.H. and Polatin, P. (1949). Pseudoneurotic forms of schizophrenia. *Psychiatry Quarterly* **23**, 248–276.

Jeste, D.V. (Ed.) (1988). Psychosis in late life. *Psychiatric Clinics of North America.* WB Saunders, Philadelphia.

Jeste, D., Harris, M., Krull, A., Kuck, J., McAdams, L. and Heaton, R. (1995). Clinical and neuropsychological characteristics of patients with late-onset schizophrenia. *Am J Psychiatry* **152**, 722–730.

Kraepelin, E. (1915). *Clinical Psychiatry* (edited and translated by A.R. Diefendorf). MacMillan, New York.

Kramer, M. (1963). Some problems for international research suggested by observations on differences in first admission rates to the mental hospitals of England and Wales and of the United States. In: *Panel Discussions of the Third World Congress of Psychiatry, Vol. 3.* Toronto University Press, Montreal, pp. 153–160.

Lesser, I.M., Jeste, D.V., Boone, K.B. *et al.* (1992). Late onset psychotic disorder, not otherwise specified: clinical and neuroimaging findings. *Biol Psychiatry* **31**, 419–423.

Lief, A. (1948). *The Commonsense Psychiatry of Dr Adolf Meyer.* McGraw-Hill Book Company, Toronto.

Moore, M.T. and Nathan, D. (1993). Encephalographic studies in schizophrenia (dementia praecox). *Am J Psychiatry* **12**, 801–812.

Pearlson, G.D., Kreger, L., Rabins, P.V. *et al.* (1989). A chart review study of late-onset and early-onset schizophrenia. *Am J Psychiatry* **146**, 1568–1574.

Pearlson, G.D., Tune, L.E. ,Wong, D.F. *et al.* (1993). Quantitative D_2 dopamine receptor PET and structural MRI changes in late-onset schizophrenia. *Schizophr Bull* **19**, 783–795.

Rabins, P.V. (1994). The genesis of phantom (deenervation) hallucinations: an hypothesis. *Int J Geriatr Psychiatry* **9**, 775–777.

Rabins, P.V. (1995). Can schizophrenia-like disorders beginning in late life tell us anything about early life onset schizophrenia? *J Mental Health* **4**, 177–181.

Rabins, P.V., Pearlson, G.D., Jayaram, G., Steele, C. and Tune, L. (1987). Increased ventricle-to-brain ratio in late-onset schizophrenia. *Am J Psychiatry* **144**, 1216–1218.

Rabins, P.V. Pauker, S. and Thomas, J. (1984). Can schizophrenia begin after age 44? *Compr Psychiatry* **25**, 290–293.

Stevens, J.R. (1992). Abnormal reinnervation as a basis for schizophrenia: a hypothesis. *Arch Gen Psychiatry* **49**, 238–243.

Stevens, J.R. (1973). An anatomy of schizophrenia? *Arch Gen Psychiatry* **29**, 147–189.

Weinberger, D.R. (1987). Implications of normal brain development for the pathogenesis of schizophrenia. *Arch Gen Psychiatry* **44**, 660–669.

4

Validity of Late Onset Schizophrenia: A European View

ANITA RIECHER-RÖSSLER, HEINZ HÄFNER AND PØVL MUNK-JØRGENSEN

University Psychiatric Outpatient Department, Basel, Switzerland

INTRODUCTION

Since the time schizophrenic diseases – then still called 'dementia praecox' – were first described by Kraepelin (1893), it has been generally accepted that most cases occur before the age of 40. On the other hand, the illness – or a similar illness – has also been described to begin at a more advanced age in some cases. There have been many efforts to differentiate these late onset psychoses from the group of the classic schizophrenias with early onset, i.e. before age 40, based on their symptomatology, risk factors and course (Riecher-Rössler, 1994, 1997; Riecher-Rössler *et al.*, 1995, 1997; see also Riecher-Rössler, this volume, Chapter 1).

Manfred Bleuler presented the first comprehensive empirical work on these psychoses and coined the term 'late onset schizophrenia' (see Riecher-Rössler, this volume, Chapter 1). According to his definition, these diseases are kinds of schizophrenic psychoses with onset after age 40 years but mainly before age 60 years. They resemble the classic early onset schizophrenia in their clinical picture, although he also found certain differences. Many authors before and after M. Bleuler have also found certain differences between late and early onset schizophrenias as regards symptomatology. Even more equivocally described from the very beginning was another difference between late and early onset cases, namely an intriguing excess of women in late onset schizophrenics.

These characteristics have again and again raised the question of whether late onset schizophrenia should be regarded as a separate diagnostic entity, aetiologically (at least partially) differing from early onset schizophrenia. The term 'late onset schizophrenia' has subsequently become widely accepted. In

1987 it was even included into the American diagnostic manual DSM-IIIR (American Psychiatric Association, 1987).

But what do we really know about this illness (group)? Are there really decisive differences between late and early onset schizophrenia patients which justify the use of an extra diagnostic label for this illness group? Do these late onset cases not rather belong instead to the same group of diseases as the classic early onset schizophrenias? The following is an attempt to answer these questions based on a comprehensive literature review and on our own studies (see also Riecher-Rössler et al., 1997).

METHODS

The literature review in Chapter 1 of this volume includes all articles and monographs published during this century in English or German either on late onset schizophrenia or on similar illness groups before this diagnostic label was coined. Based on a computerized literature search (MEDLINE; PSYCLIT) and all standard textbooks and handbooks, including the references found in these articles and books, we could identify 121 articles published until 1995. All studies were analysed concerning their methodological standards: number and selection of patients, diagnostic criteria, kind of investigation, definition of onset, exclusion criteria, representativity of the sample, restriction to first admitted or first episode patients, etc. Drawing mainly on studies with relatively sound methodology we then tried to summarize the scarce knowledge on incidence, prevalence, sex distribution, symptomatology and course.

The results of our own studies are referred to separately, as they – in contrast to most previous studies – fulfil most of the methodological standards required: we examined representative populations of first admitted using standardized diagnostic criteria and instruments and an operationalized definition of onset. In the framework of the ABC-study (Häfner et al., 1991a, 1993a,b) we have directly examined all 392 patients, who were first admitted with a schizophrenic or paranoid psychosis (ICD-9: 295, 297, 298.3+0.4, WHO 1978) during a period of 24 months from a well defined catchment area in southern Germany and who were 12–59 years old. Exclusion criteria were suspected organic brain syndromes or severe mental retardation. As concerns incidence and sex distribution, our results are based on this population; as concerns symptomatology, a representative sample of 267 of these patients were examined thoroughly with a whole set of instruments. Further details about this population are given by Häfner et al. (1991a, 1993a,b). Seventy-six of all 392, or 43 of the fully examined 267, patients had their first admission with one of the above named diagnoses ('index admission') at age 40 or later (Riecher-Rössler, 1994). Regarding the course of late onset schizophrenia, we have analysed a representative case register cohort of all 1423 Danish patients first admitted in 1976 with a diagnosis of a schizophrenic, paranoid or paranoid reactive psychosis or borderline state (ICD-8: 295, 297, 298.3, 301.83, WHO, 1967). Inclusion and exclusion criteria were the same as in the ABC-study. Seven hundred and thirty-four of the patients had their index admission at age 40 or later.

RESULTS

How sound is our knowledge?

Unfortunately the validity of the existing findings on late onset schizophrenia is seriously restricted by two major problems, namely the confusion of terms and concepts that has developed internationally regarding this illness group (see Riecher-Rössler, this volume, Chapter 1; Riecher-Rössler *et al.*, 1995) and the methodological short-comings of the empirical studies conducted so far.

As to the concept 'late onset schizophrenia', German language psychiatry has largely adopted that of Manfred Bleuler and labels as 'late onset schizophrenia' only those clinical pictures that resemble early onset schizophrenia but have their onset after age 40. They usually occur before age 60 and do not have an organic basis. Other, mainly Anglo-American, authors use the term late onset schizophrenia also for the paranoid psychoses of old age with onset after age 60. According to British tradition the latter clinical pictures have also been called 'late paraphrenia', which has led to an increasing confusion of terms and concepts (Riecher-Rössler, this volume; Riecher-Rössler *et al.*, 1995). Thus internationally there has not been a clear differentiation between late onset schizophrenia of German tradition and late paraphrenia of British tradition. As a consequence, many findings on so-called late onset schizophrenia are in fact based on populations with late paraphrenia or on mixed diagnostic groups and are only of limited validity regarding late onset schizophrenia itself.

A further problem concerns the age limit. In German psychiatry this has been fixed at age 40, in Anglo-American psychiatry partly at age 45 (in accordance with DSM-III, APA, 1980), partly even at age 60. The latter age limit mainly resulted from the already mentioned confusion between late onset schizophrenia and late paraphrenia. Furthermore it is usually not clear how 'onset' is operationalized. Usually it is simply equated with 'first admission' which – as we now know – on average occurs only about 4–5 years after the first signs of the disease (Häfner *et al.*, 1992b, 1993a,b).

As to the methodology of the studies conducted so far, Table 1 gives an overview of the studies since Kraepelin (1919) and describes their most important methodological aspects and limitations:

– The main problem is that almost all studies have so far only been done on rather selected patient groups, e.g. on patients of a certain hospital for the chronically ill, and the results can therefore not be generalized.

Table 1.   Clinical and epidemiological studies on classic late onset schizophrenia –

Authors	Patients examined[b] n Total/ late onset	Selection of patients	Diagnostic criteria of schizophrenia	Kind of investigation
Kraepelin (1919)	1054/61	?	Dementia praecox without paraphrenia	Clinical cross-sectional
Kraepelin (1913)	?/78		Paraphrenia	Cross-sectional
Kolle (1931)	889/142	Cases of Carl Schneider	Schizophrenia and paraphrenia	Clinical with follow-up
	182/33	All cases of 1 year in one hospital	Schizophrenia and paraphrenia	Clinical cross-sectional
Bleuler, M. (1943)	(a) Clinical study ?/130	Non-systematic: schizophrenics 'who became known to me'	Schizophrenia according to Bleuler	Follow-up by M. Bleuler personally
	(b) Calculations of frequencies 459/68	'Patients in asylum'	Schizophrenia according to Bleuler	Cross-sectional
	300/51	All schizophrenics of a certain hospital	Schizophrenia according to Bleuler	
Knoll (1952)	?/114	Female inpatients of a university hospital	'Delusional psychosis of menopause'[c] (paranoid schizophrenia)	Direct clinical and retrospective case-note assessment
Müller (1959)	(101)[b]/30	All schizophrenic inpatients aged > 65 years at a fixed day	'Schizophrenia according to Bleuler'	Direct, cross-sectional
Klages (1961)	?/53	All admissions with 'late onset' of a university hospital in 4 years	Schizophrenia with first rank symptoms, M. Bleuler's criteria for late onset schizophrenia	Direct interviews and different sources of information; follow-up: several years
Funding (1963)	148/5	All first admissions of a certain hospital in 14 years with onset of paranoid delusions after age 50	'Schizophrenia'	Direct examination catamnesis of 1–15 years, different sources of information
Schimmel-penning (1965)	?/117(82)[d]	All inpatients of a university hospital in 5 years	Broad (schizophrenia, schizoform psychosis, paranoid react.)	Direct, different sources of information, catamnesis of > 5 years
Retterstøl (1966)	84/14	All first admissions of a certain hospital with paranoid psychosis from two periods	Paranoid schizophrenic criteria of Langfeldt (1960)	Direct with follow-up; different sources of information

methodological problems.[a]

Onset of disorder Definition	Age limit (years)	Exclusion criteria/ exclusion diagnoses	1. Representative sample? 2. first episode/ first admitted?	Remarks
?	> 40	?	1. No 2. No	'Coined the term 'dementia praecox' because of onset in youth and poor prognosis
?	> 30	?	1. No 2. No	Mayer (1921) showed that 50 of the 78 later had developed classical dementia praecox
?	> 40	Pure paranoid disorder	1. No 2. No	Found them similar to early onset cases
First admission	> 40	Pure paranoid disorder	1. No 2. No	
?	> 40	Amnestic syndrome and physical disease with suspected brain disturbance	1. No 2. No	Cases and their relatives from several institutions and countries, 17 already dead; Coined the term 'late onset schizophrenia'
?	> 40	Amnestic syndrome and physical disease with suspected brain disturbance	1. No 2. No	as half of those with onset> 40 years old showed a 'characteristic symptom-colouring'
	> 40	Amnestic syndrome and physical disease with suspected brain disturbance	1. Hospital prevalence 2. No	
First paranoid disorder	> 40	Organic symptoms, psychoreactive psychosis	1. No 2. No	Found them to be a subgroup of schizophrenia
First psychotic symptoms	> 40	None	1. No 2. No	Only nine out of 30 had no organic brain pathology
'Onset'	40–60	Onset > 60 years, 'cerebral-organic colouring', paraphrenia, paranoid reactions	1. No 2. No	No empirical control group, but found them 'similar to early onset schizophrenia'
Beginnings of paranoid delusions	> 50 syndrome	Organic brain	1. No 2. Yes	In only five of the 148 paranoid patients could the diagnosis of schizophrenia be confirmed
First paranoid symptoms	> 40	Suspected organic psychosis, depressive delusions	1. No 2. No	In 67 patients the diagnosis of schizophrenia was not confirmed due to organic deterioration or lack of chronicity
First admission	> 40	Affective psychosis confusional state	1. No 2. Yes	Study not mainly aimed at late onset schizophrenia

continued

Table 1. *Continued.*

Authors	Patients examined[b] n Total/ late onset	Selection of patients	Diagnostic criteria of schizophrenia	Kind of investigation
Post (1966)	(93)/34	Three samples of 'persistent persecutory states', > 60 years old at admission	First rank symptoms	Partly retrospective, partly follow-up
Siegel and Rollberg (1970)	?/60	All inpatients of a university hospital in 10 years	'Schizophrenia' not specified	Clinical/case-notes, details not given
Sternberg (1972)	?/487	Outpatients of a certain clinic, > 60 years old	'Schizophrenia' (Russian diagnosis)	Details not given
Angst et al. (1973)	291/101	Consecutive admissions in 7 hospitals in five countries	Only paranoia subgroup of schizophrenia (ICD 295.3)	Exact documentation, details not given
Berner et al. (1973)[c] and Gabriel (1974a,b, 1978)[c]	311/110	Basis: all patients of a university hospital first admitted between age 40 and 65, follow-up at a mean age of 77 (only one-fifth of patients could be traced)	Late onset schizophrenia according to M. Bleuler (1943)	Direct, duration of catamnesis > 20 years in 73% of the cases
Hinterhuber (1973)	157/39	All first admissions of a university hospital in 5 years (between 1930 and 1940)	Rediagnosis of schizophrenia from case-notes according to Bleuler's (1908) criteria	Case-notes and direct, different sources of information, duration of catamnesis 30–40 years
Huber et al. (1975, 1979)	644/110; survivors: 502/70	All admissions of a university hospital in 14 years	Schizophrenia diagnosed according to K. Schneider (1957), late onset criteria according to M. Bleuler (1943)	Retrospective, mean duration of catamnesis 17.8 years (incl. prodromi 20.7 years) sources of information?
Rabins et al. (1984)	(35)/21	Non-systematic, persistent delusional disorder with onset age > 44 years	Schizophrenia according to DSM-III without age limit	25× direct with follow-up, 10× retrospective case-note analysis
Marneros and Deister (1984)	1208/170	All first admissions of a university hospital during 30 years	Schizophrenia, clinical diagnosis according to K. Schneider (1957)	Analysis of case-notes with own standardized instruments
Jeste et al. (1988)	?/36	'Typical' patients of four centres	Schizophrenia – late onset according to DSM-IIIR	Comparison of clinical data, details not given

Onset of disorder Definition	Age limit (years)	Exclusion criteria/ exclusion diagnoses	1. Representative sample? 2. first episode/ first admitted?	Remarks
Onset of paranoid symptoms	> 50	Affective disorder	1. No 2. No	34 of the 93 patients had first rank symptoms, 33 organic brain pathologies
?	> 40	Organic psychosis	1. No 2. No	No empirical control group
?	?	Organic brain pathologies allowed	1. No 2. No	Many details missing
'Onset'	> 40	?	1. No 2. No	Markedly smaller proportion of late onset cases in catatonic and schizoaffective psychosis
First admission	> 40	None	1. No 2. Yes	Many patients dead. All patients with progressive course after age 65 had marked had marked organic brain pathology
First psychotic symptoms, if onset insidious: First admission	> 40	Not from catchment area, organic psychosis, no safe diagnosis based on case-notes	1. No 2. Yes	One of the few who discusses the validity of retrospective diagnoses based on case-notes
?	> 40	Organic clinical picture, organic brain disease	1. No 2. No	Found slightly more paranoid and paranoid hallucinatory delusions in late as compared with early onset cases
Beginning of persistent delusions	> 44	Affective disorder, cognitive disturbance (Mini-Mental State)	1. No 2. No	Diagnosed 21× schizo-, phrenia 11× schizo-phreniform disorder and 3× paranoia; found late onset similar to early onset cases
First admission	> 50	Not German speaking	1. No 2. Yes	Found more delusions and hallucinations, but less thought disorder in patients with onset age > 50 as opposed to < 50
'Onset'	> 45	Organic brain disorder, affective disorder etc., accor-ding to DSM-IIIR	1. No 2. No	Four highly selected samples from four different centres; only one sample was compared with early onset cases

Continued

Table 1.   *Continued.*

Authors	Patients examined[b] n Total/ late onset	Selection of patients	Diagnostic criteria of schizophrenia	Kind of investigation
Craig and Bregman (1988)	(658)[b]/32	All schozphrenic inpatients aged > 65 of a state mental hospital during 5 years	DSM-III	Longitudinal case-note analysis
Pearlson et al. (1989)	?/54	All admissions of a hospital during 5 years with onset age > 45	DSM-IIIR schizophrenia	Longitudinal case-note analysis, comparison with 22 age-matched early onset and 54 young schizophrenic patients
Marneros et al. (1992)	148/12	Admissions of two university hospitals during 30 years	Schizophrenia according to K. Schneider (1957)	Case-notes and direct, all sources of information, mean duration of catamnesis 27 years
Häfner et al. (1993a,b)	276/(76)[f]	All first admissions of a definite catchment area during 2 years	ICD-9: 295, 297, 298.3+0.4	Direct with follow-up and follow-back, all sources of information
Howard et al.[g] (1993a); Castle and Murray[g] (1993)	470/134	All first contacts with psychiatric services (inpatient and out-patient) in definite catchment area over 20 year period	ICD-9: 295, 297.2, 298	Case-note analysis with standardized instruments, patients ascertained by case-register
Mayer et al. (1993)	1371/130	All first admissions of a hospital in 4 years (onset in the 2 years beforehand)	ICD-9: 295, 297	Clinical routine–document. (AMDP) cross-sectional
Yassa and Suranyi-Cadotte (1993)	(40)/20	All patients > 65 years old admitted to a psychogeriatric ward in 7 years	DSM-IIIR	Direct with follow-up and follow-back
Jeste et al. (1995)	64/25	Nonsystematic, patients from different medical centres and private physicians	DSM-IIIR	Direct clinical and neuropsychological assessment with follow-back

[a] Only studies on schizophrenia with late onset are considered, not studies restricted to 'late paraphrenia' or 'paranoid disorders', which do not differentiate between schizophrenic and non-schizophrenic patients. Neither have case-reports nor studies restricted to aetiological questions (e.g. CT or MRI studies) been listed in this table.
[b] The total number of patients examined has been put in brackets, if the number did not refer to the schizophrenic patients of all age groups, but the study population consisted of elderly patients of different diagnostic categories.
[c] Special category of Knoll.
[d] Only 82 were examined directly, 15 of them being late onset schizophrenia patients.
[e] Subgroup of the study by Ciompi and Müller (1976).
[f] Number in brackets, as the age boundary was 35 years in this study.
[g] Howard et al. (1993a) and Castle and Murray (1993) refer to the same sample.

Onset of disorder Definition	Age limit (years)	Exclusion criteria/ exclusion diagnoses	1. Representative sample? 2. first episode/ first admitted?	Remarks
'Onset'	> 45	Affective disorder, organic brain disease	1. No 2. No	Schizophrenia diagnosis confirmed in only 25%, 40% organic deterioation, 20% affective disorder, 15% full remission
Age at first positive symptoms	> 45	Organic brain disorder	1. No 2. No	Only one rater, no test of reliability; found less thought disorder and affective flattening in late o.c., but more persecutory delusions
'Onset'	> 45	Organic psychosis, schizoaffective psychosis, affective psychosis	1. No 2. No	Part of a bigger study on 402 of originally 950 patients with functional psychoses
First admission	> 35	Suspected organic brain pathology, mental handicap	1. Yes 2. Yes	Comparison of three age-groups: 12–24, 25–34, 35–59
First treatment or beginning of subjective distress or impairment	> 45	Organic basis of disorder early onset cases	1. Yes 2. Yes	Very broad diagnostic spectrum; found late and 'psychopathologically *not* homogenous'
'Onset'	40–63	Organic brain disorder	1. No 2. Yes	Comparison of extreme age-groups: 40–63 versus 18–23
'Active symptoms'	> 45	Evidence of organicity in tests, conditions that may mimic schizophrenia	1. No	Comparison of 20 late onset schizophrenics with seven paraphrenia patients and 13 patients with paranoia
Onset of psychotic symptoms	> 45	Psychosis secondary to substance abuse or dementia	1. No 2. No	Comparison of 25 late onset with early onset schizophrenic and 35 healthy subjects

- For the same reason reliable calculations on prevalence or incidence, which would have to be based on all patients of a whole catchment area, do not exist.
- In most studies there was no distinction between first and re-admitted patients (e.g. Roth and Morrissey, 1952; Roth, 1955; Fish, 1960; Kay and Roth, 1961; Klages, 1961; Angst et al., 1973; Huber et al., 1975; Blessed and Wilson, 1982; Pearlson et al., 1989; Quintal et al., 1991; Marneros et al., 1992; Yassa and Suranyi-Cadotte, 1993). This means that the comparison group of early onset patients had on average a much longer course of their disease and therefore more signs of chronicity. A comparison with the relatively fresh clinical picture of the late onset patients is in this case not very valid. Only a few studies were restricted to first admissions (Funding, 1963; Hinterhuber, 1973; Marneros and Deister, 1984; Jørgensen and Munk-Jørgensen, 1985; Mayer et al., 1993; Häfner et al., 1993a,b).
- In many studies there were no control groups of early onset patients. Comparisons were rather made on the basis of literature (e.g. Klages, 1961; Kay and Roth, 1961; Post, 1966; Herbert and Jacobson, 1967; Siegel and Rollberg, 1970; Larson and Nyman, 1970; Rabins et al., 1984).
- Finally it has to be mentioned that in the older studies neither standardized diagnostic systems nor standardized assessment instruments were in use (e.g. Bleuler, 1943; Kay and Roth, 1961; Retterstøl, 1966; Larson and Nyman, 1970; Huber et al., 1975). Often the analyses were retrospective only, based on case-notes and not on direct investigations (e.g. Larson and Nyman, 1970; Rabins et al., 1984).

Nevertheless the great advantage of some – mainly European – studies is that very big populations were examined thoroughly and over long periods of time (e.g. on average 17.8 years by Huber et al., 1975; or even 30–40 years by Hinterhuber, 1973). As to the results it has to be stated that, despite the differing methodology, some findings are astonishingly similar. Other results are, in contrast, very inconsistent and even contradictory, so that many questions are left to be answered. In the following an attempt is made to critically review our actual knowledge on the epidemiology, symptomatology and course of classic late onset schizophrenia with onset after age 40, and to summarize what we really know, if we mainly draw on methodologically sound studies.

What do we really know?

Epidemiology

The proportion of patients with illness onset after age 40 among those actually examined in most studies lies between 15 and 25% (e.g. Kolle, 1931; Bleuler, 1943; Fish, 1958; Astrup, 1962; Retterstöl, 1966; Hinterhuber, 1973; Huber et al., 1979; compare Riecher-Rössler et al., 1997). Results differing from this are mainly due to differing methodologies. Thus, for example, Kraepelin (1919) and Schulz (1933) found lower proportions of 5.8% and 5.3%, respectively, as they excluded the subgroup of 'paraphrenia', which is supposed to have a comparatively late disease onset. On the other hand, for example, Angst *et al.* (1973) found a very high proportion of late onset cases, 35%, as they only referred to the paranoid subtype of schizophrenia, which is also thought to start later than most other subtypes.

One of the most interesting findings is the excess of women in late onset schizophrenia. While there is an excess of men in early onset cases (Riecher *et al.*, 1989), in late onset patients the sex distribution female:male was found to be about 2:1 to 4:1 in most studies (Bleuler, 1943; Knoll, 1952; Klages, 1961; Schimmelpenning, 1965; Siegel and Rollberg, 1970; Berner *et al.*, 1973; Hinterhuber, 1973; Ciompi and Müller, 1976; Gabriel, 1978; Huber *et al.*, 1979; Craig and Bregman, 1988; Jablensky *et al.*, 1992; Howard *et al.*, 1993a; Castle and Murray, 1993). Extreme values are 1.3:1 (Shepherd *et al.*, 1989) on the one hand and 6.7:1 (Pearlson *et al.*, 1989) on the other. Only the former study, though, was based on a representative population of first admissions. The latter study, in contrast, was – as most other studies – based on a highly selected population and included re-admissions, i.e. the sex distribution could be influenced by many factors and cannot be generalized.

Own studies. In the ABC-study (Riecher *et al.*, 1991; Häfner *et al.*, 1991a, 1993a,b), which had an upper age limit at 60 years, 76 (19.4%) of all 392 patients with a schizophrenic or paranoid psychosis, or 52 (15.6%) of the 334 schizophrenic patients, were first admitted between age 40 and 60 (Riecher-Rössler, 1994). Estimations on the basis of a clinical population from the same catchment area as the ABC population suggested a further 3–4% of first admissions with this diagnostic spectrum after age 60. Population based incidence rates were found to be three to four times as high before age 40 as in the age group 40–59: whereas in the age group 12–39 the yearly incidence rate was 23 cases per 100 000 inhabitants, in the age group 40–59 it was only 6.5/100 000 (Riecher-Rössler, 1994).

As regards sex distribution only 12.8% of the male but 25.5% of the female patients had their first admission when they were 40 years or older. Restricting the analyses to schizophrenic patients only, the corresponding figures were 10.1% and 21.1%, respectively. This ratio of about 2:1 (female:male) could also be confirmed based on incidence rates (Riecher-Rössler, 1994).

In earlier studies we had already shown that the morbidity risk of women does not simply continuously decrease with increasing age (Häfner *et al.*, 1989, 1991a, 1993a,b). Rather, women have a second peak of illness onset after age 45. In order to explain this phenomenon we have conducted systematic investigations (Häfner *et al.*, 1989, 1991a, 1993a,b). At first we tested if psychosocial factors with age and sex specific distribution, like family status or occupational status, were influencing age of onset. The results were largely negative (Häfner et al., 1989; Riecher-Rössler et al., 1992). To explain the sex differences in age at onset, a biological hypothesis gained increasing evidence on the basis of our epidemiological (Häfner et al., 1989, 1991a, 1992b, 1993b) and clinical studies (Riecher-Rössler et al., 1994a,b, 1998) as well as animal experiments (Häfner et al., 1991b): the so-called oestrogen hypothesis. This suggests that oestradiol can enhance the vulnerability threshold for the outbreak of schizophrenia, probably mainly by its antidopaminergic properties known from basic and animal research (Seeman, 1981; Riecher-Rössler and Häfner, 1993). If this hypothesis were valid, women would be protected from the outbreak of schizophrenia to a certain degree from puberty until (pre-)menopause, i.e. during their period of life with a high physiological oestradiol production. Only when oestradiol levels slowly decrease – and this begins about 5 years before actual menopause, which occurs at a mean age of about 51–52 years (Labhart, 1978) – this protective factor would slowly disappear and women would 'catch up' with their morbidity risk. This could, at least partly, explain women's second peak of illness onset after age 45, and thereby also the excess of women in late onset schizophrenia.

Symptomatology

As concerns symptomatology, most earlier and also contemporary researchers found no or only marginal differences between late and early onset schizophrenic diseases (e.g. Kolle, 1931; Bleuler, 1943; Knoll, 1952; Klages, 1961; Siegel and Rollberg, 1970; Huber et al., 1975, 1977; Rabins et al., 1984; Jeste et al., 1988; Mayer et al., 1993; Davidson et al., 1993; Jeste et al., 1995). This does not only apply to authors who examined symptomatology cross-sectionally but also to those who examined longitudinally in the course of the disease.

Even Kraepelin's patients, who in the beginning (1912) had shown an excess of paraphrenic clinical pictures, were shown to develop a symptomatology 'which could not be differentiated from that of other patients with dementia praecox anymore' in the later course of the disease (Mayer, 1921). Further, Manfred Bleuler (1943), who coined the term 'late onset schizophrenia', had – as already mentioned – himself found only a subgroup of patients differing from the classic clinical picture of early onset schizophrenia.

In contrast, there are only single studies pointing to more marked differences (Pearlson et al., 1989; Howard et al., 1993a,b). However, only one of these was aimed solely at schizophrenia, and this was a retrospective analysis of case-notes only, restricted to a certain hospital. It was that of Pearlson et al. (1989), who compared 54 late onset schizophrenia patients with 22 age-matched chronic and 54 young, early onset schizophrenia patients. Late onset cases showed significantly less thought disorder and flattening of affect but

a more colourful picture of hallucinations. The frequency of acoustic hallucinations and persecutory delusions was positively correlated with age but
not with age at onset. Even these authors finally concluded that 'the
phenomenologic similarities ... outweigh the differences' (p. 1572). Howard
et al. (1993a,b), who found that late and early onset patients were 'not phenotypically homogeneous', had examined a very wide diagnostic spectrum
including the over 60 year olds with late paraphrenia and all reactive
psychoses without clear exclusion criteria. It therefore has to be assumed that
the differences described by these authors (e.g. more persecutory and
organized delusions and certain acoustic hallucinations in late onset cases)
are widely due to their sample selection.

If one considers only those studies restricted to classic late onset
schizophrenia, the few psychopathological differences described between
them and early onset patients can be summarized as follows:

Delusions and paranoid symptomatology. In accordance with Kraepelin's
earlier work, some authors describe an association between late onset and
paranoid symptomatology (e.g. Bleuler, 1943; Huber *et al.*, 1975; Angst *et al.*,
1973). Pearlson's (1989) study would, however, imply that this is not so much
due to the higher age of onset but rather due to the higher age itself. Single
authors also described the delusions of late onset patients as more concrete,
organized and psychologically understandable (e.g. Klages, 1961). Based on
this finding, Klages (1961) states 'age ... undoubtedly has a symptom-colouring, pathoplastic influence on the psychosis' (p. 89).

In the course of the disease some authors, e.g. Marneros *et al.* (1992),
found a higher frequency of delusions; Huber *et al.* (1975, 1977) found more
primary delusions.

Hallucinations. Hallucinations are described as slightly more frequent in late
onset patients (Huber *et al.*, 1975, 1977; Marneros *et al.*, 1992) and as present
in more sensory modalities (Pearlson *et al.*, 1989). Especially described are
more tactile (Klages, 1961) and olfactory hallucinations as well as hallucinations of taste (Huber *et al.*, 1975, 1977) and also a characteristic 'verbal hallucinosis' (Schimmelpenning, 1965).

Thought disorders. Thought disorders on the other hand have been described
to be less frequent by Pearlson *et al.* (1989). Jeste *et al.* (1988) only found a
lower prevalence of looseness of association, Marneros *et al.* (1992) comparably less incoherence in late onset cases.

Affect. Some authors have reported depressive prodromal episodes in late
onset patients (e.g. Stransky, 1906; Kolle, 1931; Klages, 1961; Siegel and
Rollberg, 1970). But they have not examined if or to what extent this

phenomenon is also present in early onset patients. As to the symptomatology of the illness itself, some authors since Stransky (1906) have reported a comparably well preserved affectivity in late onset schizophrenia patients. Manfred Bleuler (1943) found less affective flattening, Pearlson *et al.* (1989) less inappropriateness of affect, Huber *et al.* (1975) and Jeste *et al.* (1988) less depressive mood – Huber, though, at the beginning of the disease only and not in its further course. On the other hand, Klages (1961) and Mayer *et al.* (1993) found comparably more depressive symptoms in late onset cases. However, when Mayer *et al.* excluded paranoid psychoses and analysed only the schizophrenic psychoses, these differences disappeared. The only persisting difference then was a higher score in the 'autonomic syndrome' with more vegetative symptoms in late onset cases.

Negative symptoms. Andreasen *et al.* (1990) have described an inverse association between age and negative symptoms but they have analysed a group of under 46 year old patients only. In only one study have age differences between late and early onset cases been described, as concerns negative symptoms. This again is the study of Howard *et al.* (1993a), i.e. the differences are probably due to their patient selection.

Own studies. We have compared 43 late onset patients with 224 early onset patients (Riecher-Rössler, 1994, 1997; Riecher-Rössler *et al.*, 1997). The patients were examined in the framework of the ABC-study (Häfner *et al.*, 1993a,b). Symptomatology at admission was assessed using the Present State Examination (PSE, Wing *et al.*, 1973, 1974), the SANS (Scale for the Assessment of Negative Symptoms, Andreasen, 1981), and the PIRS (Psychological Impairment Rating Schedule, Jablensky *et al.*, 1980). For an exact assessment and operationalization of the onset of the disease we used the IRAOS (Instrument for the Retrospective Assessment of the Onset of Schizophrenia, Häfner *et al.*, 1992a). This is a semi-structured instrument which allows the assessment of the early preclinical course of schizophrenia on different levels like prodromi, first signs, symptoms and social indicators of the beginning mental disease. All interviews were conducted by specially trained psychiatrists and clinical psychologists. Diagnoses were based on the Present State Examination and confirmed by the computer program CATEGO (Wing *et al.*, 1973, 1974).

Forty-three of the 267 patients were 40 years or older when they had their first admission with a schizophrenic or paranoid psychosis (ICD-9: 295, 297, 298.3+0.4, WHO, 1978). The symptomatology of these patients was surprisingly similar to that of the 224 early onset patients. Late onset patients merely had less unspecific neurotic symptomatology and therefore slightly lower scores of total psychopathology (PSE-total score). The two age groups did not, however, show significant differences in their psychotic symptomatology.

Slightly lower scores for the late onset patients in several unspecific symptoms and syndromes like 'depersonalization', 'ideas of reference' or 'unspecific psychotic symptoms' did not reach statistical significance. Even the mean number of psychotic symptoms and the mean number of first rank symptoms were the same for both age groups. The schizophrenic 'nuclear syndrome' according to the standardized diagnostic system CATEGO, which is mainly defined by the presence of first rank symptoms, was present in 58.6% of the late onset and in 68.3% of the early onset cases – a difference which was not statistically significant. In a discriminant analysis based on different psychopathology scores, only 60% of the patients could be correctly classified as belonging to the early or late onset group (Riecher-Rössler, 1994). These results were true for the whole group of schizophrenic and paranoid patients but also if one looked at the schizophrenic patients separately. As further analyses showed, the few differences in unspecific symptoms were mainly due to pathoplastic influence of age and age-associated characteristics. They did not by any means point at late onset schizophrenia being a distinct entity or subgroup of schizophrenic disorders, which would justify a special term or diagnostic category.

One of the most intriguing findings again concerned gender differences: symptomatology of late onset women proved to be distinctly more severe than that of late onset men. The few late onset men not only showed a lower total score of psychopathology (mean PSE-total score in men: 24.6; SD14.8 / in women 39.5; SD14.5, $p < 0.01$) but also suffered less from delusions and hallucinations. Late onset women were, in contrast, in most areas almost as severely disturbed as the early onset patients of both genders.

Course

Studies on the course of late onset schizophrenia are rare, although age has been analysed as an influencing factor in various studies on the course of schizophrenia in general. The results of these latter studies are inconsistent; details are given by Watt and Szulecka (1979) or Häfner and Hambrecht (1994), for example. Neither these studies nor those on late paraphrenia, nor those on the later course of early onset patients, will be considered here (for reviews concerning these patients see Ciompi, 1987; Harris and Jeste, 1988; Gurland, 1988; Häfner and Hambrecht, 1994). This review, rather, will be restricted to the course of late onset schizophrenia itself. Methodological details of the studies have been given in Table 1.

M. Bleuler (1943) was again one of the first to examine the course of late onset schizophrenia and found that these patients, as compared to early onset patients, less often end up with severe dementia but more often with a 'mild state of deficiency' and that a comparable proportion experiences 'social healing'. Also most other early German researchers describe a relatively benign prognosis in late onset cases (e.g. Klages, 1961; Siegel and Rollberg, 1970), though early onset cases were never directly compared on an empirical basis.

On the other hand, there were several authors who did not confirm this. Thus, for example, Schimmelpenning (1965) and Berner et al. (1973) found a preponderance of uniformly chronic courses in late onset schizophrenia. In Berner's population only 13% of the patients with onset between 40 and 65 years could be said to be 'healthy' when they were re-examined at an average age of 77 years. Gabriel (1974a, 1978) assessed the psychosocial adaptation in the same population and described it as very poor in about one-third of the patients.

Hinterhuber (1973) and Huber et al. (1975, 1977) were the first to compare late onset cases with early onset cases directly on an empirical basis. Hinterhuber (1973) found a definitely poorer course in the late onset cases: after a catamnestic period of 30–40 years, only 16% of them were cured and 40% suffered from severe psychotic disturbances, while 63% of the patients with onset before age 20 had completely recovered and only 12% of them suffered from a 'severe deficiency syndrome'. Huber et al. (1975, 1977) in contrast found a milder course in late onset schizophrenia. After a catamnestic period of on average 17.8 years, they found that 30% of the late onset as opposed to only 22% of all schizophrenic patients had completely remitted. Only Hinterhuber's study, however, was restricted to first admitted.

Only a few studies on the course of classic late onset schizophrenia have been conducted by Anglo-American authors. Fish (1960), Blessed and Wilson (1982) and Rabins et al. (1984) have examined small samples of diagnostically mixed patient groups which cannot easily be interpreted. Craig and Bregman (1988) conducted a chart review of 32 patients aged 65 or older with onset of symptoms after age 45, who met DSM-III criteria for schizophrenia (except age of onset). Clinical course revealed only 25% to follow an unequivocally schizophrenic pattern, while 40.6% showed signs of organic deterioration.

Holden (1987) only described patients with late paraphrenia occurring for the first time after age 60. His study, nevertheless, must be mentioned, since he found that after a course of 10 years only 10% of these 47 patients could be still diagnosed as 'schizophreniform'. The other patients had to be classified as schizoaffective, paranoid, organic, symptomatic or affective at follow-up. This study confirms that late paraphrenia has to be considered as different from late onset schizophrenia and probably as a whole 'spectrum of overlapping conditions with paranoid delusions' (Holden, 1987, p. 635). Also more recent studies indicate that late paraphrenia is distinct from late onset schizophrenia and that an organic substrate probably exists in many cases of late paraphrenia, while gross organic pathology cannot be detected in late onset schizophrenia (Naguib, 1991; Howard et al., 1994; for review see Riecher-Rössler et al., 1995).

Own studies. Own analyses have so far only been done on case register data, i.e. on the institutional course of late onset as compared with early onset patients. We examined the 10 year course of a cohort of all 1423 Danish patients first admitted in 1976 with a clinical diagnosis of schizophrenia, paranoid or paranoid reactive psychosis or borderline state (ICD-8: 295, 297, 298.3, 301.83, WHO, 1967). Of these patients 536 at the 'index admission' belonged to the narrow diagnostic group of schizophrenia (ICD:295). Seven hundred and thirty-four (51.6%) of all patients and 212 (39.6%) of the schizophrenic patients had their index admission at age 40 or later. As the schizophrenia diagnosis is given only quite restrictively in Denmark (Munk-Jørgensen, 1985; Häfner *et al.*, 1989), 27.7% of the patients had already been admitted with another diagnosis before this index admission (Riecher-Rössler, 1994) – a fact that can explain why the proportion of late onset cases is comparatively high in this population.

Comparing the patients with index admission before age 40 with those thereafter, the institutional course was found to be much better in the late onset cases (Riecher-Rössler, 1994). This was true for the schizophrenic patients only, and also when the analyses included all patients. The mean number of hospitalizations over the 10 year course was only 2.6 (SD 2.2) in late onset patients but 4.3 (SD 3.5) in early onset cases ($p < 0.001$). Also, total duration was much lower in late onset cases (mean 286 days, SD 607) than in early onset cases (mean 506 days, SD 690, $p < 0.001$). Already after index hospitalization the late onset cases had a significantly longer 'survival time' in the community before they had to be rehospitalized, and significantly more of them did not have to be rehospitalized at all. These results were also true after correcting for the differing mortality rates of the two age groups.

But even if these differences were more marked than those concerning symptomatology, we could nevertheless show that they do not indicate late and early onset schizophrenia as being different entities or due to different pathogenetic processes. Rather, numerous influencing factors can be identified, covarying with age, which contributed to the better course of the elderly late onset patients. Thus, a multiple regression analysis showed that the better course of the late onset cases seems, among other reasons, to be due to the fact that these patients are more often married than the younger early onset patients, and being married was one of the factors found to reduce mean number and duration of hospitalizations.

Concerning gender differences we again had a very interesting result: the course of late onset women was significantly poorer than that of late onset men. Late onset women had more admissions and spent significantly more days in hospital during the 10 years observed than late onset men (Riecher-Rössler, 1994).

CONCLUSIONS

Based on a comprehensive review of the literature it could be shown that we do not have a very sound knowledge of the classic late onset schizophrenia(s) as defined by M. Bleuler (1943) and adopted by German language psychiatry, i.e. schizophrenia-like clinical pictures with onset after age 40. This is mainly due to two reasons: on the one hand the existing studies on late onset schizophrenia suffer from severe methodological limitations. On the other hand, the term and concept 'late onset schizophrenia' internationally is used unequivocally with the consequence that many findings on so-called 'late onset schizophrenia', though cited again and again, are in fact not based on classic late onset schizophrenia, but on late paraphrenia, i.e. 'spectrum of overlapping conditions with paranoid delusions' (Holden, 1987, p. 635), or on mixed populations of both diagnostic groups (Riecher-Rössler, this volume, Chapter 1; Riecher-Rössler et al., 1995). The problems of terminology and nosology have until now seriously limited international research. When researchers report on the same sort of patients using different terms (and vice versa) it is not possible to arrive at a reliable and valid description of disease entities. The result is a serious deficit in empirically sound knowledge in this area. It is therefore suggested that the term 'late paraphrenia' be abandoned to avoid further confusion. There is now enough evidence that this is not a valid entity but an umbrella diagnosis for a heterogeneous group of diseases, including many cases of organic aetiology (Riecher-Rössler et al., 1995).

Looking at classic late onset schizophrenia only and at the methodologically sounder studies, few findings really appear to be reliable. Late onset schizophrenic disorders are much rarer than the classic schizophrenic psychoses with onset before age 40. In accordance with other authors, in our own studies only about 15–16% of all schizophrenic patients had their first admission with this diagnosis between age 40 and 60. Based on all first admissions of a defined catchment area we calculated the morbidity risk for schizophrenia being about 3–4 times as high before age 40 as in the age group 40–60 years. Furthermore, late onset schizophrenia is much more frequent in women than in men: within the age group 40–60 the morbidity risk for women was about twice as high as that for men. First admission after age 60 was very rare.

As concerns symptomatology, most studies have not found essential differences between late and early onset cases. The same was true in our own study, which was one of the first to examine a representative sample of first admissions with standardized instruments, and in direct comparison to a control group of early onset patients. Late onset cases only showed a somewhat milder, unspecific neurotic symptomatology and as a consequence of this a somewhat lower score for total psychopathology. But there were no significant differences in psychotic symptoms. If one looked at the genders separately, however, the few late onset men could be shown to have a distinctly milder symptomatology than the late onset women and the early onset patients of both genders. This was true even for the psychotic area. In contrast, the late onset women's symptomatology was almost as severe as that of the early onset cases.

As to the course of late onset schizophrenia, studies are rare and their results very contradictory. Thus, conclusions can hardly be drawn. Own studies could so far only be done on a Danish cases register population, i.e. on the institutional aspects of the course. During the 10 years after first admission for a schizophrenic or paranoid disorder, late onset patients had significantly fewer and shorter hospital stays as compared to the early onset cases. Eaton *et al.* (1992) had similar results based on case register data not only from Denmark but also from other countries. As regards gender differences our results are in accordance with our results on symptomatology: the course of late onset women was poorer than that of late onset men.

In summary, it can thus be stated that late onset schizophrenia does not substantially differ from early onset schizophrenia as regards symptomatology. The course of late onset cases, however, seems to be comparably milder. But this, and also the few slight differences in unspecific symptomatology, are obviously simply due to the fact that age and numerous age-associated characteristics have a somewhat symptom-colouring pathoplastic effect and also a positive influence on the course of the disease. There are no hints on late onset schizophrenia being a separate entity or subgroup of the disease, thereby justifying the use of a separate term or even a separate diagnostic category for these late onset cases. Rather they seem to belong to the same (group of) diseases as the classic early onset schizophrenia(s) with onset before age 40. Our results also give additional support for the decision to omit late onset schizophrenia as a separate subcategory in DSM-IV (APA, 1994) as opposed to the former DSM-IIIR (APA, 1987).

The fact that most late onset patients are female and also our finding that these late onset women suffer from a comparatively more severe symptomatology and course might be explained by the above-mentioned oestrogen effect: it could be speculated that oestradiol by its neuromodulatory and probably antidopaminergic properties can delay illness onset in some women until around menopause, when physiological oestradiol levels drastically drop. These women would then be 'unmasked' as a comparatively vulnerable population and develop a relatively severe symptomatology and course of their disease. This, however, is still speculative and further studies will have to be conducted to confirm our results and possibly also this hypothesis.

ACKNOWLEDGEMENTS

This study was funded by the DFG (German Society for the Advancement of Scientific Research).

REFERENCES

American Psychiatric Association (1980). *Diagnostic and Statistical Manual of Mental Disorders, 3rd edn* (DSM-III). American Psychiatric Association, Washington, DC.

American Psychiatric Association (1987). *Diagnostic and Statistical Manual of Mental Disorders, 3rd edn revised* (DSM-IIIR). American Psychiatric Association, Washington, DC.

American Psychiatric Association (1994). *Diagnostic and Statistical Manual of Mental Disorders, 4th edn* (DSM-IV). American Psychiatric Association, Washington, DC.

Andreasen, N.C. (1981). *Scale for the Assessment of Negative Symptoms (SANS)*. The University of Iowa, Iowa City.

Andreasen, N.C., Flaum, M., Swayze, V.W., Tyrrell, G. and Arndt, M.S. (1990). Positive and negative symptoms in schizophrenia. *Arch Gen Psychiatry* **47**, 615–621.

Angst, J., Baastrup, P., Grof, P. *et al.* (1973). Statistische Aspekte des Beginns und Verlaufs schizophrener Psychosen. In: Huber, G. (Ed.), *Verlauf und Ausgang schizophrener Erkrankungen*. Schattauer, Stuttgart, New York, pp. 67–78.

Astrup, C., Fossum, A. and Holmboe, R. (1962). *Prognosis in Functional Psychoses*. Thomas, Springfield.

Berner, P., Gabriel, E. and Naske, R. (1973). Verlaufstypologie und Prognose bei sogenannten Spätschizophrenien. In: Huber, G. (Ed.), *Verlauf und Ausgang schizophrener Erkrankungen*. Schattauer, Stuttgart, New York, pp. 85–95.

Blessed, G. and Wilson, I.D. (1982). The contemporary natural history of mental disorder in old age. *Br J Psychiatry* **141**, 59–67.

Bleuler, M. (1943). Die spätschizophrenen Krankheitsbilder. *Fortschr Neurol Psychiatr* **15**, 259–290.

Bleuler, E. (1908). Die Prognose der Dementia praecox (Schizophreiegruppe). *Allg Z Psychiatr* **65**, 436–464.

Castle, D.J. and Murray, R.M. (1993). The epidemiology of late-onset schizophrenia. *Schizophr Bull* **19**, 691–700.

Ciompi, L. (1987). Review of follow-up studies on long-term evolution and aging in schizophrenia. In: Miller, N.E. and Cohen, G.D. (Eds), *Schizophrenia and Aging*. The Guilford Press, New York, London, pp. 37–51.

Ciompi, L. and Müller, C. (1976). *Lebensweg und Alter der Schizophrenen*. Springer, Berlin, Heidelberg, New York.

Craig T.J. and Bregman, Z. (1988). Late onset schizophrenia-like illness. *J Am Geriatr Soc* **36**, 104–107.

Davidson, M., Harvey, P.D., Haroutuinan, V. *et al.* (1993). Symptom severity and cognitive impairment in elderly schizophrenic patients. *Schizophr Res* **9**, 97.

Eaton, W.W., Mortensen, P.B., Herrman, H. *et al.* (1992). Long-term course of hospitalization for schizophrenia: Part I. Risk for rehospitalization. *Schizophr Bull* **18**, 217–228.

Fish, F. (1958). A clinical investigation of chronic schizophrenia. *J Mental Sci* **104**, 34–54.

Fish, F. (1960). Senile schizophrenia. *J Mental Sci* **106**, 938–946.

Funding, T. (1963). Paranoid psychoses in later life. *Acta Psychiatr Scand* **39** (suppl 169), 356–361.

Gabriel, E. (1974a). Der langfristige Verlauf schizophrener Späterkrankungen im Vergleich mit Schizophrenien aller Lebensalter. *Psychiatrica Clinica* **7**, 172–180.

Gabriel, E. (1974b). Über den Einfluss psychoorganischer Beeinträchtigung im Alter auf den Verlauf sogenannter Spätschizophrenien. *Psychiatrica Clinica* **7**, 358–364.

Gabriel, E. (1978). *Die langfristige Entwicklung der Spätschizophrenien*. Karger, Basel.

Gurland, B.J. (1988). Schizophrenia in the elderly. In: Tsuang, M.T. and Simpson, J.C. (Eds), *Handbook of Schizophrenia: Nosology, Epidemiology and Genetics*. Elsevier Science Publishers BV, Amsterdam, New York, Oslo, pp. 299–317.

Häfner, H. and Hambrecht, M. (1994). The elderly with schizophrenia. In: Chiu, E. and Ames, D. (Eds), *Functional Psychiatric Disorders in the Elderly*. Cambridge University Press.

Häfner, H., Riecher, A., Maurer, K., Löffler, W., Munk-Jørgensen, P. and Strömgren, E. (1989). How does gender influence age at first hospitalization for schizophrenia? *Psychol Med* **19**, 903–918.

Häfner, H., Riecher-Rössler, A., Maurer, K. *et al.* (1991a). Geschlechtsunterschiede bei schizophrenen Erkrankungen. *Fortschr Neurol Psychiatr* **59**, 343–360.

Häfner, H., Behrens, S., De Vry, J. and Gattaz, W.F. (1991b). An animal model for the effects of estradiol on dopamine-mediated behaviour: implications for sex differences in schizophrenia. *Psychiatry Res* **38**, 125–134.

Häfner, H., Riecher-Rössler, A., Hambrecht, M. *et al.* (1992a). IRAOS: an instrument for the retrospective assessment of onset and early course of schizophrenia. *Schizophr Res* **6**, 209–223.

Häfner, H., Riecher-Rössler, A., Maurer, K., Fätkenheuer, B. and Löffler, W. (1992b). First onset and early symptomatology of schizophrenia – a chapter of epidemiological and neurobiological research into age and sex differences. *Eur Arch Psychiatry Clin Neurosci* **242**, 109–118.

Häfner, H., Maurer, K., Löffler, W. and Riecher-Rössler, A. (1993a). The influence of age and sex on the onset and course of early schizophrenia. *Br J Psychiatry* **162**, 80–86.

Häfner, H., Riecher-Rössler, A., an der Heiden, W., Maurer, K., Fätkenheuer, B. and Löffler, W. (1993b). Generating and testing a causal explanation of the gender difference in age at first onset of schizophrenia. *Psychol Med* **23**, 925–940.

Harris, M.J. and Jeste, D.V. (1988). Late-onset schizophrenia: an overview. *Schizophr Bull* **14**, 39–55.

Herbert, M.E. and Jacobson, S. (1967). Late paraphrenia. *Br J Psychiatry* **113**, 461–469.

Hinterhuber, H. (1973). Zur Katamnese der Schizophrenien. *Fortschr Neurol Psychiatr* **41**, 527–558.

Holden, N.L. (1987). Late paraphrenia or the paraphrenias? *Br J Psychiatry* **150**, 635–639.

Howard, R., Castle, D., Wessely, S. and Murray, R. (1993a). A comparative study of 470 cases of early- and late-onset schizophrenia. *Br J Psychiatry* **163**, 1–6.

Howard, R.J., Almeida, O. and Levy, R. (1993b). Phenomenology of late-onset schizophrenia. *Schizophr Res* **9**, 100.

Howard, R.J., Almeida, O., Levy, R., Graves, P. and Graves, M. (1994). Quantitative magnetic resonance imaging volumetry distinguishes delusional disorder from late-onset schizophrenia. *Br J Psychiatry* **165**, 474–480.

Huber, G., Gross, G. and Schüttler, R. (1975). Spätschizophrenie. *Arch Psychiatr Nervenkr* **221**, 53–66.

Huber, G., Gross, G. and Schüttler, R. (1977). Schizophrene Psychosen der 2. Lebenshälfte. *Med Welt* **28**, 166–168.

Huber, G., Gross, G. and Schüttler, R. (1979). *Schizophrenie: Verlaufs- und sozialpsychiatrische Langzeituntersuchung an den 1949–1959 in Bonn hospitalisierten schizophrenen Kranken*. Springer, Berlin.

Jablensky, A., Schwarz, R. and Tomov, T. (1980). WHO collaborative study on impairments and disabilities associated with schizophrenic disorders. *Acta Psychiatr Scand* **62** (suppl 285), 152–163.

Jablensky, A., Sartorius, N., Ernberg, G. *et al.* (1992). *Schizophrenia: Manifestations, Incidence and Course in Different Cultures. A World Health Organization Ten-Country Study.* Cambridge University Press, Cambridge.

Jeste, D.V., Harris, M.J., Pearlson, G.B. *et al.* (1988). Late-onset schizophrenia. Studying clinical validity. *Psychiatric Clin North Am* **11**, 1–13.

Jeste, D.V., Harris, M.J., Krull, A., Kuck, J., McAdams, L.A. and Heaton, R. (1995). Clinical and neuropsychological characteristics of patients with late-onset schizophrenia. *Am J Psychiatry* **152**, 722–730.

Jørgensen, P. and Munk-Jørgensen, P. (1985). Paranoid psychosis in the elderly. *Acta Psychiatr Scand* **62**, 358–363.

Kay, D.W.K. and Roth, M. (1961). Environmental and hereditary factors in the schizophrenia of old age ('late paraphrenia') and their bearing on the general problem of causation in schizophrenia. *J Mental Sci* **107**, 649–686.

Klages, W. (1961). *Die Spätschizophrenie.* Enke, Stuttgart.

Knoll, H. (1952). Wahnbildende Psychosen in der Zeit des Klimakteriums und der Involution in klinischer und genealogischer Betrachtung. *Arch Psychiatr Z Neurol* **189**, 59–92.

Kolle, K. (1931). *Die primäre Verrücktheit: psychopathologische, klinische und genealogische Untersuchungen.* Thieme, Leipzig.

Kraepelin, E. (1893–1915). *Psychiatrie, ein Lehrbuch für Studierende und Ärzte,* Vols 4–8. Barth, Leipzig.

Kraepelin, E. (1919). *Dementia praecox und Paraphrenie.* Krieger, New York (reprint in English, 1971).

Labhart, A. (1978). *Klinik der inneren Sekretion.* Springer, Berlin.

Langfeldt, G. (1960). Diagnosis and prognosis in schizophrenia. *Proc R Soc Med* **53**, 1047–1052.

Larson, C.A. and Nyman, G.E. (1970). Age of onset in schizophrenia. *Human Heredity* **20**, 241–247.

Marneros, A. and Deister, A. (1984). The psychopathology of 'late schizophrenia'. *Psychopathology* **17**, 264–274.

Marneros, A., Deister, A. and Rohde, A. (1992). Schizophrenic, schizoaffective and affective disorders in the elderly: a comparison. In: Katona, C. and Levy, R. (Eds), *Delusions and Hallucinations in Old Age.* Gaskell, London, pp. 136–152.

Mayer, C., Kelterborn, G. and Naber, D. (1993). Age of onset in schizophrenia: relations to psychopathology and gender. *Br J Psychiatry* **162**, 665–671.

Mayer, W. (1921). Über paraphrene Psychosen. *Z Gesamte Neurol Psychiatr* **71**, 187–206.

Müller, C. (1959). *Über das Senium der der Schizophrenen.* Karger, Basel, New York.

Munk-Jørgensen, P. (1985). The schizophrenia diagnosis in Denmark. *Acta Psychiatr Scand* **72**, 266–273.

Naguib, M. (1991). Paraphrenia revisited. *Br J Hosp Med* **46**, 371–375.

Pearlson, G.D., Kreger, L., Rabins, P.V. *et al.* (1989). A chart review study of late-onset and early-onset schizophrenia. *Am J Psychiatry* **146**, 1568–1574.

Post, F. (1966). *Persistent Persecutory States of the Elderly.* Pergamon, Oxford.

Quintal, M., Day-Cody, D. and Levy, R. (1991). Late paraphrenia and ICD 10. *Int J Geriatr Psychiatry* **6**, 111–116.

Rabins, P., Pauker, S. and Thomas, J. (1984). Can schizophrenia begin after age 44? *Compr Psychiatry* **25**, 290–293.

Retterstøl, N. (1966). *Paranoid and Paranoiac Psychoses*. Thomas, Springfield.

Riecher, A., Maurer, K., Löffler, W., Fätkenheuer, B., an der Heiden, W. and Häfner, H. (1989). Schizophrenia – a disease of young single males? *Eur Arch Psychiatry Neurol Sci* **239**, 210–212.

Riecher, A., Maurer, K., Löffler, W. *et al.* (1991). Gender differences in age at onset and course of schizophrenic disorders – a contribution to the understanding of the disease? In: Häfner, H. and Gattaz, W.F. (Eds), *Search for the Causes of Schizophrenia. Vol. 2*. Springer, Berlin, Heidelberg, New York, pp. 14–33.

Riecher-Rössler, A. (1994). *Die Spätschizophrenie – eine valide Entität? Eine empirische Studie zu Risikofaktoren, Krankheitsbild und Verlauf.* Habilitationsschrift. Medizinische Fakultät der Universität Heidelberg.

Riecher-Rössler, A. (1997). 50 Jahre nach Manfred Bleuler. Was wissen wir heute über Spätschizophrenie(n)? *Der Nervenarzt* **68**, 159–170.

Riecher-Rössler, A. and Häfner, H. (1993). Schizophrenia and estrogens – is there an association? *Eur Arch Psychiatry Clin Neurosci* **242**, 323–328.

Riecher-Rössler, A., Fätkenheuer, B., Löffler, W., Maurer, K. and Häfner, H. (1992). Is age of onset in schizophrenia influenced by family status? Some remarks on the difficulties and pitfalls in systematic testing of a 'simple' question. *Social Psychiatry* **27**, 122–128.

Riecher-Rössler, A., Häfner, H., Stumbaum, M., Maurer, K. and Schmidt, R. (1994a). Can estradiol modulate schizophrenic symptomatology? *Schizophr Bull* **20**, 203–214.

Riecher-Rössler, A., Häfner, H., Dütsch-Strobel, A. *et al.* (1994b). Further evidence for a specific role of estradiol in schizophrenia? *Biol Psychiatry* **36**, 492–495.

Riecher-Rössler, A., Rössler, W., Förstl, H. and Meise, U. (1995). Late onset schizophrenia and late paraphrenia: a history of confusion about terms and concepts. *Schizophr Bull* **21**, 345–354.

Riecher-Rössler, A., Löffler, W. and Munk-Jørgensen, P. (1997). What do we really know about late-onset schizophrenia? *Eur Arch Psychiatry Clin Neurosci* **247**, 195–208.

Riecher-Rössler, A., Häfner, H., Dütsch-Strobel, A. and Stumbaum, M. (1998). Gonadal function and its influence on psychopathology. A comparison of schizophrenic and non-schizophrenic female inpatients. *Arch Women's Mental Health* **1**, 15–26.

Roth, M. (1955). The natural history of mental disorders in old age. *J Mental Sci* **101**, 281–301.

Roth, M. and Morrissey, J.D. (1952). Problems in the diagnosis and classification of mental disorder in old age; with a study of case material. *J Mental Sci* **98**, 66–80.

Schimmelpenning, G.W. (1965). *Die paranoiden Psychosen der zweiten Lebenshälfte.* Karger, Basel.

Schneider, K. (1957). Primäre und sekundäre Symptome bei Schizophrenie. *Fortschr Neurol Psychiatr* **25**, 487.

Schulz, B. (1933). Zur Erbpathologie der Schizophrenie. *Z Gesamte Neurol Psychiatr* **143**, 175–293.

Seeman, M.V. (1981). Gender and the onset of schizophrenia: neurohumoral influences. *Psychiatr J Univ Ottawa* **6**, 136–138.

Shepherd, M., Watt, D., Falloon, I. and Smeeton, N. (1989). The natural history of schizophrenia. A five-year follow up study of outcome and prediction in a representative sample of schizophrenics. *Psychol Med Monograph*, suppl 15.

Siegel, E. and Rollberg, I. (1970). Über Spätschizophrenien. *Wien Z Nervenheilk Grenzg* **28**, 145–151.

Spitzer, R.L., Endicott, J. and Robins, E. (1978). *Research Diagnostic Criteria for a Selected Group of Functional Disorders (3rd edn)*. New York State Psychiatric Institute, New York.

Sternberg, E. (1972). Neuere Forschungsergebnisse bei spätschizophrenen Psychosen. *Fortschr Neurol Psychiatr* **40**, 631–646.

Stransky, E. (1906). Dementia tardiva. *Mschr Psychiatr* **18**, 1–38.

Watt, D.C. and Szulecka, T.K. (1979). The effect of sex, marriage and age at first admission on the hospitalization of schizophrenics during 2 years following discharge. *Psychol Med* **9**, 529–539.

Wing, J.K., Cooper, J.E. and Sartorius, N. (1973). *Present State Examination (PSE)*. Deutsche Bearbeitung von M.v.Cranach 1978. Medical Research Council, UK.

Wing, J.K., Cooper, J.E. and Sartorius, N. (1974). *Measurement and Classification of Psychiatric Symptoms. An Instruction Manual for the PSE and CATEGO Program*. Cambridge University Press, Cambridge.

World Health Organization (1967). *International Classification of Diseases, ICD, 8th Revision*. World Health Organization, Geneva.

World Health Organization (1978). *Mental Disorders: Glossary and Guide to their Classification in Accordance with the Ninth Revision of the International Classification of Diseases*. World Health Organization, Geneva.

World Health Organization (1993). *Tenth Revision of the International Classification of Diseases, Chapter V (F): Mental and Behavioural Disorders (Including Disorders of Psychological Development). Clinical Description and Diagnostic Guidelines*. World Health Organization, Geneva.

Yassa, R. and Suranyi-Cadotte, B. (1993). Clinical characteristics of late-onset schizophrenia and delusional disorder. *Schizophr Bull* **19**, 701–707.

5

Late Onset Schizophrenia: Diagnosis in France: Myth or Reality?

JEAN-PIERRE CLÉMENT

Psychiatric Service of the University Hospital Esquirol, Limoges, France

INTRODUCTION

Henri Ey said 'La schizophrénie est à la fin' (schizophrenia is at the end) in order to emphasize the inevitably deteriorating course ('l'évolution défici- taire') (Ey, 1948–1954).

Dilip Jeste, in a recent editorial of the *American Journal of Psychiatry* (Jeste, 1997), asked the question that, since the average lifespan in the United States has increased from 47 years in 1900 (when Kraepelin described dementia praecox) to 75 years today, should we be shocked if the symptoms of schizophrenia manifest for the first time in some cases after age 45? France has the same average lifespan. So, if we consider the present international situation of the entity called 'late onset schizophrenia' in the realm of psychi- atry of the elderly, the French opinion may be viewed as original.

When we return to old manuscripts of French psychiatric literature, several authors (Esquirol, Ritti, Seglas, Lasègue, Falret, Sérieux & Capgras, Magnan, Pascal & Courbon, De Clérambault, Dide & Guiraud...) give their clinical position, which can be summarized by the words: late onset schizophrenia must be dropped from the nosography.

As is well-known, the French classification of delusions distinguishes schizophrenia from chronic systematized delusion syndromes and from chronic hallucinatory psychosis (la 'psychose hallucinatoire chronique') (Haugsten, 1996). Ey's approach (1977) also needs to be recalled. Fundamentally, long term delusions are personality impairments, consisting of three important psychotic structures:

- paranoiac ('paranoïaque'), for systematized delusional psychoses with delusions of passion and interpretation;
- paraphrenic ('paraphrénique'), for fantastic psychoses;
- schizophrenic ('schizophrénique'), with two forms – paranoid ('paranoïde') and autistic 'autistique').

Here, delusion is defined as a false fixed belief that the patient cannot prove, and that is inconsistent with the patient's family or social background and that the patient did not believe prior to becoming ill.

Faced with the international consensus which has been greatly influenced by the mental disorder classifications, such as the DSM from the APA (even if it was recently criticized concerning diagnostic criteria for schizophrenia; Maj, 1998) or the ICD given by the WHO, French clinical thinking has tried to conform.

However, the psychopathological approach has always had an important place in the perception of psychiatric disorders and particularly in the elderly. Different schools of thinking in France prefer to have a global view of the aged suffering patient. In this way, many disorders which appear for the first time in late life are considered according to different points, which include biography, life events, personality features, social support and ability to cope with new problems. Many disorders afflicting elderly individuals are considered to be maladjustment disorders, with eventually a continuous scale of pathology in a dimensional perspective where anxiety, delusion, depression and even dementia are possible levels of intensity of the psychological post-traumatic disorder. The time frame or accumulation of many events, as well as the magnitude of prolonged strain after the initial stress, need to be considered to understand the whole pathology. Of course, there are also biological factors which are reliable if they are considered as a relationship between genetics and environment (Roubertoux and Nosten, 1986; Van Os and Verdoux, 1998).

STATE OF PSYCHIATRY OF OLD AGE IN FRANCE

In France there is a little interest in the psychiatry of old age. The University Department of Psychiatry Head, Professor Léger, is a pioneer in this discipline, which is not considered as a subspeciality in the French University context. The French Society of Psychogeriatry has some members who are psychiatrists but also some geriatricians who deal with psychiatric disorders in the elderly. Every year, this society organizes a congress. In 1992, the topic of the 8th congress was 'confusional and delusional disorders of the elderly person'. The different studies submitted may be summarized as follows: the field of psychiatry has to consider the first onset of delusional disorders in the elderly differently as this occurs in the adult condition. There are a lot of risk factors which need to be discussed. There is also a clear psychopathology of the delusional state in geriatric psychiatry which has to consider vigilance, sensory functions, cognitive functioning, affectiveness and personality (Wertheimer, 1993).

Clément *et al.* (1993) studied risk factors and suggested a psychopathological point of view. This study compared 36 consecutive hospital records of admitted elderly patients with a late onset delusion to a literature review. Mean age of the sample was 77.2 ± 8.8 [range 61–91 years].

Observed clinical specificities were:

- a well constructed delusion;
- a paranoid structure but more or less systematized;
- in reference to the personal situation of the elderly individual, generally focused on his own world and body (Léger and Clément, 1991);
- themes of delusion are mainly persecution (92%), prejudice (80%), theft, erotomania and jealousy (51%) and hypochondriasis (17%);
- predominant mechanisms are interpretation (60%), imagination (80%) and sometimes hallucinations (auditory: 40%, visual: 30%);
- thought disorders are absent and Schneiderian first rank symptoms very rare;
- emotional reactions, mood changes, and behavioural disorders are usual.

Aetiopathogenic specificities were:

- social isolation and loneliness
- a low socio-economic level (78%)
- a low educational level (75%)
- sensory deficits (30% for auditory and 22% for visual)
- a previous history of cardiovascular diseases
- recent changes in lifestyle
- a pejorative family setting attitude
- feelings of insecurity and vulnerability.

Patients had no previous psychiatric disorder except for depressive episodes. Women seemed to be more vulnerable (78% of the sample). Marital status also seemed important because 70% were unmarried. 33% had no children. In 58% of cases, a recent stressful life event was recorded. Anxiety or depression often co-existed (44% and 50% respectively). 28% had an MMSE (Folstein *et al.*, 1975) under 20.

Using a correspondence factor analysis, it was observed that auditory hallucinations were favoured by isolation ($p = 0.0002$), and surprisingly visual hallucinations were favoured by auditory impairment ($p = 0.008$).

Finally, the last important result was that lonely individuals had no recent life event but a distressing past, and individuals with friends and/or family support had no distressing past but a recent stressful life event.

The psychopathological point of view is that this disorder is a maladjustment reaction when faced with a biopsychosocial situation. Delusion deals with prejudice but also with intrusion (for example, the intrusion of the spouse after retirement), in the same perspective as suggested by Howard *et al.* (1992) when they spoke about 'partition delusions'. Ideas of prejudice concern ownership, health and reputation. Delusion is related to anxiety and represents a singular adjustment condition to fight against isolation and depression. In this way of thinking, Portuguese researcher Dias Cordeiro (1989) suggested the term 'reactive narcissistic psychoses'.

Many papers published in France, even if they use English references, do not mention late onset schizophrenia (Conférence de Consensus, 1994; l'Encéphale, 1996; Séminaire de Psychiatrie Biologique, 1994). In the latest 'gold standard' French book entitled *Les schizophrénies – Aspects actuels* (Schizophrenias – current aspects) (Scotto and Bougerol, 1997), the index does not contain the word 'sujet âgé' (elderly individual), and to have some information related to our topic, it is necessary to refer to the words 'vieillissement' (ageing) and 'âge' (age). Late onset schizophrenia is distinguished from two other main types: a congenital schizophrenia with an early onset, and an adult form with an onset near 30–40 years of age. Scotto and Bougerol's late onset schizophrenia, also called 'late paraphrenia', has an onset after age 60. Delusion is the main symptom. The disorder is predominant in women and sensory deficits are frequent. Cognitive impairment is also common (Fossati and Allilaire, 1997, p. 85). In another chapter, 'ventricular enlargement is considered as non-specific to schizophrenia because it is also observed in aging' (Martinot, 1997, p. 113). And finally, in a third chapter, it is written that 'the dopaminergic mesocortical system of the schizophrenic patient should show greater vulnerability during ageing' (Costentin, 1997, p. 153).

CURRENT OPINIONS ON LATE ONSET SCHIZOPHRENIA

In order to obtain the current opinion of the French Society of Psychogeriatry members, who have some interest in psychogeriatrics, a mail survey was performed to evaluate five points.

Drawing primarily from their clinical experience but also eventually from their theoretical knowledge, respondents had to answer the following questions:

– does late onset schizophrenia exist?
   (a) after 45 and before 65? (yes or no)
   (b) after 65? (yes or no)

- does another kind of late onset psychosis (such as late onset paraphrenia or late onset chronic hallucinatory psychosis) exist?
  (a) after 45 and before 65? (yes or no)
  (b) after 65? (yes or no)
- does a late onset delusional disorder specific of old age exist?
  (a) after 45 and before 65? (yes or no)
  (b) after 65? (yes or no)
- what clinical argument allows you to affirm the existence of late onset schizophrenia in the elderly (give one to three arguments in order of importance)?
- what clinical argument allows you to reject the existence of late onset schizophrenia in the elderly (give one to three arguments in order of importance)?
- do you have personal comments?

Table 1.   Answers to the first five questions.

	LOS 45–65	LOS > 65	ALP 45–65	ALP > 65	SDD
Yes	21 (40%)	10 (19%)	43 (83%)	35 (67%)	40 (77%)
No	26 (50%)	39 (75%)	3 (6%)	14 (27%)	7 (13%)
No answer	5	3	6	3	5

LOS: late onset schizophrenia; ALP: another late psychosis; SDD: specific delusional disorder.

The results are as follows. The society has only 167 members and 52 replied (30%). The answers to the first five questions are summarized in Table 1. Twenty-one members think that late onset schizophrenia is possible between 45 and 65 years of age (26 answers were negative). Only 10 members think that late onset schizophrenia is possible after 65 (39 answers were negative). Forty-three members think that another kind of late onset psychosis is possible between 45 and 65 years of age (three answers were negative). Thirty-five members think that another kind of late onset psychosis is possible after 65 (14 answers were negative). Finally, 40 members think that a late onset delusional disorder specific to old age is possible (seven answers were negative).

Table 2 summarizes the verification of qualitative correlations for answers which showed three statistically significant results. Those replying who reject the existence of late onset schizophrenia after 65 affirm the existence of another late psychosis after this age. Those members supporting the existence of late onset schizophrenia between 45 and 65 years of age also confirm the existence of another late psychosis after 65. Finally, those who reject the existence of late onset schizophrenia between 45 and 65 years of

Table 2. Contingency tables (Fisher test) correlating replies with the existence or not of different disorders at different times.

	LOS 45–65	LOS > 65	ALP 45–65	ALP > 65
LOS > 65	$\chi^2 = 6.12$ Fisher $p = 0.006$	–	–	–
ALP 45–65	$\chi^2 = 0.00$ Fisher $p = 0.99$	$\chi^2 = 0.28$ Fisher $p = 0.82$	–	–
ALP > 65	$\chi^2 = 8.06$ Fisher $p = 0.002$	$\chi^2 = 2.75$ Fisher $p = 0.05$	$\chi^2 = 0.65$ Fisher $p = 0.20$	–
SDD	$\chi^2 = 0.14$ Fisher $p = 0.68$	$\chi^2 = 0.01$ Fisher $p = 0.61$	$\chi^2 = 0.00$ Fisher $p = 0.99$	$\chi^2 = 0.01$ Fisher $p = 0.99$

age also reject existence of late onset schizophrenia after 65. All other correlations are not significant.

When analysing arguments to accept or reject the existence of late onset schizophrenia in the elderly, it appears that the principal argument in favour of late onset schizophrenia is the presence of a dissociative process (14%) corresponding in part to the disorganized thought of the DSM-IV (APA, 1994). The second is there is 'no argument' (10%) and the third concerns the quality of the delusional disorder (10%). To reject, the first argument is the absence of a dissociative process (35%). The second is the fact that no case has been registered (18%) and the third a persistent adjustment to reality (8%).

Considering comments, many authors suggested eliminating an associated organic disorder, particularly the onset of a dementia, consider the concept as too 'Anglo-Saxon', too theoretical, as unthinkable, or think there is a problem of terminology and this is a disorder afflicting only the young population.

LITERATURE REVIEW

To prepare this chapter, a literature review showed that 'late onset schizophrenia' is always controversial, justifying the publication of this book.

Nevertheless, I enjoyed reading some remarks in English, given by various authors from different countries, on the possibility that a late-life delusional state exists with predominantly paranoid symptoms of a highly systematized quality, particularly persecutory delusions (Castle *et al.*, 1997), usually arising in the latter part of the seventh decade, that is neither schizophrenia nor dementia (Herbert and Jacobson, 1967; Pearlson *et al.*, 1989; Gurian *et al.*, 1992). Another interesting subject is the risk of the appearance of paranoid ideation in late life related to factors which include interaction among gender (Gorwood *et al.*, 1995), social isolation, early trauma, the absence of children and/or an unmarried state, stressful environmental factors late in life, sensory impairment ... but not with a specific personality structure (Almeida *et al.*, 1995a,b; Howard and Levy, 1993), formal thought disorder, affective flattening (Howard *et al.*, 1994) or clear pattern of cognitive impairment (Almeida *et al.*, 1995c; Phillips *et al.*, 1997), and also finally with a lack of a clear specific pattern of CT or MRI imaging cerebral changes (Naguib and Levy, 1987; Burns *et al.*, 1989; Hymas *et al.*, 1989).

Two recent French papers suggest two hypotheses: (i) late onset schizophrenia is a poorly diagnosed chronic hallucinatory psychosis; (ii) late onset schizophrenia and early onset schizophrenia are quite different and justify the maintenance of the chronic hallucinatory psychosis as an independent entity (Dubertret *et al.*, 1997; Claudel *et al.*, 1998).

CONCLUSIONS

If we have to keep the word 'schizophrenia' to explain the delusional disorder having an onset after 65, it would be better to say 'schizophreniform reaction' (Léger *et al.*, 1984) or as recently suggested by Howard and Rabins (1997) 'late life onset schizophrenia-like psychoses'. In accordance with the considerations of Weinberger (1987, 1995) and Murray *et al.* (1992) and with the clinical approach (Lantéri-Laura and Gros, 1984; Clément, 1994; Sutter, 1998), it is possible to conceive true schizophrenia as the consequence of aberrant brain development during fetal and neonatal life, a position which does not exclude psychogenetic hypotheses of interactions between affective environment and neurodevelopment via a genetic vulnerability. In this way, this would be not incompatible with neuropsychological findings concerning schizophrenia which state that the disorder cannot wait 60 years to be expressed.

Finally, as discussed by Grahame (1987), the French view of the concept of 'late onset schizophrenia' is that there is a perpetuation of confusion surrounding paranoid states in the elderly. The terms are used in a very broad sense, and as suggested by Holden (1987) about late paraphrenia: this is a heterogenous syndrome giving the appearance of a spectrum of overlapping conditions with paranoid delusions. Psychotic states arising in late life are accompanied by various psychiatric symptoms that are not entirely typical of early onset schizophrenia (Almeida *et al.*, 1995a).

The French psychoanalyst, Jean Bergeret, worked for a long time on the concept of borderline personality (Bergeret, 1974). He wrote a paper on the 'late psychotic psychoses' (les psychoses tardivement psychotiques) to explain that this disorder was, in fact, the result of a breakdown late in life

of a patient with a personality insufficiently elaborated according to different genital stages to realize a neurosis, but also not having encountered
during childhood the dramatic endogenous and/or exogenous conditions
required to establish a psychotic structuration (Bergeret *et al.*, 1972).

To summarize the French point of view, it is possible to investigate the
idea that there is a specific delusional disorder with a late onset in the elderly,
particularly with interpretation and imagination mechanisms, and an underlying depression in a psychodynamic perspective (Clément *et al.*, 1999) which
could be called 'adjustment disorder with depressed mood and paranoia' in
conformity with terminology of DSM-IV and ICD-10 (Clément, 1995).

ACKNOWLEDGEMENTS

This work was supported, in part, by Janssen-Cilag France, for the mailing,
and by the University Department of Psychiatry (Professor Jean-Marie
Léger, Centre Hospitalier Esquirol, Limoges, France).

I wish to thank all the Société de Psychogériatrie de Langue Française
respondents (Alla, P., Aumjaud, F., Baranger, J.P., Beauchaud, P., Bessey,
D., Boiffin, A., Bonin-Guillaume, S., Bouckson, G., Bourdon, P., Boyon, D.,
Bucking-Cadillon, D., Bussone, A., Camus, V., Caraboeuf, A., Charazac,
P.M., Darcourt, G., Delomier, Y., Ferrey, G., Fontanier, D., Glénisson, L.,
Gonzalès, J.D., Goumilloux, R., Grillet, C., Grosclaude, M., Kloul, K.,
Lacroix, P., Legrand, V., Léger, J.M., Lion, M., Lombertie, E.R., Manciaux,
M.A., Monfort, J.C., Parry, J., Paulin, S., Pellerin, J., Ploton, L., Richard, D.,
Robert, P., Rochard-Bouthier, M.F., Savijärvi, M., Sichel, J.P., Singer, L.,
Souchaud, J.L., Tardivel, Y., Tessier, J.F., Therme, J.F., Tignol, J., Trappet,
P., Verdoux, H., Vignat, J.P., Wertheimer, J.) and Jenny Cook for her
revision of my not very idiomatic English.

REFERENCES

Almeida, O.P., Howard, R.J., Levy, R. and David, A.S. (1995a). Psychotic states
    arising in late life (late paraphrenia). Psychopathology and nosology. *Br J
    Psychiatry* **166**, 205–214.
Almeida, O.P., Howard, R.J., Levy, R. and David, A.S. (1995b). Psychotic states
    arising in late life (late paraphrenia). The role of risk factors. *Br J Psychiatry* **166**,
    215–228.
Almeida, O.P., Howard, R.J., David, A.S., Morris, R.G. and Sahakian, B.J. (1995c).
    Cognitive features of psychotic states arising in late life (late paraphrenia). *Psychol
    Med* **25**, 685–698.
American Psychiatric Association (1994). *Diagnostic and Statistical Manual of Mental
    Disorders, 4th edn* (DSM-IV). American Psychiatric Association, Washington, DC.
Bergeret, J. (1974). *La personnalité normale et pathologique*. Dunod, Paris.

Bergeret, J., Broussole, P. and Jourlin, N. (1972). Les psychoses tardivement psycho-tiques. *L'Information Psychiatrique* **48**, 135–138.

Burns, A., Carrick, J., Ames, D., Naguib, M. and Levy, R. (1989). The cerebral corti-cal appearance in late paraphrenia. *Int J Geriatr Psychiatry* **4**, 31–34.

Castle, D.J., Wessely, S., Howard, R. and Murray, R.M. (1997). Schizophrenia with onset at the extremes of adult life. *Int J Geriatr Psychiatry* **12**, 712–717.

Claudel, B., Schurhoff, F., Leboyer, M. and Allilaire, J.F. (1998). Les schizophrénies à début tardif. Particularités cliniques et familiales. *Ann Méd Psychol* **156**, 191–193.

Clément, J.P. (1994). États confusionnels et délirants du sujet âgé: orientations diagnostiques et thérapeutiques. *Rev Prat (Paris)* **44**, 1443–1447.

Clément, J.P. (1995). Les psychoses d'apparition tardive. *Thérapsy* **2**, 18–20.

Clément, J.P., Marchan, F., Morgant, F. and Léger, J.M. (1993). Spécificités des délires du sujet âgé par rapport à l'adulte. *Psychologie Médicale* **25**, 626–633.

Clément, J.P., Paulin, S. and Léger, J.M. (1999). Troubles délirants. In: Léger, J.M., Clément, J.P. and Wertheimer, J. (Eds), *Psychiatrie du Sujet Agé*. Flammarion Médecine-Sciences, Paris, pp. 202–215.

Conférence de consensus: Texte des experts (1994). *Stratégies thérapeutiques à long terme dans les psychoses schizophréniques*. Frison-Roche, Paris.

Costentin, J. (1997). Aspects neurochimiques et pharmacologiques des schizophrènes. In: Scotto, J.C. and Bougerol, T. (Eds), *Les schizophrénies – Aspects actuels*. Flammarion Médecine-Sciences, Paris, pp. 141–163.

Dias Cordeiro, J. (1989). Les conduites délirantes chez l'âgé. *Psychologie Médicale* **21**, 1125–1131.

Dubertret, C., Gorwood, P. and Adès J. (1997). Psychose hallucinatoire chronique et schizophrénie d'apparition tardive: une même entité. *Encéphale* **23**, 157–167.

Ey, H. (1948–1954). *Études Psychiatriques* (3 vols). Desclée de Brouwer, Paris.

Ey, H. (1977). *La notion de schizophrénie*. Séminaire de Thuir (février–juin 1975), Desclée de Brouwer, Paris.

Folstein, M.F., Folstein, S.E. and McHughes, P.R. (1975) 'Mini Mental State'. A practical method for grading the cognitive state of patients for the clinician. *J Psychiatry Res* **12**, 189–198.

Fossati, P. and Allilaire, J.F. (1997). Psychopathologie et influence de l'environ-nement: les approches théoriques actuelles sur la vulnérabilité à la schizophrénie. In: Scotto, J.C. and Bougerol, T. (Eds, *Les schizophrénies – Aspects actuels*. Flammarion Médecine-Sciences, Paris, pp. 74–87.

Gorwood, P., Leboyer, M., Jay, M., Payan, C. and Feingold, J. (1995). Gender and age at onset in schizophrenia: impact of family history. *Am J Psychiatry* **152**, 208–212.

Grahame, P.O. (1987). Late paraphrenia or the paraphrenias. *Br J Psychiatry* **151**, 268.

Gurian, B.S., Wexler, D. and Baker, E.H. (1992). Late-life paranoia: possible associ-ation with early trauma and infertility. Int J Geriatr Psychiatry 7, 277–284.

Haugsten, T. (1996). Des mécanismes aux structures: l'évolution de la classification des délires. Ann Méd Psychol **154**, 426–436.

Herbert, M.E. and Jacobson, S. (1967). Late paraphrenia. *Br J Psychiatry* **113**, 461–469.

Holden, N.L. (1987). Late paraphrenia or the paraphrenias? A descriptive study with a 10 year follow-up. *Br J Psychiatry* **156**, 231–235.

Howard, R. and Levy, R. (1993). Personality structure in the paranoid psychoses of later life. *Eur Psychiatry* **8**, 59–66.

Howard, R. and Rabins, P. (1997). Late paraphrenia revisited. *Br J Psychiatry* **171**, 406–408.

Howard, R., Castle, D., O'Brien, J., Almeida, O. and Levy, R. (1992). Permeable walls, floors, ceilings and doors. Partition delusions in late paraphrenia. *Int J Geriatr Psychiatry* **7**, 719–724.

Howard, P., Almeida, O. and Levy, R. (1994). Phenomenology, demography and diagnosis in late paraphrenia. *Psychol Med* **24**, 397–410.

Hymas, N., Naguib, M. and Levy, R. (1989). Late paraphrenia – A follow-up study. *Int J Geriatr Psychiatry* **4**, 23–29.

Jeste, D.V. (1997). Psychiatry of old age is coming of age (Editorial). *Am J Psychiatry* **154**, 1356–1358.

Lantéri-Laura, G. and Gros, M. (1984). *La discordance.* Unicet, Levallois-Perret.

Léger, J.M. and Clément, J.P. (1991). Le point actuel sur le délire d'apparition tardive de l'âgé. *Ann Méd Psychol* **149**, 721–726.

Léger, J.M., Descalzo, A. and Tessier, J.F. (1984). Catatonie chez le vieillard: démence ou schizophrénie? *Rev Fr Psychiatrie* **2**, 3, 35–38.

L'encéphale. (1996) Schizophrénie. Recherches actuelles et perspectives. *Encéphale* **22** (suppl III).

Maj, M. (1998). Critique of the DSM-IV operational diagnostic criteria for schizophrenia. *Br J Psychiatry* **172**, 458–460.

Martinot, J.L. (1997). Imagerie neuro-anatomique et fonctionnelle des psychoses schizophréniques. In: Scotto, J.C. and Bougerol, T. (Eds), *Les schizophrénies – Aspects actuels.* Flammarion Médecine-Sciences, Paris, pp. 111–127.

Murray, R.M., O'Callaghan, E., Castle, D.J. and Lewis, S.W. (1992). A neurodevelopmental approach to the classification of schizophrenia. *Schizophr Bull* **18**, 319–332.

Naguib, M. and Levy, R. (1987). Late paraphrenia: neuropsychological impairment and structural brain abnormalities on computed tomography. *Int J Geriatr Psychiatry* **2**, 83–90.

Pearlson, G.D., Kreger, L., Rabins, P.V. *et al.* (1989). A chart review study of late-onset and early-onset schizophrenia. *Am J Psychiatry* **146**, 1568–1574.

Phillips, M.L., Howard, R. and David, A.S. (1997). A cognitive neuropsychological approach to the study of delusions in late-life schizophrenia. *Int J Geriatr Psychiatry* **12**, 892–901.

Roubertoux, P. and Nosten, N. (1986). Interactions entre génotype et environnement. *Neuro-Psy* **1**, 449–501.

Scotto, J. C. and Bougerol, T. (1997) *Les schizophrénies – Aspects actuels.* Flammarion Médecine-Sciences, Paris.

Séminaire de Psychiatrie Biologique (1994). *Comptes rendus.* Vol. 25. Gérard, A., Loo, H. and Olié, J.P. (Eds). Spécia, Paris.

Sutter, J. (1998). Le délire et l'existence schizophrénique. *Ann Méd Psychol* **156**, 289–300.

Van Os, J. and Verdoux, H. (1998). Aspects environnementaux et psychosociaux de la recherche génétique en psychiatrie. *Encéphale* **24**, 125–131.

Weinberger, D.R. (1987). Implications of normal brain development for the pathogenesis of schizophrenia. *Arch Gen Psychiatry* **44**, 660–669.

Weinberger, D.R. (1995). From neuropathology to neurodevelopment. *Lancet* **346**, 552–557.

Wertheimer, J. (1993). Point de vue à propos de la nosologie des états délirants chez la personne âgée. *Psychologie Médicale* **25**, 617–619.

Late Onset Schizophrenia
Edited by Robert Howard, Peter V. Rabins, David J. Castle
© 1999 Wrightson Biomedical Publishing Ltd

6

Paraphrenia: The Scandinavian View

KIRSTEN ABELSKOV

Psychogeriatric Department, Psychiatric Hospital, Risskov, Denmark

This chapter discusses the diagnostic position of late onset schizophrenia patients in Sweden, Norway and Denmark. Even within the Scandinavian countries, the definitions and diagnoses for these late onset patients vary. In Sweden, the diagnosis of paraphrenia is synonymous with that of paranoid schizophrenia (Ottoson, 1983). The Swedes do not recognize this as a special old age psychosis. In Norway and Denmark, Bleuler's definition of schizophrenia (Strømgren, 1964; Kringlen, 1972; Lunn, 1985) is used; that is to say, the diagnosis of schizophrenia is made on the basis of the following features: autism, thought disorder, affective disturbances, emotional bluntness and ambivalence. Hallucinations and delusions are considered as secondary symptoms. In the Norwegian and Danish psychiatric traditions, the diagnosis of paraphrenia has been used to describe a special group of patients with a delusional psychosis that begins in old age. The inclusion of these patients who had delusions and hallucinations within schizophrenia following the introduction of ICD-10 very much changed our view of this patient group. They came to be seen as belonging to a far more treatable group and one in which the diagnosis could be made confidently shortly after presentation. Bleuler's textbook *Lehrbuch der Psychiatrie* is very influential in Denmark. He states that schizophrenia that arises in old age often does so with a pure paranoid delusional form but he does not say very much about the type of delusions that can be expected (Bleuler, 1975). In 1936 the Danish psychiatrist, August Wimmer, observed that old age delusional psychoses were not a subtype of schizophrenia and he based this opinion on his study of the genetics of the disorder (Wimmer, 1936). This finding was confirmed by Thorkild Funding's study which was carried out in Risskov in the 1950s (Funding, 1961). Since Funding's second paper on paranoid psychoses in old age (Funding, 1963) very few investigations have been carried out with this

Table 1.   Schizophrenia and paranoid psychosis in first admission inpatients in
Denmark (1987–1995).

		Male	Female
(a) Schizophrenia:	ICD-8 295		
	1987	110	54
	1988	131	62
	1989	176	66
	1990	99	53
	1991	112	48
	1992	111	75
	1993	139	75
Schizophrenia:	ICD-10 F20		
	1994	189	105
	1995	158	94
(b) Paranoid psychosis:	ICD-8 297.XX + 297.19		
	1987	120 + 2	132 + 10
	1988	94 + 3	107 + 20
	1989	107 + 2	162 + 13
	1990	100 + 4	92 + 20
	1991	98 + 2	132 + 18
	1992	111 + 1	125 + 20
	1993	147 + 3	124 + 18
Paranoid psychosis:	ICD-10 F22		
	1994	83	106
	1995	91	144

group of patients in Scandinavia. A paper written in the 1980s (Jørgensen
and Munk-Jørgensen, 1985) only highlighted the main ICD-8 diagnosis for
this group and not potential subgroups. Lately our department, together with
the Geropsychology Institute in Århus, has been investigating coping strategies in a group of patients with late paraphrenia (Fromholt et al., 1999) as
defined by Naguib and Levy (1987). The patients in this study were classified within F20 and F22 of the ICD-10 system.

   In 1994 our department changed our diagnostic system from ICD-8 to
ICD-10 and thus the definition of schizophrenia as well as late paraphrenia
changed. Indeed late paraphrenia disappeared entirely and the latest Danish
textbook in psychiatry (Parnas, 1994) makes brief mention of the disappearance of this diagnosis from ICD-10. Table 1 shows the increase in first admissions with schizophrenia in both males and females and an apparent decline
in paranoid psychosis at our clinic. The number followed by the plus sign in
the table for paranoid psychosis admissions shows the number of patients
with ICD-8 paraphrenia. This number is very small, probably because the
material refers to inpatients.

   Loss of the diagnosis of paraphrenia has caused very little concern within
psychogeriatric departments in Scandinavia. There are several reasons for

this. In the late 1970s and 1980s when psychogeriatric departments mushroomed all over Scandinavia, many of these were initiated from and dominated by geriatric medicine departments. A further reason is that most old age psychiatry departments were developed to target patients with dementia and so often focused on the oldest old patients, for example, those aged at least 80. A questionnaire circulated amongst 12 Danish old age psychiatrists revealed that all except one (who was educated outside Denmark) believed that late paraphrenia was a special old age disease and indicated that they missed having a separate ICD-10 classification category for this diagnosis. The main reason given for wanting this classification was because this would promote research into the nature of the disease.

To conclude, the term 'paraphrenia' does not mean the same in Denmark and Norway as in Sweden. The diagnosis was a very useful one that was used in Denmark for a particular kind of delusional disease that began in old age, and was in general use for at least 60 years. I believe that it is important in terms of promoting research into these patients that we have a special diagnostic group or subgroup within which to record them.

REFERENCES

Bleuler, E. (1975). In: Bleuler, M. (Ed.), *Lehrbuch der Psychiatrie*, 13th edn. Springer, Berlin, pp. 428–429.

Fromholt, P., Bender, L. and Elleberg, B. (1999). Coping with a paraphrenic world in late life. *J Clin Geropsychol*, in press.

Funding, T. (1961). Genetics of paranoid psychosis in later life. *Acta Psychiatr Scand* **37**, 267–282.

Funding, T. (1963). Paranoid psychosis in later life. *Acta Psychiatr Scand* **39**, 356–361.

Jørgensen, P. and Munk-Jørgensen, P. (1985). Paranoid psychosis in the elderly. *Acta Psychiatr Scand* **72**, 358–363.

Kringlen, E. (1972). *Psykiatri*. Universitetsforlaget, Oslo.

Lunn, V. (1985). In: Welner, J., Reisby, N., Lunn, V., Rafaelsen, O. and Schulsinger, F. (Eds), *Reaktive Psykoser, Psykiatri, en textbog*. FADL, Copenhagen, pp. 377–396.

Naguib, M. and Levy, R. (1987). Late paraphrenia. Neuropsychological impairment and structural brain abnormalities on computed tomography. *Int J Geriatr Psychiatry* **2**, 83–90.

Ottoson, J-O. (1983). *Psykiatri*. Almquist and Wiksell, Uppsala.

Parnas, J. (1994). Det schizophrene spectrum. In: Hemmingsen, R., Parnas, J., Sørensen, T., Gjerris, A., Bolwig, T. and Reisby, N. (Eds), *Klinisk Psykiatri*. Munksgaard, Copenhagen, pp. 101–115.

Strømgren, E. (1964). *Psykiatri* (8th edn). Munksgaard, Copenhagen, pp. 112–116.

Wimmer, A. (1936). *Speciel Klinisk Psykiatri*. Levin and Munksgaard, Copenhagen.

7

Late Onset Psychosis in Japan

NORIYOSHI TAKEI

Department of Psychiatry and Neurology, Hamamatsu University School of Medicine, Hamamatsu, Japan

EPIDEMIOLOGICAL STUDIES OF PATIENTS WITH LATE ONSET SCHIZOPHRENIA OR SCHIZOPHRENIA-LIKE DISORDER IN JAPAN

No studies with epidemiologically sound methods have, so far, been carried out in Japan, which examine the prevalence or incidence of schizophrenia or schizophrenia-like disorder among the elderly population. Pointing out that people with schizophrenia with late onset tend to respond well to drug treatment when compared with early onset schizophrenia patients, Ishino *et al.* (1986) investigated the frequency of late paraphrenia among outpatients at the psychiatric unit of a local university hospital (Shimane University School of Medicine). They found 0.4% of late paraphrenia (only two cases) among 500 outpatients aged 60 or over, who visited the university hospital over the period 1980–1985: the two cases were both female.

In contrast, Kido (1986) studied a population of 288 inpatients who were admitted, over the period 1973–1985, to a local hospital for the elderly (Tokyoto Youikuin, Tokyo) and aged 65 or above at the time of the investigation. Among them, he identified 16 (5.6%) individuals (male/female=3/13) who had the onset of a schizophrenia-like disorder (as defined using the criteria of Post (1980), i.e. 'persistent persecutory delusional states') over the age of 60 or above. He also found 15 (male/female=2/13) inpatients with late onset of schizo-affective disorder (co-existence of schizophrenic symptoms with depressive symptoms or alternating episodes of schizophrenic and affective features). The breakdown in his study according to the classification system by Post is shown in Table 1. He also found 19 patients with organic delusional states.

Table 1.   Breakdown of 50 inpatients with late onset of schizophrenia-like disorder (Kido, 1986).

	Male	*Female*	*Total*
Organic delusional states	6	13	19
Schizo-affective disorder	2	13	15
Persistent persecutory delusional states	3	13	16
simple paranoid psychoses	0	4	4
schizophrenia-like illnesses	0	1	1
paranoid schizophrenia states	3	8	11

Kido describes that, whereas the content of persecutory delusions has a bearing on close relatives or neighbours in simple paranoid psychoses, people who, patients believe, persecute them are expansive and become vague in both types of schizophrenia-like illnesses and paranoid schizophrenia states. The difference between the latter two groups is the presence of first rank symptoms (FRS). Eleven patients with FRS were designated as paranoid schizophrenia states following Post's criteria, while only one patient with no FRS was assigned to schizophrenia-like illnesses. Kido emphasizes the presence of FRS as evidence of schizophrenic process in the elderly. He has found that the rate of FRS in organic delusional states was 32%, whereas it was 67% for schizo-affective disorder, and 69% in persistent persecutory states. Grahame (1984) has demonstrated a similar rate (56%) in a sample of 25 patients with late paraphrenia. It should be pointed out, however, that the sample examined by Kido may not be representative of the elderly population proper as the study was based upon a single hospital which specializes in physical illnesses of the elderly.

DESCRIPTIVE PSYCHOPATHOLOGICAL STUDIES

There are still many psychiatrists in Japan who have been influenced by German psychiatry and are psychopathologically orientated. Early work in German speaking countries on late onset schizophrenia-like disorder has been well introduced to Japan. M. Bleuler's concept of late schizophrenia (spätschizophrenie) is often quoted among Japanese 'psychopathologists'. He classified late schizophrenia, with onset over 40, into three groups: (a) paraphrenia-like; (b) anxious, depressive, and catatonic states; and (c) acute confusional state. The concept of non-organic psychosis in the old age group that also appears in the Japanese literature is that of Janzarik (1957, 1973), who proposed two types of psychosis. One is schizophrenia of old age (Alterschizophrenie) and the other paranoid due to lack of contact

(Kontaktmangel paranoid). The former is subclassified into five subgroups: acute delusional psychosis, chronic delusional psychosis, delusional–halluci-natory psychosis, hallucinatory psychosis, and catatonic psychosis. This group is characterized as having acute and variable symptoms. On the other hand, the latter group is described as a chronic delusional psychosis and ascribed to isolated situations such as divorce, separation or death of the spouse.

A similar attempt based on psychopathological observations of symptom profiles and the course has been made by Hamada (1980), who places emphasis on the prognosis. He divided non-organic psychoses, which first appear after the age of 40, into good-prognosis and poor-prognosis groups. Those with good prognosis are described as having a relatively younger age of onset, acute onset, and signs of consciousness, and they have prominent emotion and psychomotor disturbances with hallucinations (in particular, auditory hallucinations) and tend to exhibit FRS. In contrast, the poor-prognosis group is referred to as the core of schizophrenic process. The picture of psychosis is dominated by either delusions or hallucinations, which become simplified and partitioned over the course, and then tend to assume double orientation.

Along with the introduction of the German literature, concepts proposed by English researchers such as late paraphrenia (Roth, 1955) and persistent persecutory states (Post, 1980) have been long known among Japanese psychi-atrists. As described above, Kido (1986) applied Post's criteria for classifying a sample of his patients. It is noticeable, however, that these earlier classifi-cation systems, including German ones, have often been used by Japanese psychiatrists to determine which criterion can be assigned most suitably to each of the patients they observed. In most instances, a single case (or a few cases) reported as study designs have been relied upon among Japanese psychopathologists (Kocha et al., 1993a; Kido, 1996; Hara et al., 1996). They also tend to report unusual and unique cases which do not fit the previously well-described criteria for psychosis in old age, such as a single male case of 'episodic psychosis' (Kocha et al., 1993b). An 83-year-old male repeated five psychotic episodes, in each of which he began with the confusional state together with delusional mood, went on to develop systematized delusions (delusional–hallucinatory states) with clear consciousness, and then recovered after a period of neuro-asthenic state. However, residual symptoms ultimately emerged after a total period of 2 years and 4 months.

What is required for research strategies is to sample a relatively large number of patients who are representative of the population, which would allow one not only to create classification systems, whatever they are, but also to further explore clinical correlates, which would successfully underpin the validity of such classifications.

There is, at least, an agreement among Japanese psychopathologists that social situations surrounding old people considerably differ from those for young people (i.e. expected social functioning). The elderly tend to suffer from physical problems including impairments in auditory function, and ageing *per se* causes material changes in the brain (i.e. atrophy resulting in poor cognitive performance), all of which may together complicate the manifestation and course of psychosis in the elderly.

DIAGNOSTIC ISSUES: LIMITATIONS OF MODERN DIAGNOSTIC CRITERIA (E.G. DSM-IV) FOR PSYCHOSIS IN THE ELDERLY

Again, relying upon psychopathological observations, Kocha and Ohno (1997) have raised the question as to whether each individual with late onset psychosis can neatly be allocated to one of the categories according to DSM-IV (APA, 1994). They described a few cases who had a diversity of the symptomatological manifestations over the course and who were considered to fit the traditional concept of 'late catatonia' (Spätkatatonie; Sommer, 1910). The picture, in general, successively changes; beginning with a depressive state, affective disturbances with anxiety, irritability, or labile emotion, and shifting to catatonic syndromes ultimately with variable defective states. This type of psychosis in the elderly is said to have traditionally been considered to belong to involutional depression (Medow, 1922; Petrilowitsh, 1959) and taken as an affective disorder. Any categories, within DSM-IV, other than 'psychotic disorder not otherwise specified' were not found suitable for diagnosing such cases with late catatonia (Kocha and Ohno, 1997). Taking this as an example, they point to the possibility that psychosis in the elderly may exhibit diverse symptomatological changes over the course, and claim that it is difficult to apply to such a case the DSM-IV system for clinical and research purposes, which heavily counts on cross-sectional symptom profiles. However, whether this type of psychosis is common among the elderly population in Japan has not been clarified: only two cases have been reported (Kocha *et al.*, 1996; Kocha and Ohno, 1997).

The same group (Kocha and Ohno, 1997) have attempted to diagnose, using DSM-IV, two female cases which were clinically diagnosed as late paraphrenia and one female with late catatonia. An 84-year-old lady was found to meet the criteria for a diagnosis of DSM-IV schizophrenia, paranoid type. However, they point out the difficulty in judging the deterioration of social or vocational function in elderly psychiatric cases who are not, in general, active in the social community. They also emphasize the changes in the symptoms over the course; some cases, like the example presented in the study, are said to shift to the fixation of only auditory hallucinations while having a chronic and persistent illness course. The second case was given a DSM-IV diagnosis of delusional disorder. An 87-year-old lady premorbidly had a personality of persecutory nature. She developed persecutory delusions against her neighbours in the milieu where she was socially isolated with hearing difficulties. On admission, her psychotic symptoms were ameliorated with an improvement in her isolation.

As a result, although based upon a single case report, there is a view among Japanese psychiatrists that the concepts involved in modern diagnostic systems (e.g. DSM-IV) are not optimal to depict a feature characteristic of psychosis in the elderly population and to discriminate it from that usually seen in relatively young age of onset groups.

MODERN STUDIES OF NEUROIMAGING AND NEUROPHYSIOLOGY

In an MRI/SPECT study of five patients with late paraphrenia (mean age at onset 68 years and all females), four were found to have lacunar infarction (i.e. periventricular high intensity on MRI) (Ishibashi *et al.*, 1997; only abstract available). In three cases, a reduction of cerebral blood flow (CBF) was found in the bilateral temporo-parietal regions. One case had a decreased CBF in the periventricular white matter. There were no abnormalities found in the remaining case. However, no controls were included in this study.

Similarly, an unpublished study (only abstract available) of a single case with MRI/SPECT (Oyamada *et al.*, 1995) showed that a lady with late schizophrenia (mainly presenting auditory hallucinations) and onset at 60 years had an enlargement in the left sylvian fissures without apparent infarction. They also showed reduced CBFs in the frontal lobe, left posterior temporal lobe, and thalamus.

Taguchi *et al.* (1997) have examined differences in the neurophysiological level between three groups of late paraphrenia (P group; $N=13$), schizophrenia in the old years (S group; $N=14$), and age-matched control (C group; $N=15$). The S group developed the disorder before age 45 years. The mean age for each of the three groups was almost equal and about 66 years. It has been reported that N3 peak latency of SER (somatosensory evoked response) is prolonged in both P and S groups compared with the C group, although there was no difference between P and S groups. Low amplitude of CNV (contingent negative validation) was found most frequently in the S group, whereas the CNV amplitude for the P group was in the middle between the other two groups (S and C). Similarly, the same pattern was evident for P300 latency; there was a significantly prolonged latency in the S group compared with the C group, while the P group had an intermediate position between the S and C groups. The authors interpret these results as indicating that patients with late paraphrenia have an impairment in the functions of concentration, recognition and information processing but not to the extent that schizophrenic patients in the old years do.

FUTURE CONTRIBUTIONS OF RESEARCH IN JAPAN TO THE INTERNATIONAL COMMUNITY

Clearly, more studies are required for investigating characteristics in late onset psychosis. Although awareness of the diversity of symptom profiles and the course of psychosis in the elderly has been increased, and pathophysiological mechanisms involved in the illness have been postulated to be distinct from schizophrenia with onset in the young ages, the literature in this field is relatively sparse, especially in Japan. The number of papers published in the Japanese medical journals (written in Japanese) that are related to schizophrenia amounts to about 500–700 a year. Moreover, there is a tendency for that number to be increasing in recent years with an increase in the number of psychiatric journals in Japan.

Ageing is a major concern in Japan as the proportion of the elderly population increases. The number of people aged 65 years or over is now 22 million, 18% of the total population of Japan. The government, at last, realizes that improvements and better provisions of care systems such as care management for the elderly are primarily important. However, areas of mental health care in this population are still neglected. Psychosis in old age is devastating since sufferers may remain physically healthy but have severely impaired mental health. Persons who develop psychoses late in life are naturally expected to peacefully enjoy their life after contributing to their next generations and the community.

In countries, in particular developed countries, where the elderly population is rapidly increasing, it is of prime importance to pay more attention to their mental health, including late onset psychosis. Systematic surveys with epidemiologically sound methods are clearly needed. Single case report types of study designs may attract clinicians, although the characteristics in a population of late onset psychosis as a whole may be overlooked. Those with a milder form of illness may never present to psychiatric services and therefore it is also important to conduct community based surveys. Investigations into clinically distinct features and risk factors including genetic components and socio-environmental variables for the development of late onset psychosis merit attention not only for the improvement of care but also in the search for preventative avenues.

Further neurophysiological and neuroimaging studies may also benefit our understanding of the mechanisms involved in the illness, which may differ from those for early onset schizophrenia. This understanding will in turn prompt our knowledge about the process of schizophrenia which in general takes place in young ages.

Therefore, Japanese researchers are encouraged to carry out research with a global view to contribute to the international scientific society as the answers to the questions we have are demanded worldwide and not by an individual country.

REFERENCES

American Psychiatric Association (1994). *Diagnostic and Statistical Manual of Mental Disorders, 4th edn* (DSM-IV). American Psychiatric Association, Washington, DC.

Bleuler, M. (1943). Die spätschizophrenen Krankheitsbilder. *Fortschr Neurol Psychiatr* **15**, 259–297.

Grahame, P.S. (1984). Schizophrenia in old age (late paraphrenia). *Br J Psychiatry* **145**, 493–495.

Hamada, H. (1980). Delusional and hallucinatory state with onset after 40 years old: gender difference, age of onset and outcome. *Seishinigaku* **22**, 749–758 (in Japanese).

Hara, H., Sakurai, A., Takahashi, K. *et al.* (1996). Old age onset psychosis: a case report. *Ronen Seishinigaku Zasshi* **7**, 423–427 (in Japanese).

Ishibashi, K., Tanaka, K., Nakamura, A. *et al.* (1997). A review of MRI and SPECT studies in late paraphrenia. *Ronen Seishinigaku Zasshi* **8**, 659–660 (in Japanese).

Ishino, H. and Inao, H. (1986). Delusional state in the elderly. *Rinsho Seishinigaku* **15**, 1759–1764 (in Japanese).

Janzarik, W. (1957). Zur Problematik schizophrener Psychosen in hoehren Lebensalter. *Nervenarzt* **28**, 535–542.

Janzarik, W. (1973). Über das Kontaktmangelparanoid des höheren Alters und den Syndromcharakter schizophrenen Krankseins. *Nervenarzt* **44**, 515–526.

Kido, M. (1986). Schizophrenia-like delusional and hallucinatory states in old ages: diversity of characteristics. *Rinsho Seishinigaku* **15**, 1821–1828 (in Japanese).

Kido, M. (1996). Late paraphrenia (in Japanese). *Ronen Seishinigaku Zasshi* **7**, 972–978.

Kocha, H. and Ohno, Y. (1997). An illness with delusions and hallucinations in old ages: late schizophrenia. *Ronen Seishinigaku Zasshi* **8**, 244–249 (in Japanese).

Kocha, H., Hamada, H., Asai, M. *et al.* (1993a). Delusional and hallucinatory state in old ages. *Rinsho Seishinigaku* **22**, 849–854 (in Japanese).

Kocha, H., Hamada, H. and Mimura, M. (1993b). Late-onset episodic psychosis with old age onset. *Seishinigaku* **35**, 1159–1165 (in Japanese).

Kocha, H., Hamada, H., Satoh, T. *et al.* (1996). A case report of late catatonia. *Seishinigaku* **38**, 141–147 (in Japanese).

Medow, W. (1922). Eine Gruppe depressiver Psychosen des Rückbildungsalters mit ungünstiger Prognose (Erstarrende Rückbildungsdepression). *Arch Psychiatr Nervenkr* **64**, 480–506.

Oyamada, S., Hori, A. and Matsuda, H. (1995). A case of late-onset schizophrenia with principal symptoms of hallucinations: a SPECT study (in Japanese). *Tokyo Seiikaishi* **13**, 89–90.

Petrilowitsh, N. (1959). Zur Klinik und nosologischen Stellung der 'erstarrenden Rückbildungsdepression'. *Arch Psychiatr Z Neurol* **198**, 506–522.

Post, F. (1980). Paranoid, schizophrenia-like, and schizophrenic states in the aged. In: Birren, J.E. and Sloane, R.B. (Eds), *Handbook of Mental Health and Aging.* Prentice-Hall, Englewood Cliffs, pp. 591–615.

Roth, M. (1955). The natural history of mental disorder in old age. *J Mental Sci* **101**, 281–301.

Sommer, M. (1910). Zur Kenntnis der Spätkatonie. *Z Neurol Psychiatr* **1**, 523.

Taguchi, S., Matsunaga, H., Takimoto, Y. *et al.* (1997). Neurophysiological evaluation of late paraphrenia (SER, CNV, P300): comparison with schizophrenia in old age (in Japanese). *Osakafu Byouishi* **20**, 26–30.

Late Onset Schizophrenia
Edited by Robert Howard, Peter V. Rabins, David J. Castle
© 1999 Wrightson Biomedical Publishing Ltd

8

Late Onset Schizophrenia in a Developing Country

SUDHIR KHANDELWAL

Department of Psychiatry, B.P. Koirala Institute of Health Sciences, Dharan, Nepal

The concept of schizophrenia represents Bleuler's revision of Kraepelin's concept of dementia praecox. Kraepelin described the illness as occurring in clear consciousness and consisting of a series of states, the common characteristic of which was a peculiar destruction of the internal connections of the psychic personality. The effects of this injury predominated in the emotional and volitional spheres of mental life (Kraepelin, 1919). Kraepelin separated paraphrenia from dementia praecox on the grounds that it started in middle life and seemed to be free from changes in emotion and volition found in dementia praecox. Kraepelin had introduced the term paraphrenia in 1909 to describe patients having chronic delusions and hallucinations without the characteristic personality deterioration of dementia praecox. Roth and Morrissey (1952) noted that illness of this description was the commonest form of psychosis in old age and called this 'late paraphrenia'. Since then there has been considerable debate as to whether late paraphrenia is a distinct entity or is another name for schizophrenia of late onset, as Fish (1960) also used the term senile schizophrenia. Most of the earlier investigations on this subject were conducted in Europe, and nosological issues perhaps led to a great deal of confusion and contributed to lack of adequate research on the subject. A large number of terms came into being with overlapping descriptions. The second edition of the *Diagnostic and Statistical Manual*, DSM-II (American Psychiatric Association, 1968) included the term 'involutional paraphrenia' to describe the onset of a delusional state during the involutional period and differentiated it from schizophrenia. There was no specific age criterion for making the diagnosis of schizophrenia. The DSM-III introduced the criterion of onset before the age of 45 to make a diagnosis of schizophrenia and thus effectively ruled out schizophrenia with onset after 45. The revised third edition of DSM (DSM-IIIR) recommended the specification of late onset if the schizophrenia began after the age of 45 and so introduced the category of late onset schizophrenia. The fourth edition of DSM (DSM-IV) neither restricts the age of onset for the diagnosis of schizophrenia nor specifies the subcategory of late onset schizophrenia and hence accepts the position that schizophrenia can begin at any age. Lately evidence has begun to accumulate regarding clinical characteristics, treatment, prognosis and outcome, and neuroimaging aspects of late onset schizophrenia. Until recently, US researchers have been relatively uninterested in this clinical entity (Harris and Jeste, 1988). Interest in the USA in this area is probably a by-product of the controversy that shrouded the age exclusion criterion of DSM-III. Studies from Asia, leave alone developing countries, on this subject are notable by a conspicuous absence. The present paper summarizes findings of some studies from India, a developing country, which were primarily done to determine the sex difference in the age of onset of schizophrenic disorders. It is desirable, however, that one appreciates the peculiarities of a developing nation.

About three-quarters of the world's population lives in developing countries. Yet the picture of a developing country which emerges in one's mind is not very complimentary. According to the *World Book Encyclopedia* (1996), developing countries are the world's poor or have-not nations once called underdeveloped nations. Most of these nations are in Africa, Asia, and Latin America, and belong to the so called 'Third World'. A typical developing country has a shortage of food, few sources of power and low gross national product (GNP). These countries experience frequent periods of extreme poverty and famine. Most countries have an increasing population because death rates are decreasing and birth rates remain high due to inadequate family planning, putting enormous pressure on scarce resources of food, housing, and services. Physical capital, e.g. machinery and efficient transport systems is scarce. Social capital, like good education and health systems, and stable government is poorly developed. Diseases, illiteracy, and inadequate equipment keep agricultural and commercial production low. Essential supplies are hindered by poor road and rail networks. These factors are most harmful in rural areas where the majority of the population lives. Where does India figure in this scenario? Most of the characteristics mentioned above define India too. India is considered a developing country because of its low GNP. Excessive population, high growth rate, poor health indicators (high infant mortality and maternal mortality rates), illiteracy, unemployment, poor socio-economic conditions, and poor support network are all present in India. However, India is also characterized as one of the world's largest industrial nations. It has some excellent academic institutions of higher learning and has more scientists and skilled workers than most other countries. Its trained professionals and skilled workers are working practically in all parts of the world. India has built nuclear reactors, conducted nuclear explosions, and launched weather and communications satellites. It has scientific bases in Antarctica.

All over the world people are living longer. Declining mortality rates, improvement in health and medical services, and control over infectious diseases have initiated changes in the age structure of the world population. In the developed countries, the rise in the number of people surviving beyond the age of 65 years is more striking, where they already constitute approximately 15% of the population. The developing world has not lagged behind as far as life expectancy, longevity, and annual growth rate of the elderly people are concerned. The current population of India is estimated to be about 950 million and life expectancy is 61 years. Presently there are more than 55 million elderly people in India constituting 6.5% of the total population. By the turn of this century, this number is likely to swell beyond 75 million, representing 7.7% of the country's population. In absolute number, India faces a tremendous task of looking after its elderly people since a large number of them are likely to have significant physical and mental morbidity besides having many psychosocial problems.

Like the general health system, the development of mental health in India is still slow and unsatisfactory. Thus, for a population of more than 950 million people, there are only 3500 psychiatrists and 25,000 psychiatric beds. However, a number of important research studies have now originated from India. One of the most important research contributions has been in the area of psychiatric epidemiology where, in the short span of 25 years, a number of surveys on various mental disorders in the general population as well as special population groups including geriatric populations have appeared. The quality of research reports has steadily improved and many problems of sampling, screening, diagnosis, classification and data analysis have been successfully tackled in keeping with the world trends in psychiatric epidemiology. These epidemiological field surveys resulted in an increased awareness of the wide prevalence of mental disorders in the community. They also eliminated the myth that mental disorders were not common in rural India. In fact for a long time it was widely assumed that serious mental disorders were not common in developing countries. General population studies (Dube, 1970; Sethi et al., 1972, 1974; Verghese et al., 1973; and Nandi et al., 1975) reported that at least 1% of the population had mental disorders requiring urgent psychiatric help, and at least another 5–10% had less serious mental disorders. Studies on the prevalence of mental disorders in the elderly point towards a large proportion of this age group having a significant rate of morbidity. These surveys have yielded rates of 349/1000 among people above 50 years (Ramachandran et al., 1979) and 89/1000 among those above 60 years of age (Venkoba Rao and Madhavan, 1983). Unfortunately not much work has been done in late onset non-affective disorders in India, though some information is available about the onset of schizophrenia in late age. Not only in India – there is a paucity of Asian studies on this subject, as reflected in the literature review done by Harris and Jeste (1988).

Findings of two studies from India (Jayaswal *et al.*, 1987; Adityanjee *et al.*, 1989) on the age of onset of schizophrenia are as follows. In these studies, case records of all the patients with a clinical diagnosis of schizophrenia seen between 1981 and 1983 at the outpatient services of the Department of Psychiatry, All India Institute of Medical Sciences, New Delhi, were screened. The quality of case records was good, because patients had been studied in detail by postgraduate psychiatric residents under supervision of a consultant. As a matter of routine, the information was obtained from at least one (sometimes more) key relatives in addition to the patient himself. The age at which the immediate family members noticed psychotic symptoms for the first time was considered to determine the age of onset of schizophrenia. The age of onset of symptoms as well as the patient's age at the time of consultation was documented in each chart by a research officer especially deputed to record sociodemographic variables of psychiatric outpatients. The age at first treatment and age at first hospitalization were not studied since owing to the poor infrastructure of mental health services, underdetection and undertreatment are very common. The diagnosis of schizophrenia was based on the International Classification of Diseases (ICD-9; World Health Organization, 1978). Patients with inadequate documentation and possibility of differential diagnosis were excluded from the sample. Also excluded were the controversial subtypes of schizophrenia. Patients with a diagnosis of paraphrenia or late paraphrenia were also excluded.

A total of 539 cases were obtained after satisfying the exclusion criteria. Thus, all these cases were likely to be of a definite clinical diagnosis of schizophrenia. Of these 539 cases, 60.8% (*N*=328) were males and 39.2% (*N*=211) were females, giving a male:female ratio of 1:0.64. Twenty-four patients (2.04%) had onset of illness after the age of 40 years, 11 of which had decompensation after the age of 45. Of the 24 cases, 15 (62.5%) were females and 9 (3.75%) were males giving a male:female ratio of 1:1.67. Ten out of 11 cases with onset after the age of 45 were females. This gives a male:female ratio of 1:10 in the above 45 age group. (See Table 1.)

These results, though not strictly comparable to earlier studies, tend to support the view that under ordinary clinical conditions, the onset of schizophrenia can occur in later life. Since we excluded the controversial subtypes from the study sample, our results are lower than in previous studies (Achte, 1967; Larson and Nyman, 1970; Huber *et al.*, 1975; Lewine, 1980). However, our results confirm the previous findings of a relatively higher ratio of females in the late onset group.

So far there have been only a few incidence studies of schizophrenia in India. One such study (Wig *et al.*, 1993) with which the author was also

Table 1. Sex difference in the age of symptom-onset in schizophrenia.

Age-group	Male patients			Female patients		
	N	%	Cumulative percentage	N	%	Cumulative percentage
10–14	15	4.57	5	6	2.84	3
15–19	11	27.74	32	44	20.85	24
20–24	105	32.01	64	65	30.81	55
25–29	63	19.21	84	43	20.38	75
30–34	32	9.76	93	27	12.80	88
35–39	13	3.96	97	11	5.21	93
40–44	8	2.44	99.7	5	2.37	95
45–49	1	0.30	100	10	4.74	100
Total	328	100	100	211	100	100

From Jayaswal et al. (1987); reproduced with permission.

associated, was conducted at the Postgraduate Institute of Medical Education and Research, Chandigarh, as part of a WHO Collaborative Study on Acute Psychosis, where the Chandigarh centre monitored two geographically defined populations over a 2-year period. Using helping-agency-coverage and other methods along with a set of specified criteria, 268 first onset potentially schizophrenic cases were actively identified. Of these, 232 could be assessed in detail, which included 209 schizophrenics as per specified ICD-9 or CATEGO criteria. The annual incidence rates obtained were 4.4 and 3.8 per 10,000 for rural and urban areas respectively. The rural cohort had a higher incidence for each of the three diagnostic definitions. In the urban cohort, sex and diagnostic definition did not affect the incidence. In the rural cohort, females had a lower incidence for CATEGO S+ and a higher incidence for other diagnostic definitions. The incidence rates obtained for the total cohort for different diagnostic definitions were 1.0 for CATEGO S+, 2.7 for CATEGO S,P,O and 3.9 for broad definition.

The age, sex, locality and diagnostic definition specific rates showed some interesting findings. For CATEGO S+ definition, the highest rates were recorded for rural females in the age group 45–49 (3.32) and rural males in the age group 50–54 (3.29). For urban males, the peak incidence was recorded in the age group 20–24 (2.14), while in all other age groups the urban males recorded very low rates. The rural males recorded higher than rural females in all age groups except 35–39 and 45–49.

For broad definition, the highest rates were recorded among rural males and females in the age group 50–54 (9.87 and 9.00 respectively) and rural females in the age group 15–19 (8.21). The urban females had their peak

Table 2. Incidence of schizophrenia in India. Specific Annual Incidence Rates per 10,000.

Age-group	CATEGO S+				CATEGO S,P,O/ICD-9			
	Urban		Rural		Urban		Rural	
	M	F	M	F	M	F	M	F
15–19	1.14	1.46	1.63	0.51	2.74	3.51	5.69	8.21
20–24	2.14	1.12	1.52	0.88	6.84	3.65	5.33	2.63
25–29	0.46	0.55	1.62	0.59	4.16	4.14	1.65	4.96
30–34	0.29	0.43	1.02	0.00	2.58	2.56	2.04	5.32
35–39	0.37	1.17	0.00	0.00	1.87	4.09	0.00	1.32
40–44	0.00	0.79	1.69	1.59	0.00	2.37	5.07	1.90
45–49	0.00	1.07	0.00	3.32	0.75	1.07	0.00	6.64
50–54	0.00	1.45	3.29	0.00	1.85	2.90	9.87	9.00

For CATEGO S+	: Highest rates	: Rural female (45–49): 3.32
		: Rural male (50–54): 3.29
For broad definition	: Highest rates	: Rural female (50–54): 9.00
		: Rural male (50–54): 9.87

From Wig *et al.* (1993). Reproduced with permission.

incidence in the age group 25–29 (4.14). There were no consistent sex differences for different age groups in either the urban or rural cohort, though rural females in the age group 45–49 had an onset rate of 6.64 with no case occurring among rural males in this age group.

Overall, for CATEGO S+ definition, the incidence peaked for males in the age group 15–24 and there was a clustering of onset among females in the older age groups. For broad definition, there was again a peak onset among both rural males and females in the age group 50–54. (See Table 2.)

Thus, these findings clearly establish the fact of onset of schizophrenia in late age.

It is pertinent to highlight here some other important findings of epidemiological studies on schizophrenia from India. (i) The majority of the patients are married at some point; (ii) most patients are living with their families, i.e. spouse, children or parents; (iii) patients continue to live in the marital unit and have children; (iv) most of the patients, especially in rural areas, are gainfully employed; and (v) patients usually have onset of their illness at a later age, have shorter duration of illness, and fewer hospitalizations; (vi) patients do not abuse illicit drugs (Srinivasamurthy *et al.*, 1996).

The major limitations of these studies are that they have focused on the number of ill persons and not studied adequately the wide variety of factors associated with schizophrenia. Most of the studies have been a one time effort. Such efforts so far have been limited by the lack of in-depth analysis of patient groups and failure to develop long-term step-by-step studies.

Follow-up studies have repeatedly found better course and outcome of schizophrenia in developing countries (Kulhara, 1994; Jablensky *et al.*, 1992, 1994). The International Pilot Study of Schizophrenia (IPSS), the international, multicentred, collaborative study, was initiated in 1965 and after recruitment, patients were followed up at 1, 2 and 5 years (WHO, 1973; 1979; Sartorius *et al.*, 1977). Some of the pertinent conclusions of this study were: (i) there is a great variability in the course and outcome of schizophrenia; (ii) the outcome of schizophrenia is not as bleak as it was expected to be; more than half the patients fell into the best outcome groups; (iii) culture has an important effect on the course and outcome of schizophrenia; (iv) social variables have a greater predictive significance in terms of prognosis than the symptomatic variables.

Another study, 'Determinants of outcome of severe mental disorders' (DOSMED), was designed in 12 centres in the late 1970s to investigate further some of the findings of the IPSS (Sartorius *et al.*, 1986). Findings from DOSMED confirmed that culture was an important determinant of outcome: (i) the course of schizophrenia defined by clinical criteria is highly variable and unrelated to clinical descriptions; (ii) the short-term outcome of schizophrenia is much better than was previously believed; (iii) in developing countries the outcome of schizophrenia is much better at the 2-year follow-up: 50.3% had a single psychotic episode followed by complete or incomplete remission and 15.7% had unremitting, continuous illness; (iv) acute onset, living in a developing country, married status and good premorbid adjustment predicted a good outcome. The finding that schizophrenia has a better outcome and more favourable course in developing countries appears to be both genuine and consistent. Not only the WHO supported research work but other independent studies have lent credence to this view. In the above studies, the inclusion criterion for age was 15–44 and 15–54 respectively. It would be appropriate to assume that the findings of better outcome and course for the entire sample would also hold true for the late age group patients.

A lot needs to be done regarding various aspects of late onset schizophrenia in developing countries. We need to systematically record the incidence and prevalence rates of schizophrenia in this age group, and any differences with younger age groups are not only to be documented but also critically examined. The earlier documented better outcome for the entire group has to be studied specifically for the late onset group. The reasons for the quality of course and outcome must also be systematically analysed. So far there are no studies on the clinical features, genetic pattern, and treatment response of this subtype from the developing world. Information is needed on all the above to accept late onset schizophrenia as a distinct entity.

REFERENCES

Achte, K. (1967). On prognosis and rehabilitation in schizophrenia and paranoid psychoses. *Acta Psychiatr Scand* **43** (suppl 196), 1–217.

Adityanjee, Jayaswal, S.K., Praveenlal, K. and Khandelwal, S.K. (1989). Late onset schizophrenia: an Asian study. *Schizophr Bull* **15**, 171–173

American Psychiatric Association (1968). *Diagnostic and Statistical Manual of Mental Disorders, 2nd edn* (DSM-II). American Psychiatric Association, Washington, DC.

American Psychiatric Association (1980). *Diagnostic and Statistical Manual of Mental Disorders, 3rd edn*, (DSM-III). American Psychiatric Association, Washington DC.

Dube, K.C. (1970). A study of prevalence and biological variables in mental illness in a rural urban community in Uttar Pradesh, India. *Acta Psychiatr Scand* **46**, 327–342.

Fish, F. (1960). Senile schizophrenia. *J Mental Sci* **106**, 938–946.

Harris, M.J. and Jeste, D.V. (1988). Late onset schizophrenia: an overview. *Schizophr Bull* **14**, 39–55.

Huber, G., Gross, G. and Schuttler, R. (1975). Late schizophrenia [in German]. *Arch Psychiatr Nervenkr* **221**, 53–66.

Jablensky, A., Sartorius, N., Emberg, G. *et al.* (1992). Schizophrenia, manifestations, incidence and course in different cultures. A World Health Organization ten-country study. *Psychol Med*, Monograph suppl. 20.

Jablensky, A., Sartorius, N., Cooper, J.E. *et al.* (1994). Culture and schizophrenia. Criticisms of WHO studies answered. *Br J Psychiatry* **164**, 434–436.

Jayaswal, S.K., Praveenlal, K., Khandelwal, S.K. and Mohan, D. (1987). Sex-difference in the age at symptom onset in schizophrenia. *Indian J Psychol Med* **10**, 68–74.

Kraepelin, E. (1919). *Dementia Praecox and Paraphrenia*. [Translated by R.M. Barclay.] Churchill Livingstone, Edinburgh.

Kulhara, P. (1994). Outcome of schizophrenia: some transcultural observations with particular reference to developing countries. *Eur Arch Psychiatry Clinical Neurosci* **244**, 227–235.

Larson, C.A. and Nyman, G.E. (1970). Age of onset in schizophrenia. *Human Heredity* **20**, 241–247.

Lewine, R.R.J. (1980). Sex differences in age of onset and first hospitalization in schizophrenia. *Am J Orthopsychiatry* **50**, 316–322.

Nandi, D.N., Ajmany, S. and Ganguly, H. (1975). Psychiatric disorders in a rural community in West Bengal – an epidemiological study. *Indian J Psychiatry* **17**, 87–90.

Ramachandran, V., Sarada, M. and Ramamurthy, B. (1979). Psychiatric disorders in subjects aged over fifty. *Indian J Psychiatry* **21**, 193–199.

Roth, M. and Morrisey, J.F. (1952). Problems in the diagnosis of mental disorder in old age. *J Mental Sci* **98**, 66–80.

Sartorius, N., Jablensky, A. and Shapiro, R. (1977). Two-year follow up of the patients included in the WHO international Pilot Study of Schizophrenia. *Psychol Med* **7**, 529–541.

Sartorius, N., Jablensky, A., Korten, A. *et al.* (1986). Early manifestations and first contact incidence of schizophrenia in different cultures. *Psychol Med* **16**, 909–928.

Sethi, B.B., Gupta, S.C. and Kumar, R. (1972). A psychiatric survey of 500 rural families. *Indian J Psychiatry* **14**, 183–186.

Sethi, B.B., Gupta, S.C., Mahendru, R.K. and Kumari, P. (1974). Mental health and urban life. A study of 850 families. *Br J Psychiatry* **124**, 243–246.

Srinivasamurthy, R., Kumar, K. and Chatterji, S. (1996). Schizophrenia: epidemiology and community aspects. In: Kulhara, P. Awasthi, A. and Verma, S.K. (Eds), *Schizophrenia: The Indian Scene*. Postgraduate Institute of Medical Education and Research, Chandigarh, pp. 39–65.

Venkoba Rao, A. and Madhavan, T. (1983). Geropsychiatric morbidity survey in a semiurban area near Madurai. *Indian J Psychiatry* **24**, 258–267.

Verghese, A., Beig, A., Senseman, L.A., Sunder Rao, B.S.S. and Benjamin, V. (1973). A social psychiatric study of a representative group of families in Vellore town. *Indian J Med Res* **61**, 608–620.

Wig, N.N., Varma, V.K., Mattoo, S.K. *et al.* (1993). An incidence study of schizophrenia in India. *Indian J Psychiatry* **35**, 11–17.

World Book Encyclopedia (1996). *World Book, Vol. 5*. World Book International, London, p.144.

World Health Organization (1973). *Report of the International Pilot Study of Schizophrenia*. World Health Organization, Geneva.

World Health Organization (1978). *Mental Disorders: Glossary and Guide to their Classification in Accordance with the 9th Revision of the International Classification of Diseases*. World Health Organization, Geneva.

World Health Organization (1979). *Schizophrenia: An International Follow-up Study*. John Wiley and Sons, Chichester.

9

I Don't Believe in Late Onset Schizophrenia

NANCY C. ANDREASEN

Mental Health Clinical Research Center, Department of Psychiatry, The University of Iowa Hospitals and Clinics, Iowa City, USA

Schizophrenia, as defined by both Kraepelin and Bleuler, has a characteristic group of symptoms and a characteristic course. Both of these nosologic pioneers emphasized that schizophrenia is a catastrophic illness that profoundly changes an individual's personality and ability to function. Kraepelin stressed this when he referred to the disorder as a 'dementia' affecting young people ('dementia praecox') (Kraepelin, 1899). Bleuler stated that people with schizophrenia do not achieve a complete *restituo ad integrum* after they become ill, although he was less pessimistic than Kraepelin (Bleuler, 1950).

Both Kraepelin and Bleuler also agreed that the symptoms we now refer to as 'psychotic' (i.e. delusions and hallucinations) were not the primary defining features of schizophrenia. For Bleuler, delusions and hallucinations were not even considered to be fundamental or primary. Instead, he believed that 'loosening of the associative threads of thought' was the pathognomonic symptom of this illness, always present in every patient with schizophrenia and not present in other disorders. We now refer to 'associative loosening' as a disorder in the form of thought, as opposed to the content of thought. Bleuler also believed other symptoms to be fundamental: affective blunting, avolition, attentional impairment, autism, and ambivalence. Although Kraepelin discusses delusions and hallucinations as important features of schizophrenia, he too recognized that they could occur in other illnesses such as mood disorder or dementia, and he believed that the most important symptoms involved affect and volition.

'...There are apparently two principal groups of disorders that characterize the malady. On the one hand we observe a weakening of those emotional activities which permanently form the mainsprings of volition.... Mental activity and instinct for occupation become mute. The result of this highly morbid process is emotional dullness, failure of mental activities, loss of mastery over volition, of endeavor, and ability for independent action.... The second group of disorders consists in the *loss of the inner unity* of activities of intellect, emotion, and volition in themselves and among one another.... The near connection between thinking and feeling, between deliberation and emotional activity on the one hand, and practical work on the other is more or less lost. Emotions do not correspond to ideas. The patient laughs and weeps without recognizable cause, without any relation to their circumstances and their experiences, smile as they narrate a tale of their attempted suicide....' (Kraepelin, 1899, pp. 74–75).

These symptoms are very similar to those that we now refer to as 'negative symptoms or cognitive signs'. Increasingly, modern studies have demonstrated that negative symptoms are present at onset and closely associated with long-term morbidity (Andreasen, 1982; Andreasen and Olsen, 1982; Andreasen *et al.*, 1995a; Ho *et al.*, 1998).

In addition to agreeing about characteristic symptoms and course of schizophrenia, Kraepelin and Bleuler also agreed that the illness was potentially heterogeneous. Kraepelin wondered whether the disorder was a single illness or many different illnesses, while Bleuler subtitled his classic book on dementia praecox *'The Group of Schizophrenias'*. Nonetheless, in his emphasis on fundamental symptoms, Bleuler also suggested the presence of a unifying thread that would hold together the various forms of this group of schizophrenias (i.e. the cognitive signs that he called 'associative loosening'.

This brief history is meant to illustrate that there **is** a concept or idea of schizophrenia that many of us who study this disorder hold in our minds and use when we diagnose patients clinically or when we design research studies. This idea has to some extent been operationalized in the diagnostic criteria that we currently use (i.e. DSM-IV (American Psychiatric Association, 1994) and ICD-10 (World Health Organization, 1994)). The idea encompasses the fact that the symptoms of schizophrenia are diverse and include negative symptoms as well as positive psychotic symptoms, that people who develop schizophrenia have a deterioration in function during the time period around its onset, and that people with schizophrenia do not have a *restituo ad integrum* after they become ill and are typically unable to return to work or school or have effective interpersonal relationships.

Confusion about the concept and definition of schizophrenia is introduced, however, by controversies about the nature of the characteristic symptoms. At present there are cross-national differences concerning the nature and importance of psychotic symptoms. British psychiatrists in particular have emphasized Schneiderian ideas and the importance of 'first rank symptoms' that have shaped the Present State Examination and the development of the International Classification of Diseases. American psychiatry has renamed these symptoms as 'bizarre' and included this concept in DSM-III and IV, although very few American psychiatrists see first rank symptoms as the defining essence of schizophrenia. In both countries, however, there is an intermingling of the concepts of psychosis and schizophrenia that sometimes leads to imprecisions in communication.

REASONS FOR DISSENT

My reasons for 'not believing' in late onset schizophrenia are tied to the belief that it is important to maintain a clear concept of the disorder at the clinical or phenomenological level. At that level the illness is defined by a breadth of symptoms. Following the lead of both Kraepelin and Bleuler, I also tend to think that negative symptoms are more important than psychotic symptoms. Clinically, it is rare to encounter a person with schizophrenia who does not have negative symptoms. Schizophrenia is a syndrome defined by a group of characteristic symptoms, a characteristic onset in late adolescence or early adult life, and a relatively chronic course with significant psychosocial impairment. The term 'schizophrenia' should be limited to people who have this characteristic syndrome. It is of course clear that people may develop psychotic symptoms later in life, either in their 40s and 50s or still later, as is amply attested to by other chapters in this book. These disorders of later onset tend to have prominent psychotic features, while negative symptoms such as affective blunting are not prominent, nor is formal thought disorder typically present. Thus, at the phenomenologic level, these patients do not have characteristic schizophrenia but instead have a psychotic disorder. In terms of age of onset, they also differ from the young 'dementia praecox' patient. Therefore, I believe it is better to term their disorder a 'late onset psychosis' rather than a 'late onset schizophrenia'. Given that the clinical presentation is not even 'schizophrenia-like' in that it does not present with negative symptoms such as affective blunting or formal thought disorder, I also dissent from the group decision to refer to this late onset syndrome as 'very late onset schizophrenia-like psychosis'. We should not refer to psychoses with an earlier onset and a late onset as both being 'schizophrenia', since these two syndromes differ at many levels.

LEVELS USED TO DISSECT NOSOLOGICAL ENTITIES

Now, nearly 100 years after Kraepelin and Bleuler wrote their definitive textbooks, what are the various levels that we can use to define syndromes as separate diseases? How much evidence do we need to find a boundary between groups of patients who resemble one another in some ways but not in others?

Table 1.   Levels of identification of diseases.

Aetiology: e.g. genes, viral infections
Pathophysiology: e.g. developmental or degenerative processes
Brain structure: e.g. structures, circuits
Brain function: e.g. neurotransmitters, rCBF, metabolism
Cognitive function: e.g. memory, attention, executive function
Epidemiology: e.g. sex ratio, age-cohort effects
Clinical presentation: e.g. symptoms, age of onset, course
Response to treatment

The various levels that may be used to identify separate diseases are summarized in Table 1. The levels have been listed in order of power and importance. Many of the chapters in this book examine individual levels in this hierarchy. Identifying the aetiology of a disease is a gold standard. At the moment in the case of schizophrenia, we are very far from understanding its aetiology, probably because it is a multifactorial illness requiring multiple 'hits' in order to become manifest, much as appears to be the case with cancer. Nonetheless, when we ultimately understand schizophrenia as a disease mediated through abnormalities transmitted through genes, due to failures in gene regulation or expression, or to interactions between molecular regulation of brain function and development and environmental influences such as nutrition or exogenous toxins (e.g. psychotogenic drugs), we will have defined a discrete disease, much as has been done already for illnesses such as cystic fibrosis or Huntington's disease. If aetiology is the gold standard, pathophysiology is the 'silver standard'. As will be discussed later in this chapter, our understanding of the pathophysiology of schizophrenia has steadily increased during the past several decades and now suggests that it is primarily a neurodevelopmental disorder.

DEFINING SEPARATE DISEASES USING CLINICAL INFORMATION

To date, psychiatric researchers have used clinical information of various types as an aid in developing psychiatric nosology. This strategy is impeccably sensible and practical, since clinical information is easily accessible. Furthermore, most psychiatric researchers are clinicians, and they understand the illnesses with which patients present themselves to them primarily based on the signs and symptoms that patients have. Epidemiology and response to treatment provide insight about other clinical aspects of disorders that also help clinical investigators refine their nosology.

The two most widely used nosologies in psychiatry, DSM and ICD, identify discrete disorders based on shared phenomenology, as assessed cross-sectionally. Patients are grouped together based on the fact that they share certain signs and symptoms. Both DSM and ICD define disorders that are referred to as 'schizophrenia', and they do not specify any particular age of onset that patients with 'schizophrenia' must have. Individuals who have the characteristic symptoms, as defined in these two nosologies, are diagnosed as having schizophrenia whether their onset is age 10 or age 90.

The shared symptoms that are used to define schizophrenia in the two nosological systems include the broad range discussed above: delusions, hallucinations, disorganized speech, disorganized behaviour and negative symptoms such as alogia (poverty of speech and thought) or affective blunting. ICD gives slightly more emphasis to the importance of Schneiderian first rank symptoms than does DSM but in general the two systems are quite similar. Neither system uses other clinical information, particularly information about course and outcome, even though it is potentially quite powerful for refining nosology. This approach was taken within the standard nomenclatures for very practical reasons. They were designed in order to permit clinicians on the 'front lines' to make a diagnosis the first time they see a given patient. Although course and outcome is at present the primary 'autopsy' available in psychiatry, clinicians do not have this information when they see a patient for the first time. Consequently, longitudinal data cannot be embedded in such clinical diagnostic systems, which must be designed for easy use in cross-sectional assessments.

As is discussed in many other chapters in this book, psychotic disorders assessed cross-sectionally share many resemblances that are independent of age of onset. This observation is of course somewhat circular since psychotic disorders are defined by the presence of psychotic symptoms (i.e. delusions and hallucinations). Nonetheless, even at the clinical level, there are also subtle differences. Patients who present with an early onset tend to be relatively variable. It is a striking clinical fact that on any given day a clinician may see two 20-year-old male patients who are both diagnosed as having schizophrenia and yet who have no symptoms in common. At one extreme, we may see one schizophrenic patient who suffers from persecutory delusions and is intensely anxious with affect appropriate to the content of his delusions and who describes his experiences in a clear and articulate manner. At the other extreme, we may see a withdrawn apathetic young man who laconically describes how voices are commanding him to perform certain acts; he scarcely seems to understand their bizarre nature or to feel any internal torment. As the age of onset gets steadily older, however, patients with psychotic syndromes seem to grow more alike. As authors of other chapters have indicated, patients with late onset psychosis tend to suffer primarily from delusions, with intact affect, and no formal thought disorder. This slight difference in pattern of symptoms may suggest that late onset psychosis is a different disease from the early onset psychotic illnesses that we consistently refer to as schizophrenia.

Epidemiology provides information on another clinical level. The epidemiologic data do not suggest a definitive solution but the chapters in this book by Castle, Riecher-Rössler, Takei, Khandelwal, and McClure and Jeste are all suggestive that psychoses with different ages of onset may differ sufficiently from one another to be considered as nosologically distinct entities. As age-of-onset increases, the male/female ratio shifts, and the genetic loading for schizophrenia decreases. The prototypical early onset schizophrenic patient is male, while the prototypical 'middle' or 'late' onset patient (also referred to as late and very late onset) is female. Younger patients have a higher genetic loading for schizophrenia, while older patients may have a higher loading for affective illness. Such epidemiologic data may suggest that late onset psychoses are different from the early onset disorder originally defined by Kraepelin and that we conventionally refer to schizophrenia or 'classic schizophrenia'.

Response to treatment is another level that is sometimes used in order to determine the nosologic boundaries between disorders. Since treatments are often nosologically non-specific (i.e. aspirin, corticosteroids, or even anticonvulsants are used to treat a variety of clearly distinct medical disorders), response to treatment is not the most powerful tool for dissecting nosological entities. Nonetheless, it is frequently used to gain perspectives. Using this level in order to determine whether late onset psychosis is the same as or different from schizophrenia yields mixed insights. On the one hand, late onset psychosis responds about as well to neuroleptic medications as schizophrenia does. In some respects it may even respond better, since neuroleptics are particularly good at psychotic symptoms and less efficacious in reducing the broad range of symptoms seen in schizophrenia as negative symptoms. One major difference between treatment response in schizophrenia and late onset psychosis is that older people suffering from psychotic symptoms have greater sensitivity to tardive dyskinesia and a need for lower doses (see Chapter 17 in this volume). It is not clear, however, whether these differences are due to simple age effects or whether they are due to a nosological distinctness of psychotic illnesses that have an onset in late life or very late life (i.e. older than age 60).

THE LEVEL OF PATHOPHYSIOLOGY

The level of pathophysiology is a 'silver standard' for identifying separate nosologic entities, since it is closer to the primary processes that produce diseases than the various clinical levels discussed above. Many aspects of clinical presentation can potentially cut across a broad range of illnesses. For example, the delusions and hallucinations that occur in schizophrenia and in late onset psychotic conditions may also occur in other conditions that are clearly nosologically distinct, such as delirium, drug-induced psychosis, or manic-depressive illness. On the other hand, pathophysiology identifies the neurobiological mechanisms that actually produce these symptoms. Clearly, the pathophysiology differs for various psychotic conditions such as delirium, drug-induced psychosis, or manic-depressive illness. Therefore, a crucial question is the following: Does early onset psychosis (i.e. schizophrenia) have a different pathophysiology from late onset psychosis?

The level of pathophysiology strongly suggests that schizophrenia and late life psychosis are probably quite different disorders. The preponderance of evidence at present suggests that schizophrenia is probably due to a disruption in neurodevelopmental processes, while late life psychosis must be due to some type of neurodegenerative process.

'Neurodevelopmental' mechanisms of schizophrenia are often discussed but the term is rarely defined. The distinction between development and degeneration is challenging, because the brain appears to be in a continual process of change from the moment of conception to the moment of death. At what point does this dynamic process change from one of growth and maturation to one of deterioration and decline? How does one distinguish a neurodevelopmental disorder from a neurodegenerative disorder?

Although some use a relatively narrow operational definition (e.g. development corresponding to growth *in utero*), the correct neurobiological definition is broader and closely tied to current concepts in neurobiology. These suggest that brain development and maturation occur as a consequence of orderly processes that begin *in utero* and continue into the early 20s. As summarized in Table 2 these neurodevelopmental processes include a series of interrelated processes that begin early in fetal life and continue into adolescence and young adult life. They include neuronal formation, neuronal migration, axon formation and dendritic proliferation, synaptogenesis, myelination, pruning, apoptosis, and activity dependent changes. The consequences of

Table 2.   Neurodevelopmental processes.

Neuronal formation
Neuronal migration
Axon formation
Dendritic proliferation
Synaptogenesis
Myelination
Pruning
Apoptosis
Activity dependent changes

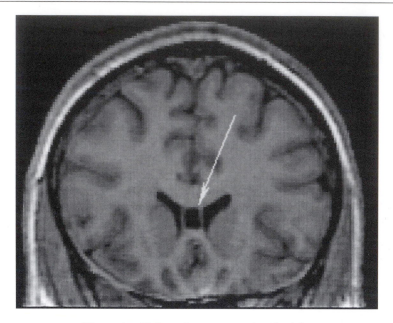

Figure 1.   Enlarged cavum septi pellucidi.

these processes can be partially tracked *in vivo* through structural imaging via the observation of neurodevelopmental anomalies such as ectopic grey matter or dysgenesis or agenesis of structures or regions, as well as the observation and measurement of patterns of gyrification (Zilles *et al.*, 1989; Swayze *et al.*, 1990, 1997; Armstrong *et al.*, 1993, 1995; Carman *et al.*, 1995; Nopoulos *et al.*, 1995a, 1996; Sisodiya *et al.*, 1996; Sisodiya and Free, 1997; Van Essen, 1997; Van Essen and Drury, 1997). Gliosis is the hallmark of neurodegenerative processes, as are indicators of neuronal loss that is not apoptotic; there is little support for these in the neuropathology literature, and this fact is one of the main lines of evidence suggesting that schizophrenia is a neurodevelopmental disorder rather than a neurodegenerative one. Figures 1 and 2 illustrate some of the neurodevelopmental abnormalities that have been observed in schizophrenia, including enlargement of the cavum septi pellucidi and grey matter heterotopia abnormalities.

Clinical definitions are sometimes used in lieu of, or as equivalent to, neurobiological definitions, which sometimes leads to confusion. Clinical definitions tend to stress a change from a higher to a lower level of function, using either cognitive or psychosocial indicators. For example, decline on standardized tests such as the WAIS (beyond that expected as a consequence of ageing) is considered to be evidence for neurodegeneration in Alzheimer's disease, and

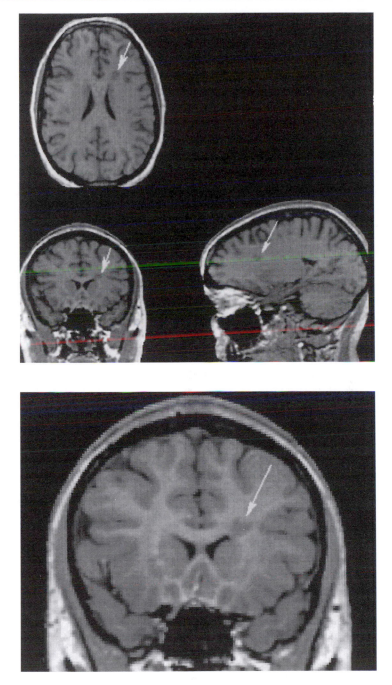

Figure 2.   Grey matter heterotopias.

Table 3. Evidence that schizophrenia is neurodevelopmental.

Neuropathology: no gliosis
Structural imaging: developmental abnormalities such as grey matter heterotopias,
enlarged cavum septi pellucidi, partial callosal agenesis
Presence of structural and functional abnormalities in first episode patients
Premorbid indicators seen in childhood and adolescence (e.g. social and physical
clumsiness)

---

this definition is sometimes applied to schizophrenia. In parallel fashion, indicators of social deterioration (e.g. decline in work function, impaired social and interpersonal skills) are also used to define 'deterioration' and by extension 'neurodegeneration'. In our definition and model, these can only provide very indirect evidence, which must be tied to observation of the entire longitudinal course of illness and available measures of brain function.

At the moment, the strongest evidence (including our own) suggests that 'real' schizophrenia is primarily a neurodevelopmental disorder. This evidence includes the presence of premorbid indicators of dysfunction prior to the onset of the full syndrome (Albee *et al.*, 1964; Goldfarb, 1967; Walker and Lewine, 1990; Murray *et al.*, 1992; Done *et al.*, 1994; Jones *et al.*, 1994; Walker *et al.*, 1994) and the presence of structural and functional brain abnormalities in first episode patients at the time of index evaluation (Schultz *et al.*, 1982, 1983; Bogerts *et al.*, 1990; DeLisi *et al.*, 1990, 1991, 1994; Lieberman *et al.*, 1992, 1993; Nopoulos *et al.*, 1995b; Andreasen *et al.*, 1997). Further, although some investigators have argued that indicators of neural integrity (e.g. the VBR) show worsening over time beyond that associated with normal ageing (DeLisi *et al.*, 1997; Nair *et al.*, 1997), most studies have been negative (Nasrallah *et al.*, 1986; Kemali *et al.*, 1989; DeGreef *et al.*, 1991; Sponheim *et al.*, 1991; Woods and Yurgelun-Todd, 1991; Jaskiw *et al.*, 1994; Vita *et al.*, 1994), and none has examined a large cohort of patients over a long time interval. This evidence is summarized in Table 3.

CONCLUSION

Late onset psychosis occurs at a time in life when the brain has clearly passed from a phase of development, proliferation, growth, and moulding to a time when the brain is losing neural tissue. Schizophrenia is in all likelihood a neurodevelopmental disorder. It is probably a misconnection syndrome in which aberrations in neural circuitry and connectivity cause garbling of signals in the brain and lead to the diversity of symptoms. Misconnections cause perceptions to be associated with inappropriate affects or interpretations (i.e. delusions), difficulty distinguishing between internal and external perceptions (i.e. hallucinations) or slowing or even freezing of the system (e.g. blocking, negative symptoms such as avolition or poverty of speech). Late life psychosis begins long after brain development has been completed, during a time when we know that neurons are losing spines and synapses and the density of neural receptors in most of the brain neurochemical systems is diminished. Presumably, late onset psychosis occurs not because of misconnections formed early in life but rather because of disconnections that have occurred due to neurodegenerative processes in a brain that was previously functioning at a healthy level. The differing age of onsets between schizophrenia and late life psychoses must be telling us something very important about the aetiology and pathophysiology of two different types of mental illness that share common signs and symptoms at the clinical level.

Why split late onset psychosis from schizophrenia? One of our most important missions in psychiatric research is to identify disorders that are discrete at the level of aetiology and pathophysiology. In order to do this, we must study them as separate conditions, using all the various levels listed in Table 1. At present, these levels do not provide definitive evidence in either direction, although the pathophysiologic level is strongly suggestive that late onset psychosis and schizophrenia are two separate conditions. If we treat them as separate conditions, we avoid the risk of pooling heterogeneous disorders that are potentially aetiologically different. Separating late onset psychosis from schizophrenia gives us a much better chance to identify the aetiology or pathophysiology for either one. Pooling them together is only likely to lead to confusion at both the clinical and research levels. Schizophrenia and late onset psychosis are probably not the same thing, and therefore they should not be 'lumped' under the single name 'schizophrenia'.

REFERENCES

Albee, G., Lane, E. and Reuter, J. (1964). Childhood intelligence of future schizophrenics and neighborhood peers. *J Psychol* **58**, 141–144.

American Psychiatric Association (1994). *Diagnostic and Statistical Manual of Mental Disorders, 4th edn* (DSM-IV). American Psychiatric Association, Washington, DC.

Andreasen, N.C. (1982). Negative symptoms in schizophrenia: definition and reliability. *Arch Gen Psychiatry* **39**, 784–788.

Andreasen, N.C. and Olson, S. (1982). Negative versus positive schizophrenia: definition and validation. *Arch Gen Psychiatry* **39**, 789–794.

Andreasen, N.C., Arndt, S., Miller, D., Flaum, M. and Nopoulos, P. (1995). Correlational studies of the Scale for the Assessment of Negative Symptoms and the Scale for the Assessment of Positive Symptoms: an overview and update. *Psychopathology* **28**, 7–17.

Andreasen, N.C., O'Leary, D.S., Flaum, M. *et al.* (1997). Hypofrontality in schizophrenia: distributed dysfunctional circuits in neuroleptic naive patients. *Lancet* **349**, 1730–1734.

Armstrong, E., Zilles, K. and Schleicher, A. (1993). Cortical folding and the evolution of the human brain. *J Human Evol* **25**, 387–392.

Armstrong, E., Schleicher, A., Omran, H., Curtis, M. and Zilles, K. (1995). The ontogeny of human gyrification. *Cerebral Cortex* **1**, 56–63.

Bleuler, E. (1950). *Dementia Praecox or the Group of Schizophrenias* [Translated by J. Zinkin]. International Universities Press, New York.

Bogerts, B., Ashtari, M., DeGreef, G., Alvir, J.M., Bilder, R.M. and Lieberman, J.A. (1990). Reduced temporal limbic structure volumes on magnetic resonance images in first episode schizophrenia. *Psychiatry Res Neuroimaging* **35**, 1–13.

Carman, G.J., Drury, H.A. and Van Essen, D. (1995). Computational methods for reconstructing and unfolding the cerebral cortex. *Cerebral Cortex* **5**, 506–517.

DeGreef, G., Ashtari, M., Wu, H., Borenstein, M., Geisler, S. and Lieberman, J. (1991). Follow-up MRI study in first-episode schizophrenia. *Schizophr Res* **5**, 204–206.

DeLisi, L.E., Gupta, S.M., Hoff, A. *et al.* (1990). Brain morphology in first episode cases of schizophrenia. *Schizophr Res* **3**, 20.

DeLisi, L.E., Hoff, A.L., Schwartz, J.E. *et al.* (1991). Brain morphology in first-episode schizophrenic-like psychotic patients: a quantitative magnetic resonance imaging study. *Biol Psychiatry* **29**, 159–175.

DeLisi, L., Hoff, A., Neale, C. and Kushner, M. (1994). Asymmetries in the superior temporal lobe in male and female first-episode schizophrenic patients: measures of the planum temporale and superior temporal gyrus by MRI. *Schizophr Res* **12**, 19–28.

DeLisi, L.E., Sakuma, M., Tew, W., Kushner, M., Hoff, A. and Grimson, R. (1997). Schizophrenia as a chronic active brain process: a study of progressive brain structural change subsequent to the onset of schizophrenia. *Psychiatry Res Neuroimaging* **74**, 129–140.

Done, D.J., Crow, T.J., Johnstone, E.C. and Sacker, A. (1994). Childhood antecedents of schizophrenia and affective illness: social adjustment at ages 7 and 11. *Br Med J* **309**, 699–703.

Goldfarb, W. (1967). Factors in the development of schizophrenic children: an approach to subclassification. In: Romano, J. (Ed.), *The Origins of Schizophrenia*. Excerpta Medica, Amsterdam, pp. 70–91.

Ho, B.C., Nopoulos, P., Flaum, M., Arndt, S. and Andreasen, N. (1998). Two-year outcome in first-episode schizophrenia: predictive value of symptoms for quality of life. *Am J Psychiatry* **155**, 1196–1201.

Jaskiw, G.E., Juliano, D.M., Goldberg, T.E., Hertzman, M., Urow-Hamell, E. and Weinberger, D.R. (1994). Cerebral ventricular enlargement in schizophreniform disorder does not progress. A seven year follow-up study. *Schizophr Res* **14**, 23–28.

Jones, P., Rodgers, B., Murray, R. and Marmot, M. (1994). Child development risk factors for adult schizophrenia in the British 1946 birth cohort. *Lancet* **344**, 1398–1402.

Kemali, A., Maj, M., Galderisi, S., Milici, N. and Salvati, A. (1989). Ventricle-to-brain ratio in schizophrenia: a controlled follow-up study. *Biol Psychiatry* **26**, 753–756.

Kraepelin, E. (1899). Dementia praecox. *Psychiatrie*. Verlag Von Johann, Leipzig.

Liberman, J., Bogerts, B., DeGreef, G., Ashtari, M., Lantos, G. and Alvir, J. (1992). Qualitative assessment of brain morphology in acute and chronic schizophrenia. *Am J Psychiatry* **149**, 784–794.

Liberman, J.A., Jody, D., Alvir, J.M.J. *et al.* (1993). Brain morphology, dopamine, and eye-tracking abnormalities in first-episode schizophrenia: prevalence and clinical correlates. *Arch Gen Psychiatry* **50**, 357–368.

Murray, R.M., O'Callaghan, E., Castle, D.J. and Lewis, S.W. (1992). A neurodevelopmental approach to the classification of schizophrenia. *Schizophr Bull* **18**, 319–332.

Nair, T.R., Christensen, J.D., Kingsbury, S.J., Kumar, N.G., Terry, W.M. and Garver, D.L. (1997). Progression of cerebroventricular enlargement and the subtyping of schizophrenia. *Psychiatry Res Neuroimaging* **74**, 141–150.

Nasrallah, H.A., Olson, S.C., McCalley-Whitters, M., Chapman, S.M. and Jacoby, C.G. (1986). Cerebral ventricular enlargement in schizophrenia: a preliminary follow-up study. *Arch Gen Psychiatry* **43**, 157–159.

Nopoulos, P.C., Flaum, M., Andreasen, N.C. and Swayze, V.W. II (1995a). Gray matter heterotopias in schizophrenia. *Psychiatry Res Neuroimaging* **61**, 11–14.

Nopoulos, P., Torres, I., Flaum, M. and Andreasen, N.C. (1995b). Brain morphology in first episode schizophrenia. *Am J Psychiatry* **152**, 1721–1724.

Nopoulos, P., Swayze, V.W. II, and Andreasen, N.C. (1996). Pattern of brain morphology in patients with schizophrenia and large cavum septi pellucidi. *J Neuropsychiatry Clin Neurosci* **8**, 147–152.

Schultz, S.C., Koller, M., Kishore, P.R., Hamer, R.M. and Friedel, R.D. (1982). Abnormal scans in young schizophrenics. *Psychopharmacol Bull* **18**, 163–164.

Schultz, S.C., Koller, M., Kishore, P.R., Hamer, R.M., Gehl, J.J. and Friedel, R.D. (1983). Ventricular enlargement in teenage patients with schizophrenia spectrum disorder. *Am J Psychiatry* **140**, 1592–1595.

Sisodiya, S.M. and Free, S.L. (1997). Disproportion of cerebral surface areas and volumes in cerebral dysgenesis. MRI-based evidence for connectional abnormalities. *Brain* **120**, 271–281.

Sisodiya, S., Free, S., Fish, D. and Shorvon, S. (1996). MRI-based surface area estimates in the normal adult human brain: evidence for structural organization. *J Anatomy* **188** (Pt 2), 425–438.

Sponheim, S.R., Iacono, W.G. and Beiser, M. (1991). Stability of ventricular size after the onset of psychosis in schizophrenia. *Psychiatry Res Neuroimaging* **40**, 21–29.

Swayze, V.W. II, Andreasen, N.C., Ehrhardt, J.C., Yuh, W.T.C., Alliger, R. and Cohen, G. (1990). Developmental abnormalities of the corpus callosum in schizophrenia. *Arch Neurol* **47**, 805–808.

Swayze, V.W. II, Johnson, V.P., Hanson, J.W. *et al.* (1997). Magnetic resonance imaging of brain anomalies in fetal alcohol syndrome. *Pediatrics* **99**, 232–240.

Van Essen, D.C. (1997). A tension-based theory of morphogenesis and compact wiring in the central nervous system. *Nature* **385**, 313–318.

Van Essen, D.C. and Drury, H.A. (1997). Structural and functional analyses of human cerebral cortex using surface-based atlas. *J Neurosci* **17**, 7079–7102.

Vita, A., Giobbio, G.M.M., Dievi, M. *et al.* (1994). Stability of cerebral appearance of the first psychotic symptoms to the later diagnosis of schizophrenia. *Biol Psychiatry* **35**, 960–962.

Walker, E. and Lewine, R. (1990). Prediction of adult-onset schizophrenia from childhood home movies of the patients. *Am J Psychiatry* **147**, 1052–1056.

Walker, E.F., Savoie, T. and Davis, D. (1994). Neuromotor precursors of schizophrenia. *Schizophr Bull* **20**, 441–451.

Woods, B. and Yurgelun-Todd, D. (1991). Brain volume loss in schizophrenia: when does it occur and is it progressive? *Schizophrenia Res* **5**, 202–204.

World Health Organization (1994). *International Classification of Diseases, 10th edn.* World Health Organization, Geneva.

Zilles, K., Armstrong, E., Schleicher, A. and Stephan, H. (1989). Gyrification in the cerebral cortex of primates. *Brain Behav Evolution* **34**, 443–450.

III

Characterizing Late Onset Schizophrenia

Late Onset Schizophrenia
Edited by Robert Howard, Peter V. Rabins, David J. Castle
© 1999 Wrightson Biomedical Publishing Ltd

10

Schizophrenia-Like Psychosis with Onset in Late Life

ROBERT HOWARD

*Section of Old Age Psychiatry, Institute of Psychiatry, De Crespigny Park,
London, UK*

SCHIZOPHRENIA-LIKE PSYCHOSIS WITH ONSET IN LATE LIFE

This chapter considers those patients who have onset of a psychotic illness characterized by core schizophrenic symptoms after their sixtieth birthday. The central paradox of schizophrenia-like psychoses with onset in late life is that although phenotypically they are remarkably similar to more typical cases with onset in early adult life and not at all like those 'organic' psychoses seen in association with conditions such as Alzheimer's disease, the information we have about risk factors for these disorders suggests a neurodegenerative aetiology. The final twist to this paradox is that neuropsychometric and brain imaging investigations have so far failed to identify evidence of progressive cognitive changes or focal brain lesions. Indeed, the deficits and structural brain changes reported are essentially similar to those seen in early adult life onset schizophrenia. The author believes that these patients are most appropriately viewed as a subtle organic phenocopy of those early adult life onset cases with a presumed neurodevelopmental aetiology. Hence the term 'schizophrenia-like' is highly appropriate in their description. Advances in brain imaging technology, in particular improvements in our ability to resolve localized vascular degenerative changes in white matter, together with more data from longitudinal neuropsychological follow-up of well-characterized cases, probably represent the most useful routes to an increased understanding of pathophysiology and aetiology. If an underlying neural substrate for the development of such a schizophrenic phenocopy can be identified in these very late onset cases, this may represent an important model for understanding the nature, anatomical location and effects of neurodevelopmental abnormalities in more typical early onset cases.

SYMPTOMATOLOGY OF SCHIZOPHRENIA-LIKE PSYCHOSIS WITH ONSET AFTER AGE 60

Initial reports of psychotic symptoms encountered in patients with onset after age 60 ('late paraphrenics' or 'senile schizophrenics') emphasized the presence of a consistent cluster of symptoms including persecutory delusions and auditory hallucinations (Fish 1960; Kay and Roth, 1961; Post, 1966; Herbert and Jacobson, 1967). Later workers noted the presence of core schizophrenic symptoms such as Schneiderian first rank symptoms (Grahame 1984; Rabins et al., 1984; Holden, 1987; Howard et al., 1994; Almeida et al., 1995), and indeed almost all the symptoms associated with schizophrenia have been reported in these patients with the exception of formal thought disorder. Development of negative symptoms appears also to be rare but may be seen after follow-up of several years. The largest single group of patients with onset after age 60 reported remains my own south London cohort. These were a group of what (in 1991) were still called late paraphrenics who were referred from specialist old age psychiatry services in the city. Hallucinatory experiences in a variety of sensory modalities were common. Non-verbal auditory hallucinations were found in 70%, third-person voices in 49.5% and voices speaking directly to the patient in 49.5% of cases. Visual hallucinations are discussed below; olfactory hallucinations with delusional elaboration were seen in 30% and hallucinations of touch or taste with delusional elaboration in 32%. The high prevalence of delusions of persecution (84.2%), reference (76.3%) and misinterpretation or misidentification (59.4%) were consistent with previous descriptions of these patients. More typically schizophrenic delusional symptoms such as delusions of control (24.8%), of alien forces penetrating or controlling the subject's body or mind (29.7%) and primary delusions (20.8%) were the next most common. Although delusions of morbid jealousy, pregnancy, altered appearance, grandiosity, religiosity and catastrophe, together with sexual and hypochondriacal delusions are often said to be important symptoms of this condition, they were individually uncommon. Features of schizophrenic formal thought disorder (Schneider, 1930) (loosening of associations, circumstantiality, etc.) were not seen in any of these patients, although two had used neologisms. This finding was consistent with Post's (1966) observation that schizophrenic disorders of speech and thinking were never seen convincingly in his patients, but contrary to Kay and Roth's (1961) finding of 'verbosity, circumstantiality and irrelevance' in 30% of their late paraphrenic patients. Although they used a younger cut-off and examined patients with onset after age 45 years, Pearlson and colleagues (1989) found formal thought disorder in only 5.6% of late onset cases, compared with 51.9% of young patients with schizophrenia and 54.5% of early onset patients who had grown old. An analysis of variance on their data indicated that the occurrence of formal thought disorder decreased as age at onset increased. So disorders of the form of thought which so characterize early onset cases of schizophrenia are infrequently seen in middle age onset cases and have disappeared if onset is in old age. Almeida, who visited many of the patients from this south London group, reported that narrowly defined negative symptoms such as shallow, withdrawn or constricted affect were only found in 8.5% of subjects and were always mild (Almeida *et al.*, 1995). Other negative symptoms such as lack of speech inflection, reduced speech output, reduced facial expression and gestures were also infrequent and never striking.

So much for the appearance of symptoms considered to be typical of schizophrenia in patients with onset after age 60 patients, but are there symptoms which are more common in, or can even be said to characterize, the later onset group? The presence of partition delusions in up to 70% of late onset cases has been noted by several authors and seems to have a specificity for the condition (Herbert and Jacobson 1967; Pearlson *et al.*, 1989; Howard *et al*, 1992). In a partition delusion there is a breakdown of the normal barrier function of a structure such as a wall or floor (usually of the patient's home), so that radiation, matter, people or animals can pass through it. Partition delusions are rare in early onset cases and while no convincing explanation for their appearance in the elderly onset group has been formulated, it has been suggested that they may reflect older peoples' preoccupation with their material surroundings and a lack of unexpectedness of bodily decay and penetration by disease in old age. For a young person with schizophrenia, the concept of bodily breakdown or penetration is unexpected and bizarre and provides rich ground for delusional growth. In older patients, however, since personal physical dependability can no longer be assumed, the location of unexpected or bizarre deterioration logically moves out to the next layer of bodily protection; the substance of the home. Persistent visual hallucinations are also much more common in patients with onset after age 60 than in more typical schizophrenia. Forty per cent of the patients in my group had reported some visual hallucinations and in 32% these were formed. About 20% of these patients experienced complex recurrent visual hallucinations of Charles Bonnet type: the so-called Charles Bonnet syndrome plus (Howard and Levy 1994). It is therefore probably fair to conclude that most if not all of the positive psychotic symptoms seen in early adult life onset schizophrenia are also seen in onset after age 60 cases. Cases of what we used to call late paraphrenia have a very different symptom profile from those established 'organic' psychoses of old age such as those associated with Alzheimer's disease or dementia with cortical Lewy bodies in which delusions and hallucinations are less organized, persistent and stable and are invariably associated with progressive cognitive deficit or fluctuations in conscious level.

EPIDEMIOLOGY

Henderson and Kay (1997) have recently reviewed the literature on both population based and psychiatric service contact based epidemiological studies of late onset psychoses. They concluded that psychotic states which are phenomenologically similar to those found in clinics occur in the community in non-trivial numbers. The point prevalence of schizophrenia-like psychoses in the elderly population is reported to be between 0.1% and 1.6% (Kay *et al.*, 1964; Parsons, 1964; Williamson *et al.*, 1964; Bollerup, 1975; Weissman *et al.*, 1985; Copeland *et al.*, 1987, 1992, 1998; Keith *et al.*, 1991) although higher figures of 2.6% (Skoog, 1993) and 4% (Christenson and Blazer, 1984) represent prevalence outliers. As regards studies of patients in contact with psychiatric services, agreement seems very good. Using first hospital admission data from England and Wales for 1966, Kay (1972) found rates of schizophrenic illness in the over-65s to be between 10 and 15 per 100,000 for males and between 20 and 25 per 100,000 for females. Holden (1987) estimated annual rates of late paraphrenia of 17–24 per 100,000 of the elderly population of Camberwell, depending upon whether or not cases with organic aetiology were included. The apparent increase in annual incidence with age after the age of 60 demonstrated by van Os and colleagues (1995) is reviewed below within risk factors, but these authors quote figures of 10–25 per 100,000.

RISK FACTORS

Genetic factors constitute the most important identified risk for young adult life onset schizophrenia. The presence of an affected first degree relative increases the risk of schizophrenia ten-fold (Gottesman and Shields, 1982). Up to the age of 60 years, the evidence that familial risk falls with increasing onset age is inconsistent (Kendler *et al.*, 1987, 1996; Sham *et al.*, 1994). Although there are few controlled studies involving patients with onset after age 60, a definite trend towards reduced familial risk emerges from the literature. In a review, Castle and Howard (1992) found that for subjects with illness onset after 40 or 45 years, reported rates of schizophrenia in relatives range from 4.4% to 19.4%, while for those with onset delayed to 50 or 60 years, rates of schizophrenia of 1.0–7.3% were reported. In a characteristically meticulous family study of 56 Stockholm late paraphrenic patients, Kay (1963) was able to trace relatives in all but seven cases. He found a morbid risk for schizophrenia among first degree relatives (Weinberg method, risk period 18–50 years) of 2.4% if only those cases who had been admitted to a psychiatric hospital were considered. If he included what he termed 'uncertain cases', i.e. those whose history was strongly suggestive of schizophrenia but who had not received an admission diagnosis, the morbid risk rose to 4.4%. The importance of examining a control group in such studies is often overlooked. The lifetime risk of schizophrenia and other mental disorders was assessed in 269 first degree relatives of 47 onset after age 60 patients and 272 first degree relatives of 42 elderly control subjects recruited from a lunch club in Camberwell with the Family History Research Diagnostic Criteria Schedule (Andreasen *et al.*, 1986). The results indicated that the first degree relatives of such patients were not at increased risk of developing schizophrenia (Howard *et al.*, 1997). Using a narrow age range at risk (15–50 years), the estimated lifetime risk of schizophrenia among the first degree relatives of both patients and controls was 1.3%. When a wider age range at risk was considered (15–90 years), the lifetime risk for patients' relatives was 2.3% and for those of controls 2.2%. Hence there was no evidence for a late life onset psychosis that 'breeds true' and for which increased risk in relatives could only be seen when later life was included in the considered lifetime period of risk. There were no significant differences in the lifetime risk of organic brain syndromes between relatives of patients and controls but the morbid risk of depression was 16.3% among relatives of patients and 4.4% among those of controls ($p=0.003$). The finding of an excess morbid risk of depression in the first degree relatives of the patients had dual significance. An aetiological link to affective disorders is intriguing and raises the possibility that at least some of these patients may have an atypical expression of a mood disorder. Secondly, convincing demonstration of an excess of any psychiatric disorder among the first degree relatives of patients lends more credence to the negative findings with respect to morbid risk of schizophrenia. Presumably, the same factors that might make it difficult to ascertain an accurate family history of schizophrenia in the situation where probands are elderly will also operate for affective disorder. Hence it is unlikely that our failure to demonstrate an increased morbid risk of schizophrenia can be attributed to those difficulties inherent in conducting family studies in elderly people who have few surviving first degree relatives.

The closest thing to a genetic marker identified for schizophrenia is the HLA antigen type A9 which has been repeatedly associated with paranoid schizophrenia. Naguib *et al.* (1987) HLA typed 31 onset after age 60 patients and reported that while there was no association with A9, the B37 antigen was associated with a relative risk of 4.38, and the frequencies of both BW55 and CW6 were significantly raised compared with controls. Other studies have shown that the frequency of another genetic marker, this time for Alzheimer's disease – ApoE $\epsilon4$, is not raised in patients with onset of schizophrenia like psychosis after age 60 patients (Howard *et al.*, 1995b).

Female gender is an important risk factor for onset after age 60 psychosis. Mary Seeman (Chapter 13) and David Castle (Chapter 12) in this book explore the interactions between gender, oestrogen status and age that might predispose to psychosis. The preponderance of women in this very late onset group is striking, and the figure of 86% in my series was very typical. Another illness which predominantly affects women and whose incidence increases with age is osteoporosis, and it may be that the female preponderance among these very late onset cases is a further important hint towards a degenerative aetiology.

Increase in age after the age of 60 appears to be associated in both males and females with a steady increase in the incidence of non-affective non-organic psychoses. van Os *et al.* (1995) followed the observation that annual first admission rates for ICD-9 paranoid schizophrenia and paranoid states rose from 8.7 per 100,000 in the 65–74 age group to 14.5 per 100,000 in the over-75s by examining first admission rates in the Netherlands and nine regional health authorities in the UK. 'Non-affective non-organic psychoses' consisted of all patients with the ICD-9 diagnoses of schizophrenia, paraphrenia and paranoid states, and specifically excluded cases of organic psychotic conditions. A sample of 8010 over-60s first admissions from the Netherlands and 1777 from the UK was ascertained. The annual incidence of psychosis increased significantly with increasing age after 60 in both samples and in both males and females, rising from 10 per 100,000 in the age group 60–65 years to 25 cases per 100,000 in the 90-plus age group. Hence ageing is an important risk factor for the development of psychosis in the seventh to tenth decades of life, suggesting that some age-related aetiological factor may be operating.

AN ORGANIC BRAIN DISEASE?

Although genetic factors seem less important in aetiology and increasing age as a risk factor suggests a degenerative process, there is little consistent evidence to suggest that these patients have a demonstrable cerebral disease. The authors of early descriptive studies agreed that when organic factors contributed to psychosis, this was generally easy to determine at the time of first presentation. Long-term follow-ups of 'functional' cases seem to have generated few surprises. While Kay and Roth (1961) found organic systemic medical conditions to coexist with 21% of their cases of late paraphrenia, they believed that such organic factors influenced the illness course in only 5%. Post (1966) reported that having excluded 12 of his original 93 subjects because of evidence of Alzheimer's disease or cerebrovascular disease, only 2% of those remaining had developed demonstrable organic brain change at follow-up. By contrast, Holden (1987) reported that 27% of 47 late paraphrenics ascertained from a retrospective case-note study had clearly developed a dementia after a 3-year follow-up. Had all these cases been seen at the time of initial presentation by an experienced old age psychiatrist, however, it is unlikely they would have all attracted a functional diagnosis.

The only available quantitative neuropathological study of such patients was by Blessed *et al.* (1966) who found that the senile plaque count in the brains of five late paraphrenic patients was no higher than seen in elderly depressives or neuropsychiatrically healthy controls. The advent of *in vivo* brain imaging techniques (reviewed in this volume by Godfrey Pearlson, Chapter 15) has tended to confirm the general conclusion that, so long as patients undergo careful screening to exclude those with a history or signs of stroke or progressive cognitive decline, and control subjects are recruited from approximately the same demographic and socioeconomic background as patients, brain imaging abnormalities affect the same areas and are of similar magnitude to those seen in younger people with schizophrenia. This is not an uncontroversial area, however. Miller *et al.* (1989, 1991, 1992) have reported an enormous excess of areas of white matter hyperintensity visualized by MRI within groups of what were initially claimed to be non-demented patients with psychosis onset after 45 years, whom these authors have termed 'late life psychosis'. Forty-two per cent of such patients (mean age 60.1 years at time of scanning) had extensive white matter lesions on MRI compared with only 8% of an age-matched healthy control group (Miller *et al.*, 1991). Further, the appearance of large patchy lesions was six times more likely in the temporal lobes and four times more likely in the frontal lobes of the patients. These authors, however, acknowledged that at least 50% of the cases had clear organic psychoses (history or signs of previous stroke, Binswanger's disease, Alzheimer's disease, brain tumour, previous brain trauma) which could have been diagnosed at presentation. Those workers who have excluded such cases to examine white matter and cortical and subcortical grey matter with MRI in patients with late onset schizophrenia (Symonds *et al.*, 1997) or late paraphrenia (Howard *et al.*, 1995a) have found no excess of focal abnormalities in the brains of patients compared with appropriately matched healthy control subjects. Of course, with advances in brain imaging we may one day be able to identify focal abnormalities that characterize even early onset schizophrenia, so the organic versus functional debate in these late onset cases is perhaps not particularly important in itself. Diffusion tensor imaging with MRI represents the next advance in our ability to detect subtle pathological changes in the white matter of patients both through comparisons of anisotropy images between patients and controls (Buchsbaum *et al.*, 1998) and construction of high anatomical resolution fibre tract maps.

DIAGNOSIS AND NOMENCLATURE

Roth and Morrissey (1952) resurrected Kraepelin's term for a psychosis characterized by hallucinations and delusions without deterioration or affective disturbance and added the prefix 'late'. They chose late paraphrenia to describe a group of patients who they believed had schizophrenia but with an illness onset delayed until after the age of 55–60 years. If this really was their belief, then perhaps they should have avoided almost half a century of controversy and confusion by calling these patients late onset schizophrenics! To add further to the confusion, in common clinical usage the 'late' is often lost, so that these patients are often called 'paraphrenics' and I am often invited to meetings in order to debate the utility of 'paraphrenia'. In spite of these problems, late paraphrenia has clinical utility, reinforces the view that these patients have a different illness from schizophrenia (which is, rather deliciously, exactly the opposite to what Roth and Morrissey intended), and European psychiatrists will probably find it difficult to forget the term although it has disappeared from official classificatory systems such as ICD. Perhaps the most pernicious aspect of late paraphrenia was the way it generated transatlantic disagreement. Psychiatrists in Europe and the USA were seeing patients with essentially the same late onsets and symptoms (Rabins *et al.*, 1984) but principally because of lack of consistent use of nomenclature, these patients appeared to be suffering from some eccentric and exclusively European illness. Peter Rabins and myself attempted to 'revisit' (the word was chosen by the *British Journal of Psychiatry*'s editor) late paraphrenia in an attempt to put the US–Europe disagreement behind us (Howard and Rabins, 1997). We bemoaned the fact that neither ICD-10 nor DSM-IV contained late onset categories for schizophrenia and suggested the diagnostic categories of late onset schizophrenia (onset age 45–59 years) and late life onset schizophrenia-like psychosis (onset after 60 years). These received a mixed welcome; I think we made the latter group's name too long but as we discovered at the 1998 Consensus meeting, it is difficult to be unambiguous in such a title without being long-winded. At the meeting, Nancy Andreasen with her quick journalist's eye for a snappy title suggested that we should call such cases 'paraschizophrenia' and, although this did not attract much support at the time, the more I think about this the more I like it!

TREATMENT

While Dilip Jeste covers treatment of late onset schizophrenia in Chapter 17 of this volume, there are a couple of additional points that relate specifically to the treatment of very late onset cases. In the UK these patients are assessed and treated in their own homes. They are reluctant to attend outpatient, day hospital or day centre facilities and hence home-based social and drug interventions are most likely to be accepted and have some chance of success. During assessment and treatment initiation it is most important that staff maintain an appearance of non-judgemental but involved concern in relation to psychotic complaints that the patient may make. Listening to complaints about the neighbours' intrusions and absorbing some of the associated anger and distress so that the patient is less likely to confront his/her neighbours or burden the local police, relatives and friends are practical measures with common-sense validity. Although these patients are often said to be eccentric and hostile, my own experience suggests that they are also often extremely lonely and will generally welcome regular community psychiatric nurse (CPN) visits to their homes. The mainstay of treatment of very late onset psychoses is, of course, the antipsychotics. Although there have been no formal prospective drug trials in these patients, naturalistic studies indicate that good treatment outcomes can be achieved with very low doses (10–25% of the young adult dose). Treatment compliance remains the most important determinant of outcome and can sometimes only be guaranteed by prescription of a depot. An advantage of this is the necessity for regular CPN visits to administer the injections which can give some timetabled structure to the nurse–patient contact. If compliance is not a problem or the patient will not accept a depot, then a good case can be made for starting with risperidone or olanzapine rather than with one of the older antipsychotics. The risks of orthostatic hypotensive incidents or the short- and long-term development of extrapyramidal motor side effects with conventional drugs are probably adequate justification for considering an atypical. Add to this the fact that these patients are often convinced that they are being poisoned or influenced in other ways by their persecutors, and the importance of their not associating prescribed medication with unpleasant effects is very obvious. A starting dose of 0.5 mg of risperidone per day, increasing in further 0.5 mg increments up to a maximum of 1.5–2.0 mg is generally well tolerated. Although there are no comparative trial data for the atypicals in elderly psychotic patients, my own clinical experience is that some patients experience more unwanted sedation with olanzapine than risperidone. Again, based on my clinical experience and from extrapolation of the use of the drug in the treatment of dopaminomimetic psychosis in Parkinson's disease, a starting dose of 2.5 mg olanzapine would be my choice, increasing to a maximum of 7.5–10 mg per day, in those patients with symptoms of Parkinson's disease or evidence of emergent extra-pyramidal side effects with other typical or atypical antipsychotic agents. Since none of the atypicals are as yet available as depot preparations, the ideal drug treatment for these patients is still awaited.

One final word about treatment concerns patient monitoring. It is very easy to start an elderly patient on an antipsychotic and then, reassured by reports that he/she is doing very well in the community, not see him/her again for several months. During this time, particularly if he/she has been receiving a depot, it is very possible that he/she will have developed potentially irreversible side effects. For this reason my own habit is to ensure that all such prescriptions are monitored by myself or junior medical staff who see each patient at least every 6 weeks. This facilitates 'fine tuning' of dose and injection interval in order to suppress psychotic symptoms with the minimum amount of medication and monitoring for the emergence of tardive dyskinesias.

REFERENCES

Almeida, O., Howard, R., Levy, R. and David, A. (1995). Psychotic states arising in late life (late paraphrenia): psychopathology and nosology. *Br J Psychiatry* **166**, 205–214.

Andreasen, N.C., Rice, J., Endicott, J., Reich, T. and Coryell, W. (1986). The family history approach to diagnosis. How useful is it? *Arch Gen Psychiatry* **43**, 421–429.

Blessed, G., Tomlinson, B.E. and Roth, M. (1966). The association between quantitative measures of dementia and of senile change in cerebral grey matter of elderly subjects. *Br J Psychiatry* **114**, 797–811.

Bollerup, T.R. (1975). Prevalence of mental disorders among 70 year olds domiciled in nine Copenhagen suburbs. *Acta Psychiatr Scand* **51**, 327–339.

Buchsbaum, M.S., Tang, C.Y., Peled, S. *et al.* (1998). MRI white matter diffusion anisotropy and PET metabolic rate in schizophrenia. *NeuroReport* **9**, 425–430.

Castle, D. and Howard, R. (1992). What do we know about the aetiology of late-onset schizophrenia? *Eur Psychiatry* **7**, 99–108.

Christenson, R. and Blazer, D. (1984). Epidemiology of persecutory ideation in an elderly population in the community. *Am J Psychiatry* **141**, 1088–1091.

Copeland, J.R., Dewey, M.E., Wood, N., Searle, R., Davidson, I.A. and McWilliam, C. (1987). Range of mental illness among the elderly in the community. Prevalence in Liverpool using the GMS-AGECAT package. *Br J Psychiatry* **150**, 815–823.

Copeland, J.R., Davidson, I.A., Dewey, M.E. *et al.* (1992). Alzheimer's disease, other dementias, depression and pseudodementia: prevalence, incidence and three-year outcome in Liverpool. *Br J Psychiatry* **161**, 230–239.

Copeland, J.R., Dewey, M.E., Scott, A. *et al.* (1998). Schizophrenia and delusional disorder in older age: community prevalence, incidence, co-morbidity and outcome. *Schizophr Bull* **24**, 153–161.

Fish, F. (1960). Senile schizophrenia. *J Mental Sci* **106**, 938–946.

Gottesman, I.I. and Shields, J. (1982). *Schizophrenia, the Epigenetic Puzzle.* Cambridge University Press, Cambridge.

Grahame, P.S. (1984). Schizophrenia in old age (late paraphrenia). *Br J Psychiatry* **145**, 493–495.

Henderson, A.S. and Kay, D.W. (1997). The epidemiology of functional psychoses of late onset. *Eur Arch Psychiatry Clin Neurosci* **247**, 176–189.

Herbert, M.E. and Jacobson, S. (1967). Late paraphrenia. *Br J Psychiatry* **113**, 461–469.

Holden, N.L. (1987). Late paraphrenia or the paraphrenias? A descriptive study with a 10-year follow-up. *Br J Psychiatry* **150**, 635–639.

Howard, R. and Rabins, P.V. (1997). Late paraphrenia revisited. *Br J Psychiatry* **171**, 406–408.

Howard, R. and Levy, R. (1994). Charles Bonnet syndrome plus: complex visual hallucinations of Charles Bonnet syndrome type in late paraphrenia. *Int J Geriatr Psychiatry* **9**, 399–404.

Howard, R., Castle, D., O'Brien, J., Almeida, O. and Levy, R. (1992). Permeable walls, floors, ceilings and doors: partition delusions in late paraphrenia. *Int J Geriatr Psychiatry* **7**, 719–724.

Howard, R., Almeida, O. and Levy, R. (1994). Phenomenology, demography and diagnosis in late paraphrenia. *Psychol Med* **24**, 397–410.

Howard, R., Cox, T., Almeida, O., Mullen, R. and Levy, R. (1995a). White matter signal hyperintensities in the brains of patients with late paraphrenia and the normal community-living elderly. *Biol Psychiatry* **38**, 86–91.

Howard, R., Dennehey, J., Lovestone, S. *et al.* (1995b). Apolipoprotein E genotype and late paraphrenia. *Int J Geriatr Psychiatry* **10**, 147–150.

Howard, R., Graham, C., Sham, P. *et al.* (1997). A controlled family study of late-onset non-affective psychosis (late paraphrenia). *Br J Psychiatry* **170**, 511–514.

Kay, D.W.K. (1963). Late paraphrenia and its bearing on the aetiology of schizophrenia. *Acta Psychiatr Scand* **39**, 159–169.

Kay, D.W.K. (1972). Schizophrenia and schizophrenia-like states in the elderly. *Br J Hosp Med* **8**, 369–376.

Kay, D.W.K. and Roth, M. (1961). Environmental and hereditary factors in the schizophrenias of old age ('late paraphrenia') and their bearing on the general problem of causation in schizophrenia. *J Mental Sci* **107**, 649–686.

Kay, D.W.K., Beamish, P. and Roth, M. (1964). Old age mental disorders in Newcastle upon Tyne. Part 1: A study of prevalence. *Br J Psychiatry* **110**, 146–158.

Keith, S.J., Regier, D.A. and Rae, S. (1991). Schizophrenic disorders. In: Robins, L.N. and Regier, D.A. (Eds), *Psychiatric Disorders in America*. The Free Press, London.

Kendler, K.S., Tsuang, M.T. and Hays, P. (1987). Age at onset in schizophrenia: a familial perspective. *Arch Gen Psychiatry* **44**, 881–890.

Kendler, K.S., Karkowski-Shuman, L. and Walsh, D. (1996). Age at onset in schizophrenia and risk of illness in relatives. Results from the Roscommon family study. *Br J Psychiatry* **169**, 213–218.

Miller, B.L., Lesser, I.M., Boone, K. *et al.* (1989). Brain white-matter lesions and psychosis. *Br J Psychiatry* **155**, 73–78.

Miller, B.L., Lesser, I.M., Boone, K., Hill, E., Mehringer, C.M. and Wong, K. (1991). Brain lesions and cognitive function in late life psychosis. *Br J Psychiatry* **158**, 76–82.

Miller, B.L., Lesser, I.M., Mena, I. *et al.* (1992). Regional cerebral blood flow in late-life-onset psychosis. *Neuropsychiatry, Neuropsychol Behav Neurol* **5**, 132–137.

Naguib, M., McGuffin, P., Levy, R., Festenstein, H. and Alonso, A. (1987). Genetic markers in late paraphrenia: a study of HLA antigens. *Br J Psychiatry* **150**, 124–127.

Parsons, P.L. (1964). Mental health of Swansea's old folk. *Br J Preventative Social Med* **19**, 43–47.

Pearlson, G.D., Kreger, L., Rabins, P.V. *et al.* (1989). A chart review study of late-onset and early-onset schizophrenia. *Am J Psychiatry* **146**, 1568–1574.

Post, F. (1966). *Persistent Persecutory States of the Elderly*. Pergamon, Oxford.

Rabins, P.V., Pauker, S. and Thomas, J. (1984). Can schizophrenia begin after age 44? *Compr Psychiatry* **25**, 290–293.

Roth, M. and Morrissey, J.D. (1952). Problems in the diagnosis and classification of mental disorders in old age. *J Mental Sci* **98**, 66–80.

Schneider, C. (1930). *Die Psychologie der Schizophrenen*. Thieme, Leipzig.

Sham, P.C., Jones, P., Russell, A. *et al.* (1994). Age at onset, sex and familial psychiatric morbidity in schizophrenia: Camberwell Collaborative Psychosis Study. *Br J Psychiatry* **165**, 466–473.

Skoog, I. (1993). The prevalence of psychotic, depressive and anxiety syndromes in demented and non-demented 85 years olds. *Int J Geriatr Psychiatry* **8**, 247–253.

Symonds, L.L., Olichney, J.M., Jernigan, T.L., Corey-Bloom, J., Healy, J.F. and Jeste, D.V. (1997). Lack of clinically significant gross structural abnormalities in MRIs of older patients with schizophrenia and related psychoses. *J Neuropsychiatry Clin Neurosci* **9**, 251–258.

van Os, J., Howard, R., Takei, N. and Murray, R. (1995). Increasing age is a risk factor for psychosis in the elderly. *Social Psychiatry Psychiatric Epidemiology* **30**, 161–164.

Weissman, M.M., Myers, J.K., Tischler, G.L. *et al.* (1985). Psychiatric disorders (DSM-III) and cognitive impairment among the elderly in a US urban community. *Acta Psychiatr Scand* **71**, 366–379.

Williamson, J., Stokoe, I.H., Gray, S., Fisher, M. and Smith, A. (1964). Old people at home: their unreported needs. *Lancet* **i**, 1117–1120.

Late Onset Schizophrenia
Edited by Robert Howard, Peter V. Rabins, David J. Castle
© 1999 Wrightson Biomedical Publishing Ltd

11

Epidemiology of Late Onset Schizophrenia

DAVID J. CASTLE

Directorate of Mental Health Services, Fremantle Hospital and Health Service, Fremantle, Western Australia

The controversies surrounding the concept of late onset schizophrenia are addressed in some detail elsewhere in this book. The historical problems associated with the acceptance of the very existence of late onset schizophrenia, as well as differing conceptualizations of how to define and classify those psychotic disorders presenting for the first time in late life, make any reading of the literature on the epidemiology of such disorders extremely problematic.

This state of affairs has been compounded *inter alia* by

- Arbitrary and inconsistent age cut-offs being introduced in a number of different sets of diagnostic criteria for schizophrenia. For example, Feighner *et al.* (1972) introduced an age of onset below 40 years as a loading factor for a diagnosis of schizophrenia; the third revision of the American Psychiatric Association's (1980) Manual (DSM-III) stipulated that schizophrenia could simply not occur for the first time after the age of 44 years; and in Roth's (1955) description of 'late paraphrenia', an onset after the age of 60 was considered to be one of the defining features.
- Confusion about nosology. For example, Kraepelin's term 'paraphrenia' was adopted by Roth (1955) to describe a rather different type of disorder, which he named 'late paraphrenia', but which the WHO (1980) called 'paraphrenia' in the ninth revision of the *International Classification of Diseases* (ICD-9); this label has now been dropped altogether from the tenth revision of the ICD.
- The fact that in many countries, there is a split between health service provision for those older than 60–65 years, leading to an ignorance amongst many 'adult' psychiatrists of psychopathology in very late life.

- The belief, seemingly held by many clinicians, that psychotic symptoms manifesting in very late life are almost always consequent upon dementing processes.

These factors have contributed to late onset cases of schizophrenia and related disorders simply being ignored in many studies of incidence and prevalence of such disorders. For example, the 'ABC' study of Häfner *et al.* (1993) in Mannheim, Germany, had a cut-off at 59 years, whilst the World Health Organization's 'Determinants of Outcome of Severe Mental Illness' study (Jablensky *et al.*, 1992) did not consider any patients presenting for the first time after the age of 54 years. Furthermore, the adoption of certain sets of diagnostic criteria for schizophrenia results in the exclusion of late onset cases, as outlined above. With this in mind, we turn first to those few studies that have determined rates of psychotic phenomena in individuals in middle and late life, and which have avoided the use of any specific set of diagnostic criteria. Such studies inform us about the relationship between psychotic symptoms and age, and thus give some insight into the particular vulnerabilities of the ageing brain to such phenomena.

STUDIES OF PARANOID IDEATION IN THE ELDERLY

There are few studies which have specifically ascertained the prevalence of paranoid ideation in a general population sample of elderly patients. In one such study, Christenson and Blazer (1984) ascertained a stratified one-in-ten sample of residents over the age of 65 years, in Durham County, North Carolina; those resident in any type of institution (hospitals, nursing homes) were excluded. Of the 997 respondents interviewed using the Mini-Mult, an abridged version of the MMPI, 40 (4%) were considered to have generalized persecutory ideation. These individuals were more likely than non-paranoid individuals to be unmarried ($p < 0.05$) but the two groups did not differ from each other in terms of age, race, gender, or education. There was a positive correlation between paranoid ideation and sensory deficits ($p < 0.001$), and with cognitive impairment ($p < 0.0001$).

In a more recent study, Henderson *et al.* (1998) used the Australian Electoral Roll to select a representative sample of individuals over the age of 70 years, living in the community, and interviewed them using the Canberra Interview for the Elderly (CIE), which contains items on auditory hallucinosis and paranoid ideation. Of the 935 completed interviews, 65 persons reported at least one psychotic symptom (22 hallucinations only; 23 delusions only); of these, 25 had concomitant dementia, leaving 40 cognitively intact individuals reporting delusions and/or hallucinations, a rate of 4.3%.

Forsell and Henderson (1998) analysed a community sample of 1,420 individuals aged 75 years and over (range 75–102 years) who had been extensively investigated by physicians, including the administration of the Comprehensive Psychopathology Rating Scale (CPRS; Asberg *et al.*, 1978), which includes interview and observer-based items pertaining to paranoid ideation. Thus assessed, the presence of paranoid ideation was 6.3%. The major risk factors for paranoid ideation were cognitive impairment, being divorced, being female, having depressive symptoms, having no friends or visitors, and being an immigrant. Individuals with paranoid ideation were also more likely to be on psychotropic medications, and to be using community care resources.

Of course, such studies inevitably underestimate true prevalence, in that individuals who manifest psychotic symptoms are often suspicious and reluctant to talk about their symptoms to others. Furthermore, the psychotic symptoms often occur in individuals who are in any event socially isolated and thus unlikely to come to the attention of health professionals. Also, many individuals with an onset of psychotic symptoms in late life are well preserved in terms of other domains of functioning, and can thus carry on caring for themselves and hence not come to the attention of, for example, social services.

HALLUCINATIONS IN THE ELDERLY

We turn now to those few studies that have attempted a population based ascertainment of hallucinations in late life. One such study is the Epidemiological Catchment Area (ECA) survey in the USA, which used a lay-administered diagnostic instrument, the Diagnostic Interview Schedule (DIS) to interview a representative sample of the general population in five sites across the USA. The diagnostic groupings and rates of specific disorders generated by the DIS have been criticized on the grounds of lack of validity but the data on rates of hallucinations in the interviewees are useful to consider in their own right, as they provide some insight into this particular symptom, so commonly a feature of psychotic disorders, in relation to the ageing brain. Thus, Tien (1991) reported rates of hallucinosis in the ECA sample, by age and sex. These data reveal a rate of visual hallucinosis of around 20 per 1000 per year in males and 13 per 1000 per year in females between ages 18 and 80, with a steep rise to 40 per 1000 per year in males after age 80. For auditory hallucinosis, males showed an early peak (25–30 years), and females a later peak (40–50 years).

A specific type of hallucination occurring in late life is that form of visual hallucination occurring in the setting of impaired visual acuity. Named after Charles Bonnet (1760), the Genoese naturalist and philosopher who so carefully described the plight of his grandfather, who developed visual hallu-cinosis in clear consciousness after surgery for cataract, this eponymous syndrome has now become accepted in the literature. The author is aware of no studies that have adequately assessed rates of this syndrome in those elderly individuals with visual impairment, and the fact that case reports still appear in the journals, suggests that it is rare. The precise mechanisms involved are complex, and though the diagnosis should not be made in the setting of dementia or obvious cerebral pathology, it seems that there is considerable aetiological heterogeneity (see Damas-Mora *et al.*, 1982).

PSYCHOTIC PHENOMENA IN DEMENTIA

The fact that cognitive dysfunction was the strongest predictor of paranoid ideation in the study of Henderson *et al.* (1998) and of Forsell and Henderson (1998), as outlined above, should hardly surprise us. Indeed, it is well known that many individuals with dementia exhibit psychotic symptomatology at some stage of their illness process. Indeed, Wragg and Jeste (1989) reviewed 21 studies which had ascertained the prevalence of psychotic symptoms in patients with Alzheimer's disease. The sampling frames (general hospital, psychiatric wards, neurology wards, neurobehavioural referrals), diagnostic criteria for Alzheimer's disease (pathological, clinical, DSM-III), mode of assessment of psychotic symptoms (clinical assessment, own scale, Brief Psychiatric Rating Scale (BPRS), Schedule for Affective Disorders in Schizophrenia – Change version (SADS-C)), and stage of illness varied markedly from study to study, yet most found high rates of delusions and hallucinations. The prevalence of delusions ranged from 10% to 73%, with an aggregation in the range 30–38% (median 33.5%). Hallucinations report-edly occurred in 21–49% of patients (mean 28%); visual phenomena were more common than auditory (medians 22% and 13% respectively). Patients in acute general hospital settings were particularly likely to experience hallu-cinations. Non-specific psychotic phenomena were reported at some time during the course of illness in 20–58% of patients (median 34.5%).

It is important to note here that patients with late and very late onset schizophrenia do not have a longitudinal course of illness, which suggests they were merely mis-diagnosed and really have dementia. Indeed, the long-term follow-up study of Roth (1955), which compared the outcome of patients with dementia and late onset affective disorder with those with late paraphrenia (onset of a schizophrenia-like illness usually after age 60 years), showed a very much worse outcome for the dementia group. Having said this, there is some evidence that some patients labelled as having 'late paraphrenia' do appear to have a rather poor long-term outcome, as evidenced by the follow-up study of Holden (1987). This study followed 37 cases initially diagnosed as having late paraphrenia for 10 years or to death. Of these, 13 (35%) progressed to dementia within 3 years, and these were considered by the author to have an 'organic' form of illness.

PROPORTIONS OF SCHIZOPHRENIA PATIENTS WITH A LATE ONSET OF ILLNESS

We now turn to those studies that have assessed the rates of psychotic illnesses *per se* in elderly populations. Harris and Jeste (1988) reviewed the then published literature on the prevalence and incidence of treated samples of patients with late onset psychotic disorders. Inevitably, studies differed markedly in terms of diagnostic criteria employed, age cut-offs, and mode of ascertainment (e.g. hospitalized samples versus case registers). In a sensible approach to these data, Harris and Jeste conceded the difficulty in establishing prevalence rates, and rather computed weighted mean proportions of the disparate findings (weightings being based on sample size). Thus, they found a weighted mean proportion of schizophrenia patients with a first onset after the age of around 40 to be 23.5%. In an analysis of those studies specifically of late onset cases (mostly after age 40), the weighted means were 57.5% in the fifth decade, 30.2% in the sixth decade, and 12.3% after age 60; this translates as 13%, 7%, and 3% of all schizophrenia patients.

PREVALENCE STUDIES

Few studies have ascertained prevalent cases of schizophrenia and related disorders in late life in a community based sample. The ECA study cited above (Keith *et al.*, 1991) did attempt to do so in the context of an examination of rates of psychiatric disorders in a community sample of individuals of all adult ages. One-year prevalence rates for schizophrenia of 0.6% for individuals between ages 45 and 64 years, and 0.2% in those over age 65 years, were reported. However, the diagnostic validity in this study is questionable, as outlined above.

In a study of 612 community-living Chinese aged 65 years and over in Singapore, Kua (1992) used the GMS-AGECAT criteria and reported a prevalence of 0.5% for schizophrenia/paranoia. However, Copeland *et al.* (1992) used the same methodology in a sample of 1,070 subjects in Liverpool, UK, and found a prevalence for these disorders of only 0.1%.

In a further study, Copeland and colleagues (1998) made use of the Medical Research Council (UK) – Ageing in Liverpool – Health Aspects (MRC-ALPHA) sample of 5,222 individuals aged 65 years old and over, ascertained through general practitioner lists. Use was made of the GMS-

AGECAT computerized diagnostic system, with a proportion of cases also being interviewed by a psychiatrist. The prevalence of DSM-IIIR schizophrenia was 0.12% (95% CI 0.04–0.25), and of delusional disorder 0.04% (95% CI 0.00–0.14).

INCIDENCE STUDIES

In the MRC-ALPHA study of Copeland *et al.* (1998), outlined above, incidence rates for schizophrenia and delusional disorder were also ascertained, with estimates of 3.0 per 100,000 per year (95% CI 0.00–110.70) for schizophrenia, according to DSM-IIIR criteria.

Castle and Murray (1993) reported rates for non-affective psychotic disorders across all ages at onset, using data from the Camberwell Cumulative Case Register, a register of all contacts with the psychiatric services, from a defined inner-city London catchment area. Somewhat surprisingly, there was a high proportion of patients with a late onset form of illness (28% after 44 years and 12% after 64 years). Also of interest was that a high proportion of late onset and very late onset cases met stringent DSM-IIIR criteria for schizophrenia (52% of those with an onset after 44 years, compared with only 38% with an onset before that age). Rates of illness were as high as 12.6 per 100,000 population per year for those DSM-IIIR-defined cases with a first onset of illness after 44 years (this is nearly half the rate for those patients with an onset before 25 years).

In a somewhat different approach, van Os *et al.* (1995) examined the association between ageing and the incidence of schizophrenia-like psychoses manifesting for the first time after the age of 60 years. These authors used first admission data for patients admitted to hospitals for the first time in both The Netherlands and England and Wales, and found evidence in both data sets that increasing age was itself a risk factor for such disorders, with an average 11% increase in incidence with each 5 year increase in age.

The studies reviewed by Harris and Jeste (1988) were exclusively of treated samples of patients; the same is true of the Camberwell Register data, and the hospitalization data reported by van Os and colleagues. This inevitably biases the results in that many elderly patients with paranoid ideation do not seek help, or indeed see the need to seek help. This assertion is borne out by the data of Christenson and Blazer (1984), reported above, who found that, of the community-living individuals they assessed as having paranoid ideation, only half saw any need to seek help from health professionals, and even fewer had actually had contact with the psychiatric services. A handful of studies have tried to address this bias by ascertaining cases in the general population. For example, Parsons (1964) reported a prevalence rate of late paraphrenia of 1.7% amongst persons over age 65 years, resident in a Welsh town, whilst Williamson *et al.* (1964) reported a prevalence of 1% in a Scottish sample of elderly individuals. Whilst population based sampling has advantages over reliance solely on hospitalization rates, methodologically they are problematic in terms of reliability of diagnosis – problems in ensuring exclusion of individuals with dementia, as well as the inevitable reluctance of paranoid individuals to comply with questionnaires or talk to interviewers. Thus, it is likely that all these reported rates are underestimates, and there is conceivably extensive hidden morbidity in this area.

CONCLUSION

The epidemiology of late onset schizophrenia remains an under-studied area, made difficult by a number of methodological problems and ideological prejudices. However, those data that do exist suggest that the first onset of a schizophrenia-like illness after mid-life is a reality, and that a proportion of such cases have an illness consequent, in part at least, upon degenerative brain processes.

REFERENCES

American Psychiatric Association (1980). *Diagnostic and Statistical Manual of Mental Disorders*, 3rd edn (DSM-III). American Psychiatric Association, Washington, DC.

Asberg, M., Montgomery, S.A. and Perris, C. (1978). A comprehensive psychopathological rating scale. *Acta Psychiatr Scand* **271**, 5–27.

Bonnet, C. (1760). *Essai analytique sur les facultes de l'ame*. Philibert, Copenhagen.

Castle, D.J. and Murray, R.M. (1993). The epidemiology of late-onset schizophrenia. *Schizophr Bull* **19**, 691–700.

Christenson, R. and Blazer, D. (1984). Epidemiology of persecutory ideation in an elderly population in the community. *Am J Psychiatry* **141**, 59–67.

Copeland, J.R.M., Davidson, I.A., Dewey, M.E. *et al.* (1992). Alzheimer's disease, other dementias, depression, and pseudo-dementia: prevalence, incidence and three-year outcome in Liverpool. *Br J Psychiatry* **161**, 230–239.

Copeland, J.R.M., Dewey, M.E., Scott, A. *et al.* (1998). Schizophrenia and delusional disorder in older age: community prevalence, incidence, comorbidity and outcome. *Schizophr Bull* **24**, 153–161.

Damas-Mora, J., Skelton-Robinson, M. and Jenner, F.A. (1982). The Charles Bonnet syndrome in perspective. *Psychol Med* **12**, 251–261.

Feighner, J.P., Robins, E., Guze, S.B., Woodruff, R., Winokur, G. and Monoz, R. (1972). Diagnostic criteria for use in psychiatric research. *Arch Gen Psychiatry* **26**, 57–63.

Forsell, Y. and Henderson, A.S. (1998). Epidemiology of paranoid symptoms in an elderly population. *Br J Psychiatry* **172**, 429–432.

Häfner, H., Riecher-Rössler, A., an der Heiden, W., Maurer, K. Fätkenheuer, B. and

Löffler, W. (1993). Generating and testing a causal explanation of the gender difference in age at first onset of schizophrenia. *Psychol Med* **23**, 925–940.

Harris, J.M. and Jeste, D.V. (1988). Late-onset schizophrenia: an overview. *Schizophr Bull* **14**, 39–55.

Henderson, A.S., Korten, A.E., Levings, C. *et al.* (1998). Psychotic symptoms in the elderly: a prospective study in a population sample. *Int J Geriatr Psychiatry* **13**, 484–492.

Holden, N.L. (1987). Late paraphrenia or the paraphrenias? A descriptive study with a 10-year follow-up. *Br J Psychiatry* **150**, 635–639.

Jablensky, A., Sartorius, N. and Ernberg, G. (1992). Schizophrenia: manifestations, incidence, and course in different cultures. *Psychol Med*, Monograph suppl 20.

Keith, S.J., Regier, D.A. and Rae, D.S. (1991). Schizophrenic disorders. In: Robins, L.N. and Regier, D.A. (Eds), *Psychiatric Disorders in America*. Free Press, New York.

Kua, E.H.A. (1992). Community study of mental disorders in elderly Singaporean Chinese using the GMS-AGECAT package. *Austr NZ J Psychiatry* **26**, 502–506.

Parsons, P.L. (1964). Mental health of Swansea's old folk. *Br J Preventative Social Med* **19**, 43–47.

Roth, M. (1955). The natural history of mental disorders in old age. *J Mental Sci* **101**, 281–301.

Tien, A.Y. (1991). Distribution of hallucinations in the population. *Social Psychiatry Psychiatric Epidemiology* **26**, 287–292.

van Os, J., Howard, R., Takei, N. and Murray, R. (1995). Increasing age is a risk factor for psychosis in the elderly. *Social Psychiatry Psychiatric Epidemiology* **30**, 161–164.

Williamson, J., Stokoe, I.H., Gray, S., Fisher, M. and Smith, A. (1964). Old people at home: their unreported needs. *Lancet* **i**, 1117–1120.

World Health Organization (1980). *International Classification of Diseases, 9th edn.* World Health Organization, Geneva.

Wragg, R.E. and Jeste, D.V. (1989). Overview of depression and psychosis in Alzheimer's disease. *Am J Psychiatry* **146**, 577–587.

Late Onset Schizophrenia
Edited by Robert Howard, Peter V. Rabins, David J. Castle
© 1999 Wrightson Biomedical Publishing Ltd

12

Gender and Age at Onset in Schizophrenia

DAVID J. CASTLE

Directorate of Mental Health Services, Fremantle Hospital and Health Service, Fremantle, Western Australia

Whilst the nosological status of late life psychosis has been, and remains, a controversial area, one of the most consistent and robust findings of almost all studies in the area has been that females are over-represented amongst samples of patients whose first manifestation of illness occurs after mid-life. Table 1 details a selection of studies in different settings, with different methodologies, and employing different diagnostic criteria, which attest to the veracity of this conclusion.

It would seem that this robust finding of female proneness to late onset psychosis, can inform our understanding of psychoses in general, and more specifically, shed light on the aetiology of late life psychosis. In order to make sense of the gender differential, however, we need to consider potential confounding factors, and then place the findings into the context of psychosis across the life span.

DETERMINANTS OF AGE OF ONSET IN PSYCHOTIC ILLNESSES

The finding of a later onset of schizophrenia and related disorders in females is not readily explained in terms of differences in role-expectation or help-seeking behaviours between the sexes, having been reported in a number of different cultures, with very different societal role expectations, and diverse models of mental health service delivery (see Angermeyer *et al.*, 1988; Hambrecht *et al.*, 1992). Furthermore, the finding is robust, irrespective of the way in which 'onset' is defined (first signs of mental disturbance, first onset of illness, beginning of index episode, first hospitalization: see Riecher *et al.*, 1989).

Table 1. Selected series of late onset schizophrenia patients reporting gender ratio.

Reference	Number of cases	Ascertainment method	Diagnosis	Age (years)	Ratio female:male
Kay (1963)	57	Hospital admissions	Late paraphrenia[a]	>60	5.3:1
Herbert & Jacobsen (1967)	47	Hospital admissions	Systematized delusion ± hallucinations; not demented	>65	22.5:1
Huber et al. (1975)	644	Hospital admissions	Late onset schizophrenia; not organic	>40	1.8:1
Bland (1977)	6064	First admissions	ICD-8 schizophrenia	>40	1.6:1
Blessed & Wilson (1982)	320	Hospital admissions	Late paraphrenia[a]	>65	6:1
Grahame (1984)	25	Consecutive referrals	Late paraphrenia[a]	>60	3.2:1
Rabins et al. (1984)	35	Hospital admissions	Persistent delusional state; absence of mood or cognitive disorder	onset >44	10.7:1
Jørgensen & Munk-Jørgensen (1985)	106	First admissions	ICD-8 schizophrenia, paranoid state, reactive psychosis, other psychoses	>60	2.2:1
Holden (1987)	37	Case-register	Late paraphrenia[a] (13 cases considered 'organic' at follow-up)	>60	7:1 to 3:1[b]
Castle & Murray (1993)	477	Case-register	ICD-9 schizophrenia and related disorders, paraphrenia, atypical psychoses	>44	2.3:1
				>60	4.4:1
Almeida et al. (1995)	47	Referrals from a number of psychiatric settings	Late paraphrenia[a]	>65	9:1

[a]Akin to Roth's (1955) criteria.
[b]Dependent on whether 'organic' cases included.

There are, however, a number of psychosocial parameters that may potentially confound the finding of later onset of illness in women. One of these is marital status, in that males with schizophrenia are more likely than females to be unmarried, and unmarried individuals are likely to have an earlier onset of illness, than those who are married (Häfner *et al.*, 1993; Jablensky and Cole, 1997). Other factors reportedly associated with an early illness onset, and which are also more common in males than females with schizophrenia, include poor premorbid social and occupational adjustment (Foerster *et al.*, 1991) and premorbid personality disorder (Jablensky and Cole, 1997).

In terms of biological variables, associations have been found between early illness onset and a family history of schizophrenia (Sham *et al.*, 1994; Alda *et al.*, 1996); and with those obstetric complications implicated in the aetiology of schizophrenia (Verdoux *et al.*, 1997). Again, these factors might confound the finding of an earlier onset of illness amongst males. Indeed, in one of the few studies to examine the potential confounding and interaction effects of such factors, Jablensky and Cole (1997) used data on 778 men and 653 women in 10 countries to estimate the contributions of gender, family history, premorbid personality, and marital status, on age at onset. They reported strong main effects for marital status and premorbid personality, a weak effect for family history, and no effect for gender.

However, the causal associations here are complex, and difficult to tease apart definitively. Castle *et al.* (1998) assessed contributions to early illness onset in 477 patients with schizophrenia and related disorders, ascertained through a case-register. A contribution to early onset of illness from the following factors (significant at the 5% level) was confirmed: being single; poor premorbid employment history; poor premorbid social adjustment; and premorbid personality disorder. There was a trend (10% level) towards earlier onset being predicted by a family history of schizophrenia, developmental problems, and obstetric complications.

Using multiple regression to explore the independent effects of these parameters, and their effect on the gender differential, we found that the influences of poor premorbid social adjustment and personality disorder disappeared once single marital status was controlled for, leaving single marital status and poor premorbid work adjustment as the main variables associated with early illness onset. These factors operated in the same manner for both men and women (i.e. there was no significant statistical interaction). In the combined male/female analysis, male sex was found to be an independent predictor of early onset even after controlling for all other variables (although the strength of the association was marginally reduced). Thus, it appears that the later onset of illness in females with schizophrenia and related disorders cannot be explained by confounding variables, suggesting that the reasons behind the differences should be sought in factors associated with inherent differences between the sexes.

Another way of looking at this issue is to assess age at onset in highly familial samples of patients. There are a number of studies which have taken this approach (e.g. Alda *et al.*, 1996), and these consistently report that in such samples, there is no significant age at onset difference between the sexes. The implications of these findings are discussed below, but first we place the gender differential in age at onset in the context of gender differences in psychotic disorders across the life span.

GENDER AND PSYCHOTIC DISORDERS ACROSS THE LIFE SPAN

Many authors conclude that schizophrenia affects men and women roughly equally but that women tend to have a later mean onset of illness than males. However, this bland conclusion fails to accommodate the subtleties of the epidemiological findings, and reliance merely on mean ages at onset is a simplification which is not truly responsive to the data themselves. Furthermore, many studies have simply excluded those patients with an onset of illness in later life. For example the 'ABC' study by Häfner *et al.* (1993) excluded patients with an onset of illness after the age of 59 years, whilst the 10-country WHO 'Determinants of Outcome for Severe Mental Disorders' study (Jablensky *et al.*, 1992) had an age cut-off at 54 years. This problem has been compounded by the fact that certain sets of diagnostic criteria for schizophrenia included an age cut-off, and studies employing those criteria simply did not take account of later onset patients. Examples include the criteria of Feighner *et al.* (1972), which stipulate an onset of illness before 40 years as one of the criteria loading for a diagnosis of schizophrenia. The schizophrenia diagnostic criteria published in the third edition of the American Psychiatric Association's *Diagnostic and Statistical Manual* (APA, 1980) precluded a diagnosis of schizophrenia if the onset of illness was after 44 years of age; this criterion has been dropped from subsequent editions of the Manual but its impact has been pervasive.

What is also problematic is that the male:female ratio in non-affective psychotic disorders is profoundly influenced by the diagnostic criteria employed, with males more likely to fulfil those sets of criteria that emphasize severe symptoms and long illness duration. For example, Lewine *et al.* (1984) found that none of the females in their study met the Feighner diagnostic criteria for schizophrenia. In a register based catchment area study, Castle *et al.* (1993) found that both age at onset and diagnostic criteria employed affected the male:female ratio. For example, in patients with an onset under 45 years, ICD-9 (WHO, 1980) criteria for schizophrenia and related disorders resulted in a female:male ratio of 0.71:1, whilst DSM-IIIR criteria excluded more females than males, with a resultant sex ratio of

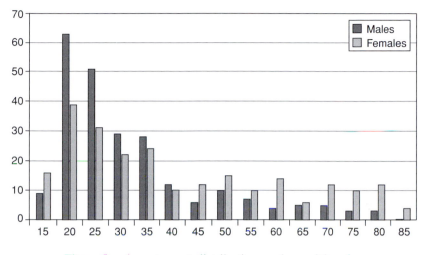

Figure 1.   Age at onset distribution, males and females.

0.45:1. In contrast, females exceeded males amongst those patients with an onset of illness after 44 years, in a ratio of around 2:1, irrespective of stringency of diagnosis.

Thus, we need to turn to studies that have considered non-affective psychotic disorders across the life span, and which have not employed restrictive diagnostic criteria, in order fully to appreciate the complexity of the age distributions. Figures 1 and 2 (a) and (b) show data from two such studies. Figure 1 represents a population based catchment area sample of 470 patients with schizophrenia and related disorders, ascertained over a period of 20 years through the Camberwell Cumulative Case Register (see Castle *et al.*, 1993). Figures 2 (a) and (b) show first admission data (for males and females, respectively) for 9,439 individuals with ICD-8/9 schizophrenia and related disorders extracted from the Queensland (Australia) Mental Health Statistics System (McLachlan *et al.*, 1998).

It is very clear from both these sets of data that, far from there being a simple shift of the mean onset of illness to the right in females, the distributions of onset for males and females are very different in shape. Indeed, even speaking of means in this context is both erroneous and misleading. One approach that is more responsive to the data is to assess whether the distributions can be interpreted in terms of admixture analyses, looking for statistical evidence that the 'fit' of distributions differs between the sexes. In the Camberwell data set (Figure 1), Castle *et al.* (1998) employed SKUMIX to investigate this matter and found that the male distribution could be best explained by a model with two age distributions, with modal ages of onset

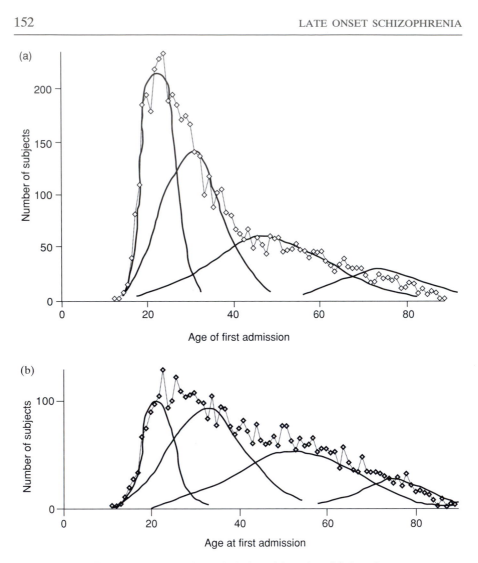

Figure 2.   Age at first admission. (a) males; (b) females.

of 21 and 39 years. Females, on the other hand, showed evidence of three distributions, with modal onsets at 22, 37, and 62 years.

   In the much larger Queensland sample (5,168 males, 4,271 females), McLachlan and colleagues (1998) used normal mixture analysis to show a four-component model best explained the distributions. For males, 27% fell into the early onset component (mean onset 22 years), 36% the second component (mean 30 years), 31% the third component (mean 49 years), and 6% the fourth component (mean 73 years). For females, the comparable proportions and mean ages for the four components were: 18% (22 years), 32% (32 years), 43% (52 years), and 8% (75 years). These distributions are represented graphically in Figures 2 (a) and (b).

Both these sets of findings underline the complexity of age-at-onset distributions in psychotic disorders. They also converge in the finding that an early onset of illness is particularly a characteristic of schizophrenia in males, that there is a mid-life 'peak' predominated by females, and that in very late onset cases there is again a female excess. We now turn to a brief overview of gender differences in the clinical expression of schizophrenia and related disorders.

SEX DIFFERENCES IN CLINICAL EXPRESSION OF SCHIZOPHRENIA

It is useful to consider gender differences in the clinical expression of schizophrenia and related disorders at different stages of the developmental trajectory. Thus, whilst the positive symptoms of these disorders (delusions and hallucinations) manifest themselves for the first time only in adulthood, it has been shown that a proportion of such individuals show deviations from normal development early in life (e.g. Foerster et al., 1991; Jones et al., 1994). In terms of gender, such deviations from normal tend to be a feature of males rather than females who later manifest psychotic illnesses. For example, Aylward et al. (1984) performed a meta-analysis of studies reporting premorbid IQ in schizophrenia patients and found that low premorbid IQ was a characteristic of males but not females who later manifested schizophrenia. It has also been shown that poor premorbid social and occupational functioning is more common amongst males than females who later manifest schizophrenia (see Castle and Murray, 1991).

In terms of clinical expression of symptoms, it has long been recognized that females with psychotic illnesses tend to manifest more affective symptoms than their male counterparts and that they are less likely to show negative symptoms. Such findings might have been influenced to some extent by the inclusion of females with affective psychoses, and by medication effects. However, Goldstein and Link (1988) investigated expression of illness in 169 patients (65 female) with DSM-III defined schizophrenia, and confirmed that, even in a group meeting these stringent criteria for the illness, females were more likely than males to exhibit affective symptoms. It has been found that males are more likely to manifest negative symptoms and to exhibit poor premorbid adjustment.

Consideration of the longitudinal course of illness can inform explanatory models. In terms of gender effects, males with schizophrenia have consistently been shown to have a poorer outcome than their female counterparts.

This is true whether one considers rehospitalization rates, social functioning, or employment parameters (Seeman, 1986; Angermeyer *et al.*, 1990; Goldstein, 1995).

Considerable excitement has been generated by the fairly consistent finding that patients with schizophrenia show more structural brain abnormalities than unaffected controls. Again, it is only more recently that gender effects have been considered in this regard and most studies have not been designed to assess gender effects. In those studies which have reported gender effects, results have been conflicting. However, Lewine (1995), who recently reviewed the relevant literature, concluded that '...although the picture remains inconsistent, when gender differences are found, there is usually greater brain morphological divergence from control subjects in men with schizophrenia. These anomalies appear to be lateralised to the left hemisphere...'.

Finally, we consider aetiological parameters. The most robust of all aetiological factors in schizophrenia is genetic. Only recently has consideration been given to possible differences in genetic loading in males and females with schizophrenia but in those studies that have considered this, it has been consistently reported that it is females who have a higher familial loading (reviewed by Goldstein, 1995).

Other factors implicated in the aetiology of schizophrenia include obstetric complications and early head injury. Verdoux *et al.* (1997) performed a meta-analysis of studies exploring the role of obstetric complications in schizophrenia and reported a positive association which was most marked for males. Data on early head injury are less compelling and confounding factors are difficult to exclude comprehensively. However, Nasrallah and Wilcox (1989) reported a differential male vulnerability amongst schizophrenia patients to early head injury.

Another 'environmental' aetiological parameter to excite recent attention has been the potential causal association between *in utero* exposure to influenza and later schizophrenia. It should be stressed that such findings remain tentative but such evidence as does exist suggests that any 'schizophrenogenic effect' of maternal influenza is more likely to be aetiologically relevant in females rather than males who later manifest schizophrenia (McGrath and Castle, 1995).

PSYCHOTIC PHENOMENA IN MEN AND WOMEN ACROSS THE LIFE SPAN

We now turn to a consideration of those few studies that have assessed psychotic phenomena, rather than specific diagnostic groups, in men and women across all ages. The study of Tien (1991) is particularly informative.

This study was based on the large Epidemiological Catchment Area (ECA) sample of the general population in five sites in the USA. Apart from reporting diagnostic issues, the study also allowed an analysis of the incidence of hallucinations by age and sex. Thus, for visual phenomena, males were slightly more prone than females until the age of 60 years (around 20 per 1000 per year, versus 13 per 1000 per year for females), whereafter the rate in females exceeded that in males; the sex differential was particularly dramatic after the age of 80 years (around 40 per 1000 per year for females). In terms of auditory hallucinations, the distribution was more complex. In males, there was a peak in the 25–30 year age group (around 25 per 1000 per year), whilst females showed a later peak (40–50 years; around 35 per 1000 per year) and a second peak after the age of 70 years (35 per 1000 per year).

Delusional beliefs in the general population are particularly difficult to assess, as one would expect that individuals with such beliefs would be reticent about reporting them. However, Verdoux *et al.* (1998) assessed delusional ideation amongst general practice attenders without any psychiatric history (207 males, 237 females; mean age 51.6, range 18–95 years) using a self-report measure. Responses were subjected to a principal components analysis, with seven dimensions explaining 55% of the variance. The dimensions encompassing 'persecution', 'thought disturbance', 'grandiosity', and 'abnormal beliefs' were negatively associated with age. The only dimension positively correlated with age was 'religiosity'. Overall, highest mean dimension scores were found in subjects aged 18–29 years for 'thought disturbances' and 'grandiosity'; 30–49 years for 'persecution'; and 80–95 years for 'religiosity'. In terms of gender, young males were most likely to exhibit grandiosity but the other dimensions were not modified by gender.

In a study particularly of elderly individuals, Christenson and Blazer (1984) interviewed a one-in-ten stratified random sample of individuals over the age of 65 years, resident in Durham County, North Carolina. They found that 40 of the 997 subjects (4%) exhibited generalized persecutory ideation but there were no significant differences between males and females; the possibility of a type II error with a small sample such as this cannot be excluded.

In a study with more statistical power, Forsell and Henderson (1998) investigated paranoid ideation in 1,420 community-living elderly patients, using the Comprehensive Psychopathological Rating Scale (Asberg *et al.*, 1978). They found a prevalence of paranoid ideation of 6.3%. Cognitive dysfunction, as measured by the Mini-Mental State Examination (MMSE; Folstein *et al.*, 1975), was the strongest predictor of paranoid ideation, but even after controlling for this in a logistic regression analysis, female gender was positively associated with paranoid ideation, with an odds ratio (adjusted) of 2.5 (95% CI 1.2–5.3).

SEX DIFFERENCES IN THE AGEING BRAIN:
IMPLICATIONS FOR PSYCHOSIS

Whilst it has been well established in neuropathological studies that the human brain shows age-related decreases in weight and volume, and that there is a loss of cortical neurones as part of normal involutional processes, it is only more recently that neuroimaging studies have allowed systematic consideration of age-related changes in specific cortical regions and in subcortical structures. For example, Jernigan *et al.* (1991) performed MRI scans on 55 individuals (21 female) with no history of dementia, ranging in age from 30 to 79 years (mean 53.8, SD 14.1). They found significant age-related decreases in the volume of the caudate nucleus and in anterior diencephalic structures, whilst there was little noticeable change in thalamic volume. There were also volume reductions in cortical grey matter, most marked in association cortex and mesial temporal lobe structures; it appeared that anterior cingulate cortex was relatively spared.

Murphy *et al.* (1996) performed a study particularly to assess gender differences in age-related brain changes. These investigators performed MRI scans on 69 healthy right handed individuals (34 female) divided into two age groups, namely 20–35 years and 60–85 years. They found that, whilst male brains showed greater age-related loss of whole-brain and frontal and temporal lobe volume than their female counterparts, females showed more extensive volume loss with age in parietal lobe and hippocampus. There were also differences in right–left asymmetry with age between men and women, with the left hemisphere being particularly affected in females.

A study of brain metabolism, measured by PET, also showed a differential effect of age in men and women (Murphy *et al.*, 1996). Thus, women showed more age-related metabolic decline in thalamus and hippocampus than their male counterparts; the hippocampal metabolism in females became less than in males around the age of 70 years.

Of particular interest to the consideration of psychotic disorders in the elderly is the effect of age on the dopamine system, given the involvement of that system in the pathogenesis of psychotic symptoms. It has been shown that the density of both dopamine D_1 and D_2 receptors declines with age but little consideration has been given to gender effects. In one of the few studies to analyse dopamine receptor density by age in males and females separately, Wong *et al.* (1984) reported loss of D_2 receptors in caudate, putamen, and frontal cortex in men and women aged 19–73 years. The rate and pattern of loss differed between the sexes: males showed an exponential decline in D_2 receptors, whilst for females the decline was essentially linear. A more recent study of dopamine D_2 receptor density in 33 men and 21 women (age 19–82 years; mean 40.2, SD 16.7), also using PET, confirms the sex differential, with men showing a rate of decline in D_2 receptors twice that of women (Pohjalainen *et al.*, 1998).

What is also important is that the decline in D_2 receptor density begins at a young age (under 20 years, and earlier for males than females). The cross-over in rate of decline between men and women occurs at around the age of 30 years (extrapolation from figures presented by Wong *et al.*, 1984). Put simply, males start with a relative excess of D_2 receptors compared with women but lose them earlier and more rapidly, such that in later life it is females who have a relative excess of these receptors. Furthermore, loss of D_2 receptors has been shown to be associated with both motor tasks and tests of frontal lobe functioning, including abstraction and mental flexibility and attention and response inhibition (Volkow *et al.*, 1998). Similar impairments have been shown in individuals with schizophrenia, reinforcing the message that consideration of dopamine system changes with age can potentially inform our consideration of ageing and psychotic illnesses.

INTERPRETATION: A CONTRIBUTION FOR SEX HORMONES?

The explanation for the differential age at onset of schizophrenia between men and women has been sought in a number of different domains. Lewine (1981) has usefully divided the competing hypotheses into two main areas, namely a 'timing' effect, where onset is either 'brought forward' in males and/or 'delayed' in females; or a typological approach, where men and women are seen as being differentially vulnerable to more-or-less discrete subtypes of illness, with different mean ages at onset.

Within each of these models, explanatory hypotheses encompass psychosocial and biological domains. For example, the 'timing' model includes consideration of role-stress differences between the sexes, and differences in help-seeking behaviour between males and females and their families. Whilst such influences may have some part to play, it is difficult to envisage them being major determinants of the sex differential in age at onset, given the fact that the differential has been found in a number of different countries with vastly different cultural expectations and mental health services (Hambrecht *et al.*, 1992). Furthermore, as detailed above, controlling for psychosocial confounding factors does not obviate the sex differential in age at onset. A more parsimonious 'timing' effect could be attributed to the sex hormones. Thus, it has been proposed that the testosterone surge at adolescence in males might serve to 'trigger' the onset of psychosis at that age. However, testosterone levels have not been shown to have a direct relationship to schizophrenia onset (Seeman and Lang, 1990).

More credence can be given to a potential protective effect of oestrogens during the reproductive period in females. Indeed, laboratory and clinical investigations have attested to oestrogen possessing anti-dopaminergic properties. Thus, animal experiments have revealed that oestradiol reduces the behavioural changes induced by the dopamine antagonist haloperidol (catalepsy) and the dopamine agonist apomorphine (oral stereotypies, grooming behaviours) (see Riecher-Rössler and Häfner, 1993). Furthermore, studies of women with schizophrenia have suggested that there is a worsening of psychotic symptomatology at the time of low oestrogens during the menstrual cycle. And oestrogens themselves might actually serve to reduce psychotic symptomatology, at least in the immediate term (Kulkarni *et al.*, 1996).

Such findings have led Häfner and colleagues (1993) to propose that the 'second peak' in schizophrenia in women in their 40s is a direct result of the decline of oestrogen levels at the menopause. However, this conclusion does not account for the fact that males also seem to exhibit a 'peak' of onset of illness at that age (admittedly a smaller peak: see above). Furthermore, oestrogen cannot account for the differential male proneness amongst children who later manifest schizophrenia to premorbid dysfunction (as outlined above), nor can sex hormones readily explain the massive female preponderance in very late onset schizophrenia. Finally, the finding that sex differences in onset of illness disappear in highly familial samples (see above) also suggests that factors other than oestrogen play a profound effect on the determination of timing of onset of illness. One proposed explanation for the latter finding has been a vulnerability locus for psychosis on the X-chromosome that determines age at onset of psychosis (DeLisi, 1989) but such a locus has not been found in genetic linkage studies.

A TYPOLOGICAL APPROACH

It has been proposed elsewhere that a plausible model for explaining gender differences in age at onset of schizophrenia, and which encompasses a number of the other gender differences outlined above, is that there exist a number of subtypes of illness to which males and females are differentially prone. The putative subtype with perhaps most support from research is that of an early onset male-predominant illness akin to Kraepelin's 'dementia praecox', and with a neurodevelopmental aetiology. Females appear less prone to this form of illness by virtue of their inherent lower vulnerability to neurodevelopmental disorders (see Castle and Murray, 1991; Murray *et al.*, 1992)

To test this hypothesis, Castle *et al.* (1994) and Sham *et al.* (1996) performed a latent class analysis of the Camberwell Register sample (details of the sample have been provided above). The existence of a subtype of illness with many of the features of dementia praecox, including a marked preponderance of males, an early onset of illness (mostly under 25 years), poor premorbid adjustment and negative symptoms was confirmed. In terms of aetiological factors, a family loading for schizophrenia and obstetric complications were both positively associated with this subtype.

We also found that a proportion of the later onset patients have a form of illness with links to affective disorder, with strong affective flavouring, and a family loading for affective disorder; we called this subtype 'schizo-affective'. Females predominate in this group, perhaps a reflection of their vulnerability to affective disorders overall.

However, this putative subtype does not encompass all of those patients with a first manifestation of psychosis in middle life. What we do know is that such patients generally have better premorbid adjustment than their early onset counterparts, that they manifest paranoia but generally do not exhibit prominent disorganization symptoms, and that their longitudinal course is relatively benign, with little by way of personality disintegration. That this group forms a relatively robust subtype of schizophrenia is fairly well established (e.g. Tsuang and Winokur, 1974; Farmer et al., 1983). In our latent class analysis, evidence was also found for a subtype with many of these features; intriguingly, an association with winter birth in the setting of a low familial morbid risk for schizophrenia was also found, suggesting that environmental aetiological factors might be important in such individuals (Castle et al., 1994).

VERY LATE ONSET PATIENTS

This typology does not adequately account for the very late onset or 'late paraphrenia' patients, amongst whom, as we have seen, females predominate (see Table 1). It is suggested that the very late onset group of patients have a form of illness consequent upon a rather different set of aetiological factors, and that brain degenerative processes are a critical determinant. The reason why females are so over-represented amongst such patients is not entirely clear. As outlined above, it is not as though they are simply 'catching up' with their earlier-onset male counterparts. Nor is it conceivable that they have an underlying predisposition to a psychotic illness, manifestation of which was being 'masked' by oestrogens, and which manifests itself upon withdrawal of this masking factor: indeed, the mean onset in this group is way beyond that of the menopause.

What is more likely is that this group is itself heterogeneous in terms of underlying predisposition but that degenerative brain changes lead to symptoms becoming manifest for the first time only in very late life. Support for this notion comes from a number of disparate sources. It is well established that a significant proportion of dementia patients experience delusions and hallucinations. In reviewing studies reporting on psychotic symptoms in Alzheimer's disease, for example, Wragg and Jeste (1989) calculated a median prevalence for delusions of 33.5% (persecutory delusions being particularly common) and for hallucinations 28% (visual hallucinations, 22%; auditory, 13%). Extrapolation from dementia patients to those with late paraphrenia is not entirely satisfactory but the general population study of Forsell and Henderson (1998) showed the strongest predicator of paranoid ideation in the elderly to be cognitive dysfunction.

Using a different strategy, van Os *et al.* (1995) reported increasing age to be a risk factor for psychosis in the elderly, with a linear trend being shown in the association between increasing age and first admission rates for non-affective non-organic psychosis. Again, subtle degenerative brain changes are probably implicated.

In neuroimaging studies, particularly of late paraphrenia patients, an excess of white- and grey-matter abnormalities has been detected, although the extent to which these could be attributed to vascular risk factors, and the non-specificity of the findings (similar changes have been seen in affective disorder patients), make the interpretation difficult (see Castle and Howard, 1992).

Finally, although Roth's (1955) landmark study showed how the long-term follow-up of patients with late paraphrenia is far more benign than those with dementia, it is increasingly clear that the outcome for such patients is not uniformly good. For example, Holden (1987) followed up 47 patients with late paraphrenia over a period of 10 years or until death and found evidence that a subgroup of 13 patients (28% of the whole) progressed to dementia within 3 years; he considered this to be an 'organic' form of the illness.

A more recent study (Almeida *et al.*, 1995), which included extensive clinical and neuropsychological assessments in 47 late paraphrenia patients, also found evidence of clinical and cognitive heterogeneity. Around half the patients showed widespread cognitive impairment, encompassing performance, memory and executive functions. The remaining patients, in contrast, exhibited only very subtle impairment, mostly in terms of executive functioning. The latter group also showed more severe psychotic symptoms and were more likely to exhibit Schneiderian first rank symptoms of schizophrenia. However, they were less likely to show neurological impairment and negative symptoms.

Thus, it seems reasonable to propose that the first manifestation of a schizophrenia-like illness in very late life is mediated to some extent at least (and to a variable extent individual to individual) by degenerative brain changes, be these at the level of actual neuronal loss or at the level of specific receptor densities (e.g. the dopamine D_2 receptor). It is likely that such changes interact with underlying risk factors (e.g. genetic loading; paranoid premorbid personality traits; sensory impairment: see Castle and Howard, 1992). The female excess amongst late paraphrenia patients could, then, be seen as a reflection of differential brain changes with age, in men and women.

As outlined above, it appears that not only are male and female brains different from early in life but they age differently. These factors can inform our understanding of gender differences in psychotic disorders across the life span, and should certainly be considered in any explanations of gender differences in late onset schizophrenia.

ACKNOWLEDGEMENTS

I am most grateful to Professor John McGrath and Ms Joy Welham of the Queensland Centre for Schizophrenia Research, for permission to publish Figures 2 (a) and (b).

REFERENCES

Alda, M., Ahrens, B., Lit, W. *et al.* (1996). Age of onset in familial and sporadic schizophrenia. *Acta Psychiatr Scand* **93**, 447–450.

Almeida, O.P., Howard, R.J., Levy, R. and David, A.S. (1995). Cognitive and clinical diversity in psychotic states arising in late life (late paraphrenia). *Psychol Med* **25**, 699–714.

American Psychiatric Association (1980). *Diagnostic and Statistical Manual for Mental Disorders, 3rd edn* (DSM-III). American Pssychiatric Association, Washington, DC.

Angermeyer, M.C., Goldstein, J.M. and Kuhn, L. (1988). Gender differences in age at onset in schizophrenia: an overview. *Eur Arch Psychiatry Neurol Sci* **237**, 351–364.

Angermeyer, M.C., Kuhn, L. and Goldstein, J.M. (1990). Sex and the course of schizophrenia: differences in treated outcomes. *Schizophr Bull* **16**, 293–307.

Asberg, M., Perris, C., Schalling, D. and Sedvall, G. (1978). The CPRS: development and application of a psychiatric rating scale. *Acta Psychiatr Scand* **271** (Suppl.), 5–27.

Aylward, E., Walker, E. and Bettes, B. (1984). Intelligence and schizophrenia: a meta-analysis. *Schizophr Bull* **10**, 430–459.

Bland, R.C. (1977). Demographic aspects of functional psychoses in Canada. *Acta Psychiatr Scand* **55**, 369–380.

Blessed, G. and Wilson, I.D. (1982). The contemporary natural history of mental disorder in old age. *Br J Psychiatry* **141**, 59–67.

Castle, D.J. and Howard, R. (1992). What do we know about the aetiology of late onset schizophrenia? *Eur Psychiatry* **7**, 99–108.

Castle, D.J. and Murray, R.M. (1991). The neurodevelopmental basis of sex differences in schizophrenia. *Psychol Med* **21**, 565–575.

Castle, D.J. and Murray, R.M. (1993). The epidemiology of late onset schizophrenia. *Schizophr Bull* **19**, 691–700.

Castle, D.J., Wessely, S. and Murray, R.M. (1993). Sex and schizophrenia: effects of diagnostic stringency, and associations with premorbid variables. *Br J Psychiatry* **162**, 658–664.

Castle, D.J., Sham, P., Wessely, S. and Murray, R.M. (1994). The subtyping of schizophrenia in men and women: a latent class analysis. *Psychol Med* **24**, 41–51.

Castle, D.J., Sham, P.C. and Murray, R.M. (1998). Differences in distribution of ages of onset in males and females with schizophrenia. *Schizophr Res* **33**, 179–183.

Christenson, R. and Blazer, D. (1984). Epidemiology of persecutory ideation in an elderly population in the community. *Am J Psychiatry* **141**, 59–67.

DeLisi, L.E. (1989). The significance of age of onset for schizophrenia. *Schizophr Bull* **15**, 209–215.

Farmer, A.E., McGuffin, P. and Spitznagel, E.L. (1983). Heterogeneity in schizophrenia: a cluster-analytic approach. *Psychiatry Res* **8**, 1–12.

Feighner, J.P., Robins, E., Guze, S.B., Woodruff, R., Winokur, G. and Munoz, R. (1972). Diagnostic criteria for use in psychiatric research. *Arch Gen Psychiatry* **26**, 57–63.

Foerster, A., Lewis, S.W., Owen, M.J. and Murray, R.M. (1991). Premorbid adjustment and personality in psychosis: effect of sex and diagnosis. *Br J Psychiatry* **158**, 171–176.

Folstein, M.F., Folstein, S.E. and McHugh, P.R. (1975). 'Mini-Mental State': a practical method for grading the cognitive state of patients for the clinician. *J Psychiatr Res* **12**, 189–198.

Forsell, Y. and Henderson, A.S. (1998). Epidemiology of paranoid symptoms in an elderly population. *Br J Psychiatry* **172**, 429–432.

Goldstein, J.M. (1995). Gender and the familial transmission of schizophrenia. In: Seeman, M.V. (Ed.), *Gender and Psychopathology*. American Psychiatric Association, Washington, DC, pp. 201–226.

Goldstein, J.M. and Link, B.G. (1988). Gender and the expression of schizophrenia. *J Psychiatr Res* **22**, 141–155.

Grahame, P.S. (1984). Schizophrenia in old age (late paraphrenia). *Br J Psychiatry* **145**, 493–495.

Häfner, H., Riecher-Rössler, A., an der Heiden, W., Maurer, K., Fätkenheuer, B. and Löffler, W. (1993). Generating and testing a causal explanation of the gender difference in first onset of schizophrenia. *Psychol Med* **23**, 925–940.

Hambrecht, M., Maurer, K., Häfner, H. and Sartorius, N. (1992). Transnational stability of gender differences in schizophrenia. *Eur Arch Psychiatry Neurol Sci* **242**, 6–12.

Herbert, M.E. and Jacobsen, S. (1967). Late paraphrenia. *Br J Psychiatry* **113**, 461–469.

Holden, N.L. (1987). Late paraphrenia or the paraphrenias? A descriptive study with 10-year follow-up. *Br J Psychiatry* **150**, 635–639.

Huber, G., Gross, G. and Schüttler, R. (1975). Spätschizophrenie. *Arch Psychiatr Nervenkr* **221**, 53–66.

Jablensky, A. and Cole, S.W. (1997). Is the earlier age at onset of schizophrenia in males a confounded finding? *Br J Psychiatry* **170**, 234–240.

Jablensky, A., Sartorius, N. and Ernberg, G. (1992). Schizophrenia: manifestations, incidence and course in different cultures. *Psychol Med*, Monograph suppl 20.

Jernigan, T.L., Archibald, S.L., Berhow, M.T., Sowell, E.R., Foster, D.S. and Hesselink, J.R. (1991). Cerebral structure on MRI: Part 1: Localisation of age-related changes. *Biol Psychiatry* **29**, 55–67.

Jones, P., Rodgers, B., Murray, R. and Marmot, M. (1994). Child developmental risk factors for adult schizophrenia in the British 1946 birth cohort. *Lancet* **344**, 1398–1402.

Jørgensen, P. and Munk-Jørgensen, P. (1985). Paranoid psychoses in the elderly. *Acta Psychiatr Scand* **72**, 358–363.

Kay, D.W.K. (1963). Late paraphrenia and its bearing on the aetiology of schizophrenia. *Acta Psychiatr Scand* **39**, 159–169.

Kulkarni, J., de Castella, A., Smith, D., Taffe, J., Keks, N. and Copolov, D. (1996). A clinical trial of the effects of estrogen in acutely psychotic women. *Schizophr Res* **20**, 247–252.

Lewine, R.R.J. (1981). Sex differences in schizophrenia: timing or subtypes? *Psychol Bull* **90**, 432–444.

Lewine, R.R.J. (1995). Gender, brain, and schizophrenia. In: Seeman, M.V. (Ed.), *Gender and Psychopathology*. American Psychiatric Association, Washington, DC, pp. 131–158.

Lewins, R.R.J., Burbach, D. and Meltzer, H.Y. (1984). Effect of diagnostic criteria on the ratio of male to female schizophrenic patients. *Am J Psychiatry* **141**, 84–87.

McGrath, J. and Castle, D.J. (1995). Does influenza cause schizophrenia? A five-year review. *Austr NZ J Psychiatry* **29**, 23–31.

McLachlan, G., Welham, J. and McGrath, J. (1998). Heterogeneity in schizophrenia: a mixture model based on age-of-onset, gender and diagnosis. *Schizophr Res* **29**, 21.

Murphy, D.G.M., DeCarli, C., McIntosh, A.R. *et al.* (1996). Sex differences in human brain morphometry and metabolism: an *in-vivo* quantitative magnetic resonance imaging and positron emission tomography study on the effect of aging. *Arch Gen Psychiatry* **53**, 585–594.

Murray, R.M., O'Callaghan, E., Castle, D.J. and Lewis, S.W. (1992). A neurodevelopmental approach to the classification of schizophrenia. *Schizophr Bull* **18**, 319–332.

Nasrallah, H.A. and Wilcox, J.A. (1989). Gender differences in the etiology and symptoms of schizophrenia: genetic versus brain injury factors. *Ann Clin Psychiatry* **1**, 51–53.

Pohjalainen, T., Rinne, J.O., Nagren, K., Syvalahti, E. and Hietala, J. (1998). Sex differences in the striatal dopamine D2 receptor binding characteristics *in vivo*. *Am J Psychiatry* **155**, 768–773.

Rabins, P., Paulker, S. and Thomas, J. (1984). Can schizophrenia begin after age 44? *Compr Psychiatry* **25**, 290–293.

Riecher, A., Maurer, K., Löffler, W., Fätkenheuer, B., an der Heiden, W. and Häfner, H. (1989). Schizophrenia: a disease of single young males? *Eur Arch Psychiatry Neurol Sci* **239**, 210–212.

Riecher-Rössler, A. and Häfner, H. (1993). Schizophrenia and oestrogens: is there an association? *Eur Arch Psychiatry Neurol Sci* **242**, 323–328.

Roth, M. (1955). The natural history of mental disorder in old age. *J Mental Sci* **101**, 281–301.

Seeman, M.V. (1986). Current outcome in schizophrenia: women vs men. *Acta Psychiatr Scand* **73**, 609–617.

Seeman, M.V. and Lang, M. (1990). The role of oestrogens in schizophrenia gender differences. *Schizophr Bull* **16**, 185–194.

Sham, P.C., Jones, P., Russell, A. *et al.* (1994). Age at onset, sex, and familial psychiatric morbidity in schizophrenia. Report from the Camberwell Collaborative Study. *Br J Psychiatry* **165**, 466–473.

Sham, P.C., Castle, D.J., Wessely, S., Farmer, A.E. and Murray, R.M. (1996). Further exploration of a latent class typology of schizophrenia. *Schizophr Res* **20**, 105–115.

Tien, A.Y. (1991). Distribution of hallucinations and delusions in the population. *Social Psychiatry Psychiatric Epidemiology* **26**, 287–292.

Tsuang, M.T. and Winokur, G. (1974). Criteria for subtyping schizophrenia: clinical differentiation of hebephrenic and paranoid schizophrenia. *Arch Gen Psychiatry* **31**, 43–47.

van Os, J., Howard, R., Takei, N. and Murray, R.M. (1995). Increasing age as a risk factor for psychosis in the elderly. *Social Psychiatry Psychiatric Epidemiology* **30**, 161–164.

Verdoux, H., Geddes, J.R., Takei, N. *et al.* (1997). Obstetric complications and age at onset in schizophrenia: an international collaborative meta-analysis of individual patient data. *Am J Psychiatry* **154**, 1220–1227.

Verdoux, H., van Os, J., Maurice-Tison, S., Gay, B., Salamon, R. and Bourgeois, M. (1998). Is early adulthood a critical developmental stage for psychosis proneness? A survey of delusional ideation in normal subjects. *Schizophr Res* **29**, 247–254.

Volkow, N.D., Gur, R.C., Wang, G .-J. *et al.* (1998). Association between decline in brain dopamine activity with age and cognitive and motor impairment in healthy individuals. *Am J Psychiatry* **155**, 344–349.

Wong, D.F., Wagner, H.N., Dannals, R.F. *et al.* (1984). Effects of age on dopamine and serotonin receptors measured by positron tomography in the living human brain. *Science* **226**, 1393–1396.

World Health Organization (1980). *Ninth Revision of the International Classification of Diseases*. World Health Organization, Geneva.

Wragg, R.E. and Jeste, D.V. (1989). Overview of depression and psychosis in Alzheimer's disease. *Am J Psychiatry* **146**, 577–587.

Late Onset Schizophrenia
Edited by Robert Howard, Peter V. Rabins, David J. Castle
© 1999 Wrightson Biomedical Publishing Ltd

13

Oestrogens and Psychosis

MARY V. SEEMAN

*The Centre for Addictions and Mental Health, Clarke Division, Department of
Psychiatry, University of Toronto, Ontario, Canada*

Oestrogen withdrawal in both women and men may be a risk factor for the
emergence of psychosis. This makes oestrogen depletion a possible contrib-
utor to the development of psychosis in late life. New research findings about
the mechanisms of action of oestrogen in the brain make its decline in late
life loom large as one facet, perhaps a major facet, in late life onset of
psychosis. Oestrogen effects are known to be tissue-specific; oestrogen
withdrawal occurring in specific brain cells may promote psychosis, just as
its withdrawal in bone cells leads to osteoporosis or its withdrawal in
endothelial cells leads to cardiovascular events. In other words, central
nervous system (CNS) effects of oestrogen withdrawal are analogous to, but
need not always be associated with, effects in bone and vasculature.

The ageing of ovaries in women begins to decrease circulating oestrogen
serum levels and, presumably, brain tissue levels as well by the late thirties.
Ovaries, however, are not the body's only source of oestrogen. In both
women and men, oestrogen is synthesized and secreted from the adrenals
until such time as they, too, begin to age and discontinue production, probably by the early sixties. Additional sources of oestrogen are the body's subcu-
taneous fat stores which make sex steroids from their parent compound,
cholesterol. For this reason, very thin people are at relatively greater risk for
osteoporosis than the rest of the population and perhaps, too, more vulnerable to the development of late life psychosis, although this needs to be
systematically investigated.

A further brain source of oestradiol (the most active CNS oestrogen) is by
local enzymatic conversion from the male hormone testosterone. This occurs
via aromatase, an enzyme whose abundance declines, as does everything else,
with increasing age. The precise rate of decline in humans is unknown.

Additionally, it has been found recently that a variety of neurosteroids are enzymatically synthesized from cholesterol in the glial cells of the rodent central nervous system. The end products of cholesterol side-chain cleavages include catechol oestrogens and their sulphated conjugates (Smith, 1994). Local steroid production of this kind is probably also operant in humans and almost certainly decreases with age. Thus, most endogenous sources decline over time but do so earlier in women than in men.

Oestrogens and anti-oestrogens entering the brain also come from dietary, herbal, and air-borne environmental sources. Polychlorinated biphenyls (PCBs) and insecticides (such as DDT) exhibit substantial oestrogenic activity (MacLusky, 1988). Histamine H_2 receptor antagonists (cimetidine, ranitidine) produce oestrogen-like effects. Certain antifungals are aromatase inhibitors, i.e. they interfere with the conversion of testosterone to oestradiol in the brain. Chemicals with similar effects are used in agriculture. A number of plants (soybeans, chickpeas, cherries, alfalfa, peas, beans) synthesize phyto-oestrogens, substances that bear a structural resemblance to oestrogen. Phyto-oestrogens may also grow in fungi on bread or grain products. Such substances may exert oestrogenic or anti-oestrogenic effects but animal studies suggest a net oestrogenic effect (MacLusky, 1988). Exposure to these substances may down-regulate oestrogen receptors and cause effective non-responsivity to endogenous oestrogen. Non-responsivity and age-related oestrogen decline may – as in Alzheimer's and perhaps in Parkinson's disease – both be important mediators of late onset schizophrenia.

Although it has been known for many years that steroid hormones, oestradiol in particular, act as 'multi-modal' messengers in the brain (McEwen, 1991a), renewed interest has been sparked by the recent discovery of a second oestrogen receptor (ERβ) (Kuiper et al., 1996) whose distribution in the brain is different from that of the first (ERα) (Shugrue et al., 1997; Österlund et al., 1998) and more abundant in areas that have been implicated in schizophrenia.

OESTROGENS AND SCHIZOPHRENIA

Oestrogens have been indirectly associated with schizophrenia (Seeman, 1981; Seeman and Lang, 1990; Häfner et al., 1991b; Häfner et al., 1993) because of the proximity of peak onset age with puberty (Galdos et al., 1993), reports of symptomatic worsening during low oestrogen phases of the menstrual cycle and improvement during the high phase (Hallonquist et al., 1993; Riecher-Rössler and Häfner, 1993; Gattaz et al., 1994; Riecher-Rössler et al., 1994; Seeman, 1996) and during pregnancy (Seeman and Lang, 1990), reports of frequent relapse postpartum (Kendell et al., 1987) and of increasing severity of symptoms at menopausal ages in women (Seeman, 1998). The incidence curves for schizophrenia also point to a possible role for oestrogen modulation: a one-to-one sex ratio prior to puberty, an increased male to female ratio at adolescence and early adulthood, and a reversed sex ratio at menopause and thereafter (Castle *et al.*, 1991).

More directly, oestrogen has been given to women with schizophrenia and has been able to hasten the response to neuroleptics in the acute phase of illness (Kulkarni *et al.*, 1996). Lindamer *et al.* (1997) report improvement of psychotic symptoms in a menopausal woman with schizophrenia upon administration of oestrogen replacement. There are reports of oestrogen and/or progesterone administration being helpful in recurrent premenstrual aggravation of psychotic symptoms (Korhonen *et al.*, 1995; Levitte, 1997). Recent work in our clinic has shown that early puberty significantly correlates with late onset of schizophrenia in young women whereas the opposite trend is true for young men (Cohen, 1998), suggesting a 'protective' role for female hormones with respect to fending off onset in genetically vulnerable young adults. Such relative protection has been debated for many years, based not only on women's later onset (Häfner *et al.*, 1991a, 1998) but also on their relatively more robust response to neuroleptics (Seeman, 1983; Lieberman *et al.*, 1993; Szymanski *et al.*, 1996) and other treatments (Haas *et al.*, 1990) and their generally better outcomes, especially in the first 15 years after onset (Salokangas, 1983; Seeman, 1986; Harrison *et al.*, 1996)

A rationale for improved neuroleptic response in women has been the interaction of oestrogens and dopamine, generally thought to dampen dopamine pathways over and above the dopamine blockade of neuroleptic medications (Häfner *et al.*, 1991a; Di Paolo, 1994). Since neuroleptic-induced dopamine blockade in the hypothalamus leads first to a rise in prolactin production in the pituitary, with a subsequent inhibition of oestrogen secretion by the ovaries and a resultant relative hypo-oestrogenism, women's advantage with respect to neuroleptic response is dependent on both prolactin and oestrogen levels and, indeed, is not always found (Salokangas, 1995; Pinals *et al.*, 1996). It is still unclear whether women require lower doses than men when taking the newer neuroleptics, some of which appear to be less dependent for their effectiveness on dopamine blockade but, by the same token, less likely to cause prolactin rises and subsequent oestrogen declines (Szymanski *et al.*, 1996; Meltzer *et al.*, 1997).

Oestrogen levels may also help to explain why certain neuroleptic side effects are more common in women (because drug dose is enhanced by oestrogen). Women's greater susceptibility to tardive dyskinesia after the menopausal years can be attributed to oestrogen withdrawal. This is analogous to the commonly seen dyskinesias brought on by antipsychotic drug withdrawal or dose reduction. There is another possible explanation. Female hormones ebb and flow during menstrual cycles, which means that brain oestrogen receptors are periodically flooded and drained. It is difficult to know the downstream effects of such rhythmical alterations, especially since these may be frequently interrupted by anovulatory cycles, pregnancy, and lactation. If the analogy is made with off and on antipsychotic drug treatment, it may well contribute to tardive dyskinesia susceptibility. From both a symptom and a side effect point of view, it is much safer to maintain low dose medication than to frequently start and stop. Perhaps this adds another piece to the puzzle as to why schizophrenia in women does not die down and become quiescent at approximately age 40, the way it so often does in men (Seeman, 1997, 1998).

Rationales for the 'protectiveness' of oestrogens in schizophrenia have been based on much more than their effect on dopamine pathways, although the dopamine hypothesis of schizophrenia remains a powerful explanatory model for the emergence and evolution of this illness (Seeman, 1995).

OESTROGENS AND COGNITION

More recently, oestrogens have come into prominence for their ability to delay and lessen the severity of cognitive slippage (Kampen and Sherwin, 1994; Sherwin, 1998). Several case-control studies (Henderson et al., 1994; Paganini-Hill and Henderson, 1996) have suggested that women who use oestrogen as a replacement therapy postmenopausally are less likely to develop Alzheimer's disease (AD) than women who do not. Still more recent prospective studies have also observed a protective effect of oestrogen (Kawas et al., 1997). In the Kawas et al. (1997) Baltimore Longitudinal Study of Aging, a follow-up period of 16 years yielded 34 women with incident AD. Nine had used replacement hormone treatment; the others had not. After adjusting for education, the relative risk for AD in oestrogen users compared with non-users was found to be less than one-half. This conclusion was supported by Tang et al., 1996. Paganini-Hill and Henderson (1994) have suggested that both dose and duration of use may help protection. A randomized controlled trial is now in progress.

OESTROGENS AND NEUROTRANSMITTER SYSTEMS

Oestrogenic influences on neurotransmitter levels can operate through genomic effects on neurotransmitter receptor protein (McEwen, 1991a, b) or through direct membrane effects on the electrical firing rate of neurotransmitter-secreting cells (Schumacher, 1990; Xiao and Becker, 1998). The genomic effect is slow (hours to years); the membrane effect is rapid (minutes to hours). In rats, oestrogen increases levels of choline acetyltransferase, the enzyme needed to synthesize acetylcholine (Luine, 1985; Birge, 1997). This is certainly important in Alzheimer's disease and probably also in schizophrenia since cholinergic and cognitive functions have long been linked (Bartus *et al.*, 1982); in fact, in schizophrenia, the administration of anticholinergics to counteract extrapyramidal side effects of neuroleptics is known to exacerbate memory problems.

It has also been established that oestrogens increase the density of serotonin 5-hydroxytryptamine 2A ($5HT_{2A}$) receptors in rat cerebral cortex and nucleus accumbens (de Vry, 1995; Sumner and Fink, 1995; Birge, 1997). They do not alter 5-hydroxytryptamine 1A ($5HT_{1A}$) mRNA levels in rat hippocampus or cingulate cortex but decrease $5HT_{1A}$ mRNA in the medial amygdala, piriform cortex, and perirhinal cortex, suggesting a possible route to modulation of emotional memory, mood, and cognitive function (Österlund and Hurd, 1998). In schizophrenia, the status of serotonin receptors remains unclear.

Metabolites of progesterone potentiate gamma-aminobutyric acid (GABA) inhibition, producing an anxiolytic affect which is enhanced in the presence of oestrogen (Smith, 1994). On the other hand, progesterone attenuation of the effects of excitatory amino acids is cancelled out by oestrogens which exert a primarily activating role in the central nervous system. Oestrogens potentiate excitatory amino acids such as glutamate and aspartate (Smith, 1994).

Oestrogens can also block inhibitory neurotransmission. Their action on the dopaminergic system, referred to earlier, is complex (Smith, 1994; Pohjalainen *et al.*, 1998) and phasic, causing alterations in pre- and postsynaptic dopamine receptors (DiPaolo, 1994) and differential distribution of the isoforms of the dopamine D_2 receptor mRNA (Guivarc'h *et al.*, 1995).

OESTROGEN EFFECTS

On membrane stability

Because of their mainly activational influences, oestrogens are 'proconvulsants' in susceptible individuals (Butterbaugh, 1987), decreasing seizure threshold and increasing the magnitude of seizure activity. In experimental animals, this appears to be a direct consequence of depolarization of cellular membranes. Subthreshold seizure activity has been implicated as a possible mechanism of action of neuroleptics and may be one way in which oestrogens potentiate neuroleptics in schizophrenia. Progesterone, on the other hand, raises the seizure threshold (Smith, 1994), an effect opposite to that of oestrogen and probably responsible for catamenial or premenstrual epilepsy.

On sensory perception

In both human and animal studies, increases in oestrogen correlate with increases in perception in many sensory modalities including hearing, olfaction, visual signal detection and two-point discrimination (Smith, 1994). It is possible that decreased sensory discrimination facilitates the emergence of hallucinations and delusional attribution, especially in the elderly when all modes of perception begin to be impaired.

On attention

Levels of circulating oestrogens are associated with increased alertness in animals, reduced distractibility, and shorter reaction times (Smith, 1994).

On blood flow

Oestrogens increase blood flow to the brain and within the brain, which speeds metabolism and increases the general efficiency of neural networks as well as increasing the efficiency of drug delivery (Gur *et al.*, 1982; Birge, 1997).

On glucose utilization

Oestrogens stimulate glucose transport and metabolism, allowing nerve cells to do their work (Namba and Sokoloff, 1984; Bishop and Simkins, 1992; Birge, 1997).

SITES OF ACTION OF OESTROGEN

It is thought that neuronal responsiveness to steroid stimulation may result from both genetic and membrane effects at multiple distributed sites involving large neural circuitry (Carson-Jurica *et al.*, 1990; Schumacher, 1990; McEwen, 1992; Smith, 1994; Tsai and O'Malley, 1994; Brann *et al.*, 1995; Xiao and Becker, 1998). Network effects may differ depending on the particular configuration of a specific circuit. Importantly, hormonal effects on neural network properties appear to be state-dependent in experimental animals. In other words, net results differ depending on the light/dark cycle, the glucose level, the noise level, the presence of an animal of the opposite sex, and the stress level (Smith, 1994). If this is the case in rodents, how much more complex must it be in humans.

GENOMIC EFFECTS OF OESTROGEN: WHICH GENES?

Among the many genes that have been implicated as being under the influence of oestrogen are genes responsible for neuronal development, migration, growth, survival, dendritic spine formation and density, antioxidant activity, synaptic plasticity, neurodegeneration, apoptosis secondary to glucose deprivation or other toxic stimuli (Murphy *et al.*, 1987; Nakano *et al.*, 1987; Toran-Allerand *et al.*, 1988; Gould *et al.*, 1990; Niki and Nakano, 1990; Matsumoto, 1991; Rogers *et al.*, 1991; McEwen, 1992; Shugrue and Dorsa, 1993; Sohrabji *et al.*, 1994; Woolley and McEwen, 1994; Behl *et al.*, 1995; Toran-Allerand, 1996; Birge, 1997; Woolley *et al.*, 1997; Xu *et al.*, 1998).

OESTROGEN MEDIATED GENE TRANSCRIPTION

We do not yet know which genes are most relevant to schizophrenia but whichever they turn out to be, their expression has to be activated in the relevant neurones of the brain to set off and maintain the symptoms of schizophrenia. Steroid hormones are among the most important known epigenetic regulators. In a tissue-specific manner, they control dosage effects of genes. They activate them or silence them. As this applies to schizophrenia, the relevant genes might be neurotransmitter receptor genes; they may be growth factor genes controlling neurodevelopment, apoptosis, or atrophy; they may be regulatory genes modulating intracellular signalling; they may be stress response genes.

HOW OESTROGENS ACTIVATE GENES

The brain is the target for circulating oestrogens emanating from peripheral tissues or from the local metabolism of other steroids such as testosterone. The way in which oestrogen hormones modify gene expression is by binding to their own receptors – a family of DNA-binding proteins synthesized on cytoplasmic microsomes – and transversing the nuclear membrane almost immediately to take up residence within the cell nucleus (Carson-Jurica *et al.*, 1990). The human oestrogen receptor (ERα) has been characterized both at the cDNA level and at the genomic level (Carson-Jurica *et al.*, 1990) and it has been shown that it is transcribed from two different promoters, a proximal and a distal promoter separated by a 2 kilobase intron (Freyschuss and Grandien, 1996). A third ERα mRNA isoform has recently been isolated, transcribed from a third, more distal, promoter region (Grandien, 1996). The expression of these three ERα mRNAs appears to be regulated in a tissue-specific manner which suggests tissue-specific promoter usage (Grandien *et al.*, 1995). Differential promoter usage is an important mechanism for tissue specificity and for developmentally regulated gene expression. It seems to be a common feature among many members of the nuclear hormone receptor family (Freyschuss and Grandien, 1996).

Until the recent discovery of a new oestrogen receptor (ERβ) (Kuiper *et al.*, 1996) and its localization in brain regions associated with learning, memory, and emotion (Shugrue *et al.*, 1997; Österlund *et al.*, 1998), it was difficult to understand how oestrogen replacement therapy could improve cognitive functions since ERα is sparsely distributed in key cognitive regions such as neocortex, hippocampus, and basal forebrain nuclei. It is now thought that oestrogens can work through both these receptors and that the two receptors can even co-exist within the same cell.

Once oestrogen enters the cell nucleus and binds to the ER expressed in that cell, a conformational change occurs in the now activated receptor. This alteration exposes the receptor's DNA binding domain (two 'zinc fingers' or amino acid loops containing four cysteine molecules, each coordinating one zinc molecule and linked together by a straight chain of amino acids (Carson-Jurica *et al.*, 1990)). Once exposed, the DNA binding domain of the receptor attaches to specific sequences of nucleotides in the nuclear DNA, thus regulating the transcription of a gene. Genetic transcription is one way through which oestrogens modify the structure and function of brain cells. The latency of such genomic effects is thought to be anywhere between hours to years (McEwen, 1991b, 1992) and so could account for both the organizational and also some of the activational effects of oestrogens.

NUCLEAR OESTROGEN RECEPTORS

Oestrogens are lipid based molecules, derived from the parent compound cholesterol. They slip through the cell's fatty outer membrane unaided and into the cell nucleus where they do their work. There are a variety of oestrogens. In the central nervous system, oestradiol (E2) is the most abundant. Different neurons may express one or the other of the two oestrogen receptors discovered up to now, but it is also possible that one cell may express more than one, each individually activated by different promoter mechanisms. Oestrogen receptors have six structural domains of overlapping function. One domain binds with the incoming oestrogen (Tsai and O'Malley, 1994). When this happens, a structural change takes place which first induces two receptors to couple (i.e. they form a dimer complex). Then the dimer's now exposed DNA binding domain seeks, finds, and binds to a consensus palindromic segment of DNA referred to as the oestrogen response element (ERE). The ERE is a 13 base pair piece of DNA (McCarthy, 1994) that, when fastened to the receptor's DNA binding domain, allows two further domains of the receptor (transactivating domains) to activate the promoter region of a target gene. The strength of the activation of the gene is modulated by specific adapter proteins or other transcription factors which are cell specific (Mitlak and Cohen, 1997). Thus far, at least ten co-activator proteins or basal factors have been identified, all capable of forming combinatorial complexes with EREs and, in turn, tempering oestrogen receptor function.

It should also be noted that gene response to oestrogen in a target tissue is not necessarily related to its affinity for or its occupancy of oestrogen receptors. Oestrogen-responsive genes with no recognizable oestrogen response element have been identified (Das *et al.*, 1997). It is now recognized that oestrogens and anti-oestrogens can exert their effect even when both Erα and Erβ are 'knocked out'. This may occur via membrane receptors or via what have been called 'orphan' nuclear receptors. Another possible mechanism is the formation of heterodimeric complexes by Erα and Erβ or through other as yet unidentified mechanisms (Das *et al.*, 1997).

SELECTIVE OESTROGEN RECEPTOR MODULATORS

Newly synthesized molecules, the selective oestrogen receptor modulators (SERMS), act both as tissue-specific oestrogen agonists and also as antagonists in the sense that, to various extents and by a variety of intermediary means, they can either inhibit or enhance oestrogen-induced activation of ERE-containing genes (Kauffman and Bryant, 1995). Raloxifene, one of the new SERMS, forms a raloxifene response element (RRE) which does not itself bind directly to the DNA domain of the gene but activates it via an intermediate molecule, 17-epiestriol (Yang *et al.*, 1996). Other oestrogen by-products may similarly take oestrogen's place in turning on target genes through unfamiliar pathways, and this may especially happen in non-reproductive tissues such as the brain, which has been little studied. A recently identified pathway is via a response element called the AP1 site (both oestrogen and tamoxifen, an early SERM, work through this site in uterine tissue). Raloxifene does not interact with the AP1 site and, therefore, does not lead to uterine proliferation as do both oestrogens and tamoxifen. Tamoxifen is anti-oestrogenic in breast tissue; raloxifene is anti-oestrogenic in breast and uterine tissue and pro-oestrogenic in bone. This kind of selectivity shows the promise of SERMS for central nervous tissue modulation. For instance, the neurone-specific growth-associated protein gene GAP-43, whose expression is modulated by oestrogen (Shugrue and Dorsa, 1993), contains sequences that resemble those of the RRE (raloxifene response element). This suggests that raloxifene may have beneficial (pro-oestrogenic) effects in nervous tissue.

MEMBRANE OESTROGEN RECEPTORS

Oestrogen also produces non-genomic effects by binding to neuronal membrane receptors (in distinction to nuclear receptors). This effect is rapid, with a latency of seconds to minutes, and it disappears rapidly as well (McEwen, 1991b; Brann *et al.*, 1995). The neurotransmitter effects of oestrogen referred to earlier are likely to be mediated by membrane receptors since nuclear oestrogen receptors have not been found in the areas of the brain where these effects take place (Fink *et al.*, 1996).

Oestrogen effects on dendritic spines in the CA1 region of the hippocampus are another example. Oestrogen given to an ovariectomized rat produces an increase in the number of spines on apical dendrites of CA1 pyramidal neurones (Gould *et al.*, 1990; Woolley and McEwen, 1994; Woolley *et al.*, 1998). Cyclic changes in spine density can be seen throughout the oestrus cycle of rats, suggesting the formation and destruction of synapses in quick time presumably, therefore, mediated via membrane receptors. Oestrogens, then, increase neuronal connections, helping to create networks that maintain attention and preserve memory functions.

OESTROGENS AND SCHIZOPHRENIA

The organizational effects of oestrogens in fetal life may be important in ensuring the integrity of neural networks that protect against the early development of schizophrenia. At the other end of life, oestrogens may be important in protecting these same circuits against degeneration. As reviewed above, oestrogens have many CNS protective effects which act throughout life and which may modulate schizophrenia onset and expression at adolescence or adulthood as well as in old age. Oestrogens increase blood flow and glucose utilization; they are neurotrophic – making dendrites grow; they are anti-apoptotic, i.e. delaying programmed nerve cell death. They also reduce amyloid plaque formation (Xu *et al.*, 1998). And they modulate several neurotransmitter systems.

Oestrogens also increase membrane excitability, i.e. lower the seizure threshold; they buffer the neurotoxic effects of glucocorticoids released during stress and oxidants such as glutamate and free radicals. Once nerve impairment occurs, they foster repair, and protect against or delay the secondary atrophy that can ultimately lead to the disruption of neural circuit integrity, a disruption that may finally be responsible for the emergence of psychosis.

HOW OESTROGEN WITHDRAWAL CAN CREATE THE CONTEXT FOR THE ONSET OF LATE LIFE PSYCHOSIS

We know, from the example of various cancers and of Alzheimer's disease, that the ageing process can lead to a chain of events that 'turn on' existing

Table 1.   Oestrogen effects.

Neuronal effects: genomic via oestrogen receptors?	Non-specific effects: genomic/ membrane?	Neurotransmission membrane?	Effects in rodents
Neuronal migration	Glucose utilization	Acetylcholine	Attention
Neuronal differentiation	Blood flow	Serotonin	Memory
Apoptosis	Oxidative stress	Dopamine	Perception
Neuronal injury	Glucocorticoid-	Glutamate	Activity
Neuronal inflammation	mediated stress	GABA	
Neuronal atrophy	Progesterone	NMDA	
Synaptic density	potentiation		
Dendritic spine growth	Membrane excitability		
Myelinization	Amyloid plaques		

disease genes. This is presumably what happens in late onset schizophrenia and related psychoses. One event in that chain is probably the withdrawal of oestrogens from specific neurones, thus reducing blood flow and needed nutrients, glucose in particular. Oestrogen withdrawal also exposes neurones to oxidative stress and to glucocorticoid-mediated stress. It reduces synaptic density and dendritic spine growth. Oestrogen depletion decreases protection against neurone atrophy, neurone injury, and neurone inflammation, all of which occur with increasing age. Lack of oestrogen adversely affects attention, memory, sensory perception and motor activity, all of which may bring psychotic symptoms to the foreground. Various effects on neurotransmitter systems are difficult to predict but, hypothetically, they interfere with neuronal harmony in the same way as may happen at the onset of adolescent schizophrenia. In other words, neuronal circuit integrity is destroyed in early onset schizophrenia when developing neurones fail to make crucial connections. The integrity of the same circuits is destroyed in late onset schizophrenia when atrophying neurones fail to maintain these same connections. Gonadal hormones may or may not prove to be of overriding importance to the maintenance of central nervous system equilibrium but there is mounting evidence that they play a significant role.

Table 1 summarizes the various putative protective effects of oestrogens on neural circuits potentially involved in the production of psychotic symptoms. As we learn more about which specific genes are activated or silenced by oestrogens, we will have new leads on susceptibility genes in schizophrenia. Equally importantly, as selective oestrogen receptor modulators become increasingly specific, we will have another family of drugs for prevention and treatment of psychosis (Grese et al., 1998).

REFERENCES

Bartus, R.T., Dean, R.L., Beer, B. and Lippa, A.S. (1982). The cholinergic hypothesis of memory dysfunction. *Science* **217**, 208–217.

Behl, C., Widman, M., Trapp, T. and Holsboer, F. (1995).17-Beta estradiol protects neurons from oxidative stress-induced cell death *in vitro*. *Biochem Biophys Res Commun* **216**, 473–482.

Birge, S.J. (1997). The role of estrogen in the treatment of Alzheimer's disease. *Neurology* **48**, (suppl 7), S36–S41.

Bishop, J. and Simpkins, J.W. (1992). Role of estrogens in peripheral and cerebral glucose utilization. *Rev Neurosci* **3**, 121–137.

Brann, D.W., Hendry, L.B. and Mahesh, V.B. (1995). Emerging diversities in the mechanism of action of steroid hormones. *J Steroid Biochem Molec Biol* **52**, 113–133.

Butterbaugh, G.G. (1987). Postictal events in amygdala-kindled female rats with and without estradiol replacement. *Explor Neurol* **95**, 697–713.

Carson-Jurica, M.A., Schrader, W.T. and O'Malley, B.W. (1990). Steroid receptor family: structure and functions. *Endocrine Rev* **11**, 201–220.

Castle, D.J., Wessely, S., Der, G. and Murray, R.M. (1991). The incidence of operationally defined schizophrenia in Camberwell 1965–85. *Br J Psychiatry* **159**, 790–794.

Cohen, R.Z. (1998). Puberty and schizophrenia. Master's Thesis. Institute of Medical Science, University of Toronto.

Das, S.K., Taylor, J.A., Korach, K.S., Paria, B.C., Dey, S.K. and Lubahn, D.B. (1997). Estrogenic responses in estrogen receptor-a deficient mice reveal a distinct estrogen signaling pathway. *Proc Natl Acad Sci USA* **94**, 12786–12791.

de Vry, J. (1995). 5HT1A receptor agonists: recent developments and controversial issues. *Psychopharmacology* **121**, 1–26.

Di Paolo, T. (1994). Modulation of brain dopamine transmission by sex steroids. *Rev Neurosci* **5**, 27–42.

Fink, G., Sumner, B.E.H., Rosie, R., Grace, O. and Quinn, J.P. (1996). Estrogen control of central transmission: effect on mood, mental state, memory. *Cell Molec Neurobiol* **16**, 325–344.

Freyschuss, B. and Grandien, K. (1996). The 5'flank of the estrogen receptor gene: structural characterization and evidence for tissue and species specific promotor utilization. *J Molec Endocrinol* **17**, 197–206.

Galdos, P., van Os, J. and Murray, R.M. (1993). Puberty and the onset of psychosis. *Schizophr Res* **10**, 7–14.

Gattaz, W.F., Vogel, P., Riecher-Rössler, A. and Soddu, G. (1994). Influence of the menstrual cycle phase on the therapeutic response in schizophrenia. *Biol Psychiatry* **36**, 137–139.

Gould, E., Woolley, C.S., Frankfurt, M. and McEwen, B.S. (1990). Gonadal steroids regulate dendritic spine density in hippocampal pyramidal cells in adulthood. *J Neurosci* **10**, 1286–1291.

Grandien, K. (1996). Determination of transcription startsites in the human estrogen receptor gene and identification of a novel, tissue-specific, estrogen receptor–mRNA isoform. *Molec Cell Endocrinol* **116**, 207–212.

Grandien, K., Bäckdahl, M., Ljungren, Ö., Gustafsson, J-Å. and Berkenstam, A. (1995). Estrogen target tissue determines alternative promoter utilization of the human estrogen receptor gene in osteoblasts and tumor cell lines. *Endocrinology* **136**, 2223–2229.

Grese, T.A., Pennington, L.D., Sluka, J.P. *et al.* (1998). Synthesis and pharmacology of conformationally restricted raloxifene analogues: highly potent selective estrogen receptor modulators. *J Med Chem* **41**, 1272–1283.

Guivarc'h, D., Vernier, P. and Vincent, J.D. (1995). Sex steroid hormones change the differential distribution of the isoforms of the D2 dopamine receptor messenger RNA in the rat brain. *Neuroscience* **69**, 159–166.

Gur, R.C., Gur, R.E., Orbist, W.D. *et al.* (1982) Sex and handedness differences in cerebral blood flow during rest and cognitive activity. *Science* **217**, 659–661.

Haas, G.L., Glick, I.D., Clarkin, J.F., Spencer, J.H. and Lewis, A.B. (1990). Gender and schizophrenia outcome: a clinical trial of inpatient family intervention. *Schizophr Bull* **16**, 277–292.

Häfner, H., Behrens, S., De Vry, J. and Gattaz, W.F. (1991a). An animal model for the effects of estradiol on dopamine-mediated behavior: implications for sex differences in schizophrenia. *Psychiatry Res* **38**, 125–134.

Häfner, H., Behrens, S., De Vry J. and Gattaz, W.F. (1991b). Oestradiol enhances the vulnerability threshold for schizophrenia in women by an early effect on dopaminergic transmission. *Eur Arch Psychiatry Clin Neurosci* **241**, 65–68.

Häfner, H., Riecher-Rössler, A., an der Heiden, W., Maurer, K., Fätkenheuer, B. and Löffler, W. (1993). Generating and testing a causal explanation of the gender difference in age at first onset of schizophrenia. *Psychol Med* **23**, 925–940.

Häfner, H., an der Heiden, W., Behrens, S. *et al.* (1998). Causes and consequences of the gender difference in age at onset of schizophrenia. *Schizophr Bull* **24**, 99–113.

Hallonquist, J., Seeman, M.V., Lang, M. and Rector, N. (1993). Variation in symptom severity over the menstrual cycle of schizophrenics. *Biol Psychiatry* **33**, 207–209.

Harrison, G., Croudace, P., Mason, C., Glazebrook, C. and Medley, I. (1996). Predicting the long-term outcome of schizophrenia. *Psychol Med* **26**, 697–705.

Henderson, V.W., Paganini-Hill, A., Emanuel, C.K., Dunn, M.E. and Buckwalter, J.G. (1994). Estrogen replacement therapy in older women. *Arch Neurol* **51**, 896–900.

Kampen, D.L. and Sherwin, B.B. (1994). Estrogen use and verbal memory in healthy postmenopausal women. *Obstetrics Gynecol* **83**, 979–983.

Kauffman, R.F. and Bryant, H.U. (1995). Selective estrogen receptor modulators. *DrugLine* **8**, 531–539.

Kawas, C., Resnick, S., Morrison, A. *et al.* (1997). A prospective study of estrogen replacement therapy and the risk of developing Alzheimer's disease. *Neurology* **48**, 1517–1521.

Kendell, R.E., Chalmers, J.C. and Platz, C. (1987). Epidemiology and puerperal psychoses. *Br J Psychiatry* **150**, 662–673.

Korhonen, S., Saarijarvi, S. and Aito, M. (1995). Successful estradiol treatment of psychotic symptoms in the premenstrual phase: a case report. *Acta Psychiatr Scand* **92**, 237–238.

Kuiper, G.G.J.M., Enmark, E., Pelto-Huikko, M., Nilsson, S. and Gustafson, J. (1996). Cloning of a novel estrogen receptor in rat prostate and ovary. *Proc Natl Acad Sci USA* **93**, 5925–5930.

Kulkarni, J., de Castella, A., Smith, D., Taffe, J., Keks, N. and Copolov, D. (1996). A clinical trial of the effects of estrogen in acutely psychotic women. *Schizophr Res* **20**, 247–252.

Levitte, S.S. (1997). Treatment of premenstrual exacerbation of schizophrenia. *Psychosomatics* **38**, 582–584.

Lieberman, J., Jody, D., Geisler, S. *et al.* (1993). Time course and biologic correlates of treatment response in first-episode schizophrenia. *Arch Gen Psychiatry* **50**, 369–376.

Lindamer, L.A., Lohr, J.B., Harris, M.J. and Jeste, D.V. (1997). Gender, estrogen, and schizophrenia. *Psychopharmacol Bull* **332**, 221–228.

Luine, V.N. (1985). Estradiol increases choline acetyltransferase activity in specific basal forebrain nuclei and projection areas of female rats. *Experimental Neurol* **80**, 484–490.

MacLusky, N.J. (1988). Developmental actions of gonadal steroids. *Progr Clin Biol Res* **281**, 243–263.

Matsumoto, A. (1991). Synaptogenic action of sex steroids in developing and adult neuroendocrine brain. *Psychoneuroendocrinology* **19**, 415–427.

McCarthy, M.M. (1994). Molecular aspects of sexual differentiation of the rodent brain. *Psychoneuroendocrinology* **19**, 415–427.

McEwen, B.S. (1991a). Steroid hormones are multifunctional messengers to the brain. *Trends Endocrinol Metab* **2**, 62–67.

McEwen, B.S. (1991b). Non-genomic and genomic effects of steroids on neural activity. *Trends Pharmacol Sci Rev* **12**, 141–147.

McEwen, B.S. (1992). Steroid hormones: effect on brain development and function. *Hormone Res* **37** (suppl 3), 1–10.

Meltzer, H.Y., Rabinowitz, J., Lee, M.A. *et al.* (1997). Age at onset and gender of schizophrenic patients in relation to neuroleptic resistance. *Am J Psychiatry* **154**, 475–482.

Mitlak, B.H. and Cohen, F.J. (1997). In search of optimal long-term female hormone replacement: the potential of selective estrogen receptor modulators. *Hormone Res* **48**, 155–163.

Murphy, L.J., Murphy, L.C. and Friesen, H.G. (1987). Estrogen induction of N-myc and c-myc proto-oncogene expression in rat uterus. *Endocrinology* **120**, 1882–1888.

Nakano, M., Sugioka, K., Naito, I., Takekoshi, S. and Niki, E. (1987). Novel and potent biological antioxidants on membrane phospholipid peroxidation: 2-hydroxy estrone and 2-hydroxy estradiol. *Biochem Biophys Res Commun* **142**, 919–924.

Namba, H. and Sokoloff, L. (1984). Acute administration of high doses of estrogen increases glucose utilization throughout brain. *Brain Res* **291**, 391–394.

Niki, E. and Nakano, M. (1990). Estrogens as antioxidants. *Methods Enzymol* **186**, 330–333.

Österlund, M.K. and Hurd, Y.L. (1998). Acute 17β-estradiol treatment down-regulates serotonin 5HT1A receptor mRNA expression in the limbic system of female rats. *Molec Brain Res* **55**, 69–172.

Österlund, M., Kuiper, G.G.J.M., Gustafsson, J.A. and Hurd, Y.L. (1998). Differential distribution and regulation of estrogen receptor-α and -β mRNA within the female rat brain. *Molec Brain Res* **54**, 175–180.

Paganini-Hill, A. and Henderson, V.W. (1994). Estrogen deficiency and risk of Alzheimer's disease in women. *Am J Epidemiology* **140**, 256–261.

Paganini-Hill, A. and Henderson, V.W. (1996). Estrogen replacement therapy and risk of Alzheimer's disease. *Arch Internal Med* **156**, 2213–2217.

Pinals, D.A., Malhotra, A.K., Missar, D., Pickar, D. and Breier, A. (1996). Lack of gender differences in neuroleptic response in patients with schizophrenia. *Schizophr Res* **22**, 215–222.

Pohjalainen, T., Rimme, J.O., Nagren, K., Syvalahti, E. and Hietala, J. (1998). Sex differences in the striatal dopamine D2 receptor binding characteristics *in vivo*. *Am J Psychiatry* **155**, 768–773.

Riecher-Rössler, A. and Häfner, H. (1993). Schizophrenia and oestrogens – is there an association? *Eur Arch Psychiatry Clin Neurosci* **242**, 323–328.

Riecher-Rössler, A., Häfner, H., Stumbaum, M., Maurer, K. and Schmidt, R. (1994). Can estradiol modulate schizophrenic symptomatology? *Schizophr Bull* **20**, 203–214.

Rogers, L.C., Junier, M.P., Farmer, S.R. and Ojeda, S.R. (1991). A sex-related difference in the developmental expression of class β-tubulin messenger RNA in rat hypothalamus. *Molec Cell Neurosci* **2**, 130–138.

Salokangas, R.K. (1983). Prognostic implications of the sex of schizophrenic patients. *Br J Psychiatry* **142**, 145–151.

Salokangas, R.K.R. (1995). Gender and the use of neuroleptics in schizophrenia. Further testing of the oestrogen hypothesis. *Schizophr Res* **16**, 7–16.

Schumacher, M. (1990). Rapid membrane effects of steroid hormones: an emerging concept in neuroendocrinology. *Trends Neurosci* **13**, 359–362.

Seeman, M.V. (1981). Gender and the onset of schizophrenia: neurohumoral influences. *Psychiatr J Univ Ottawa* **6**, 136–138.

Seeman, M.V. (1983). Interaction of sex, age, and neuroleptic dose. *Compr Psychiatry* **24**, 125–128.

Seeman, M.V. (1986). Current outcome in schizophrenia: women vs men. *Acta Psychiatr Scand* **73**, 609–617.

Seeman, M.V. (1996). The role of estrogen in schizophrenia. *J Psychiatry Neurosci* **21**, 123–127.

Seeman, M.V. (1997). Psychopathology in women and men: focus on female hormones. *Am J Psychiatry* **154**, 1641–1647.

Seeman, M.V. (1998). Narratives of twenty to thirty years of schizophrenia outcome. *Psychiatry* **61**, 249–261.

Seeman, M.V. and Lang, M. (1990). The role of estrogens in schizophrenia gender differences. *Schizophr Bull* **16**, 185–194.

Seeman, P. (1995). Dopamine receptors: clinical correlates in psychopharmacology. In: Bloom, F.E. and Kupfer, D.J. (Eds), *The Fourth Generation of Progress*. Raven Press, New York.

Sherwin, B.B. (1998). Estrogen and cognitive functioning in women. *Proc Soc Experimental Biol Med* **217**, 17–22.

Shugrue, P.J. and Dorsa, D.M. (1993). Gonadal steroids modulate the growth-associated protein GAP-43 (neuromodulin) mRNA in postnatal rat brain. *Devel Brain Res* **73**, 123–132.

Shugrue, P.J., Lane, M.V. and Merchenthaler, I. (1997). Comparative distribution of estrogen receptor-α and -β mRNA in the rat central nervous system. *J Comparative Neurol* **388**, 507–527.

Smith, S.S. (1994). Female sex steroid hormones: from receptors to networks to performance – actions on the sensorimotor system. *Progr Neurobiol* **44**, 55–86.

Sohrabji, F., Miranda, R.C. and Toran-Allerand, C.D. (1994). Estrogen differentially regulates estrogen and nerve growth factor receptor mRNAs in adult sensory neurons. *J Neurosci* **14**, 459–471.

Sumner, B.E.H. and Fink, G. (1995). Estrogen increases the density of 5-hydroxytryptamine-2A receptors in cerebral cortex and nucleus accumbens in the female rat. *J Steroid Biochem Molec Biol* **54**, 15–20.

Szymanski, S., Lieberman, J., Pollack, S. *et al.* (1996). Gender differences in neuroleptic nonresponsive clozapine-treated schizophrenics. *Biol Psychiatry* **39**, 249–254.

Tang, M-X., Jacobs, D., Stern, Y. *et al.* (1996). Effect of oestrogen during menopause on risk and age at onset of Alzheimer's disease. *Lancet* **348**, 429–432.

Toran-Allerand, C.D. (1996). The estrogen/neurotrophin connection during neural development: is co-localization of estrogen receptors with the neurotrophins and their receptors biologically relevant? *Devel Neurosci* **18**, 36–48.

Toran-Allerand, C.D., Ellis, L. and Pfenninger, K.H. (1988). Estrogen and insulin synergism in neurite growth enhancement *in vitro*: mediation of steroid effects by interactions with growth factors? *Devel Brain Res* **41**, 87–100.

Tsai, M.J. and O'Malley, B.W. (1994). Molecular mechanisms of action of steroid/thyroid receptor superfamily members. *Ann Rev Biochem* **63**, 451–486.

Woolley, H. and McEwen, B.S. (1994). Estradiol regulates hippocampal dendritic spine density via an N-methyl-D-aspartate receptor-dependent mechanism. *J Neurosci* **14**, 7680–7687.

Woolley, C.S., Welland, N.C., McEwen, B.S. and Schwartzkroin, P.A. (1997). Estradiol increases the sensitivity of hippocampal CA1 pyramidal cells to NMDA receptor-mediated synaptic input: correlation with dendritic spine density. *J Neurosci* **17**, 1848–1859.

Xiao, L. and Becker, J.B. (1998). Effects of estrogen agonists on amphetamine-stimulated striatal dopamine release. *Synapse* **29**, 379–391.

Xu, H., Gouras, G.K., Greenfield, J.P. *et al.* (1998). Estrogen reduces neuronal generation of Alzheimer β-amyloid peptides. *Nature Medicine* **4**, 447–451.

Yang, N.N., Venugopalan, M., Hardikar, S. and Glasebrook, A. (1996). Identification of an estrogen response element activated by metabolites of 17β-estradiol and raloxifene. *Science* **273**, 1222–1225.

14

The Neuropsychology of Schizophrenia in Late Life

OSVALDO P. ALMEIDA

Department of Psychiatry and Behavioural Science, University of Western Australia, Perth, Western Australia

INTRODUCTION

Kraepelin used the term 'dementia praecox' to emphasize his observation that patients who suffer from schizophrenia often show marked impairment of cognitive function after the onset of their illness. More recent studies have confirmed that schizophrenia is associated with decline from previous levels of functioning. Frith *et al.* (1991) assessed 283 patients and 35 controls living in the same catchment area. An estimate of their premorbid IQ with the NART showed no difference between the groups, although current IQ was, on average, 16 points lower among those with schizophrenia. Other studies have produced similar results (Nelson *et al.*, 1990; Hyde *et al.*, 1994), reinforcing the evidence for a decline of cognitive abilities among these patients.

Attempts have also been made to establish which domains of functioning are impaired. Many studies emphasize the importance of impaired executive functioning among people with schizophrenia (Weinberger, 1987; Gold *et al.*, 1992; Elliott *et al.*, 1995), while others highlight the presence of memory, attention or visuospatial deficits (Spring *et al.*, 1989; Morrinson-Stewart *et al.*, 1992; Tamlyn *et al.*, 1992; Fleming *et al.*, 1997). Braff *et al.* (1991) used a comprehensive neuropsychological test battery (extended Halstead–Reitan Battery) to assess 40 schizophrenic outpatients and 40 controls. The patients with schizophrenia showed multiple neuropsychological deficits on tests of conceptual reasoning, psychomotor speed, new learning and incidental memory, and both motor and sensory perceptual abilities. These results indicate that patients with schizophrenia, as a group, show a pattern of generalized impairment and are likely to be impaired relative to controls on most cognitive tests.

However, most studies of schizophrenia are limited by the fact that they only include relatively young adults, and it is still unclear whether these findings can be extended to elderly patients. This chapter aims to review the neuropsychology of schizophrenia in the elderly, its association with dementia, and the relationship between early and late onset cases.

WHAT HAPPENS TO PEOPLE WITH SCHIZOPHRENIA WHEN THEY GROW OLD?

Few studies have attempted to follow-up schizophrenic patients into old age. Waddington and Youssef (1996) evaluated 101 chronically ill, long-term inpatients who satisfied Feighner's criteria for schizophrenia. Subjects were evaluated with the AIMS (Guy, 1988) and with a simple 10 question mental test (Waddington et al., 1987). The authors reported a modest deterioration in cognitive functioning over a decade, particularly among those with oro-facial dyskinesia. However, these results have a number of limitations. Subjects selected for the study suffered from a very debilitating type of illness and were chronically institutionalized – they are unlikely to represent the population of patients with schizophrenia. Another important problem is that follow-up information was available for only 41 of the 101 initial assessments and it is unclear how well these represent the initial sample of patients. In addition, the neuropsychological assessment used in this investigation was very crude and unlikely to be sufficiently sensitive to change over time.

Mockler et al. (1997) addressed the issue of ageing in schizophrenia in a different way. They assessed 62 chronic schizophrenia patients with the Wechsler Adult Intelligence Scale-Revised (WAIS-R) and the NART in a cross-sectional study of five different age cohorts (18–29, 30–39, 40–49, 50–59,

Table 1. Cognitive performance of patients with chronic schizophrenia according to their age group.

	Age group					
	18–29 N=13	30–39 N=17	40–49 N=11	50–59 N=15	60–69 N=6	p
Duration of illness (years)	4.9	13.9	23.8	24.9	41.0	< 0.001
WAIS-R (IQ)	82.1	79.8	87.4	78.7	76.2	0.161
Verbal IQ	84.5	83.3	89.9	82.9	77.5	0.173
Performance IQ	81.1	79.2	87.5	74.7	76.7	0.094
NART–WAIS-R IQ	12.2	14.4	17.5	13.7	12.8	0.641

Based on Mockler et al. (1997).

and 60–69). Table 1 summarizes their main findings. There was no difference between the various age groups with regard to current IQ. In addition, there was no sign of functional decline in the older groups, which suggests that schizophrenia is not associated with progressive intellectual deterioration. Again, these results should be interpreted with caution, as the number of patients in each group was relatively small and subjects were not actually followed up over time. Other studies looking at the outcome of schizophrenia have been unable to clarify this issue, with some reporting deterioration of function (Davidson *et al.*, 1995), whilst others reported improvement or stability (Goldberg *et al.*, 1993). It is interesting to note that recent case reports and small scale clinical trials suggest that the use of atypical antipsychotics is associated with improvement of cognition in patients with schizophrenia (Stip *et al.*, 1996). Fujii *et al.* (1997) examined the cognitive function of 10 subjects with treatment-resistant schizophrenia before and after 1-year treatment with clozapine. There was significant improvement on WAIS-R scores (both verbal and performance), as well as on the performance of patients on the Wisconsin Card Sorting Test. These preliminary results indicate that the intellectual abilities of patients with schizophrenia do not necessarily deteriorate with time – in fact, they may even improve with treatment.

Neuropathological studies would, of course, provide the ultimate answer as to whether patients with schizophrenia are particularly prone to some sort of neurodegeneration. Two recent reports have, in fact, thrown some light onto this contentious issue. Purohit *et al.* (1998) examined 100 consecutive autopsy brain specimens of people with schizophrenia aged 52–101 years and compared them with 47 subjects with other neuropsychiatric disorders and 50 age-matched controls. The degree of senile plaques and neurofibrillary tangles was very similar in the three groups, suggesting that schizophrenia is not associated with Alzheimer's disease pathology or other obvious forms of neurodegeneration. Similarly, Arnold *et al.* (1998) used a stereological counting method to quantify the presence of neurofibrillary tangles, amyloid plaques, and Lewy bodies in 23 elderly subjects with chronic schizophrenia, 14 elderly controls with no neuropsychiatric disease, and 10 patients with Alzheimer's disease. They also used a number of cellular reactions to ascertain the presence of ubiquitinated dystrophic neurites, astrocytosis, and microglial infiltrates in the ventromedial temporal lobe, the frontal lobe, and the calcarine cortices. No differences were found between patients with schizophrenia and normal controls, while both groups displayed far fewer lesions than did subjects with Alzheimer's disease (Table 2). Furthermore, there was no significant association between cognitive performance on the MMSE and densities of any of the neuropathological markers.

In summary, the results of neuropsychological and neuropathological studies indicate that schizophrenia is **not** associated with cognitive decline or

Table 2.   Density values of PHF-tangles and amyloid plaques among patients with schizophrenia, subjects with no neuropsychiatric disorder, and patients with Alzheimer's disease.

	Schizophrenia N=23	*Controls* N=14	*Alzheimer's disease* N=10
PHF-tangles			
Entorhinal	0.76	0.55	3.23
Subiculum	0.67	0.48	5.98
CA1	0.63	0.96	4.03
Midfrontal	0	0	5.20
Orbitofrontal	0	0	2.93
Calcarine	0	0	0.52
Amyloid plaques			
Entorhinal	4.15	2.12	4.18
Subiculum	1.11	1.14	2.64
CA1	1.17	0.92	3.58
Midfrontal	4.30	3.52	6.63
Orbitofrontal	4.89	3.73	8.55
Calcarine	1.72	1.20	3.04

Based on Arnold *et al.* (1998).

with signs of neurodegeneration. We may still be unsure about what schizophrenia is, but we can now say with a reasonable degree of certainty what it is not.

NEUROPSYCHOLOGY OF SCHIZOPHRENIA WITH ONSET IN LATE LIFE

There is only scant information about the neuropsychology of very late onset cases of schizophrenia. This may partially be because these cases are relatively uncommon, and also due to the widespread belief that psychotic symptoms arising in late life are the result of neurodegenerative disorders such as Alzheimer's disease or cerebrovascular disease.

Almeida *et al.* (1995) tried to clarify the cognitive profile of the psychotic states arising in late life that did not fulfil criteria for other neuropsychiatric disorders. They assessed the performance of 40 patients and 33 age-matched controls on a number of cognitive tasks that included the NART, CAMCOG (the cognitive section of the CAMDEX – Roth *et al.*, 1986), WAIS-R, Recognition Memory Test, verbal fluency, and computerized tests (CANTAB) designed to evaluate recall memory, working memory, attention shift ability, and planning. Table 3 presents the qualitative results of patients' performance relative to controls. Their performance was worse than that of

Table 3. Summary of the cognitive performance of patients with late life psychosis relative to age-matched controls.

NART	↔
CAMCOG	↓
WAIS-R	↓
Recognition Memory Test for Faces	↓
Delayed-matching-to-sample	↓
Verbal fluency	↓
Extra-dimensional shift ability	↓
Spatial working memory	↓
Tower of London Planning Task	↓

↔ No difference relative to controls; ↓ impaired relative to controls.
Based on Almeida *et al.* (1995).

controls in all tasks, even though the groups were well matched for premorbid IQ and schooling.

Elliott *et al.* (1995) used a similar set of cognitive tests to evaluate a group of 32 chronic non-elderly schizophrenia sufferers. They found that the performance of schizophrenic patients was impaired relative to controls on most cognitive tasks, a finding that was later replicated by Pantelis *et al.* (1997) with a different group of patients. Furthermore, comparing the results of these studies with those reported by Almeida *et al.* (1995) for late onset cases, it is easy to see that, regardless of the age of onset, people with schizophrenia display a similar pattern of generalized cognitive impairment (Table 4). This confirms previous findings in late life psychosis (Naguib and Levy, 1987; Miller *et al.*, 1991) as well as in schizophrenia research (see above). However, the generalized cognitive impairment found among patients is both quantitatively and qualitatively different from the deficits observed in dementia of Alzheimer's or Lewy body type (Sahakian *et al.*, 1988; Sahgal *et al.*, 1992a,b; Tombaugh and McIntyre, 1992), as the deficits seem to spare patients' learning capacity (Almeida *et al.*, 1995).

THE RELATIONSHIP BETWEEN PSYCHOTIC SYMPTOMS AND COGNITIVE DYSFUNCTION

The findings of the studies described above are, to some extent, disappointing. They show no obvious specificity and, as a consequence, provide no great insight into the possible mental mechanisms involved in the causation of psychosis. Testing patients with schizophrenia with comprehensive neuropsychological batteries does not seem to be the answer!

Table 4.   Cognitive performance of early (EOS) and late
(LOS) onset schizophrenic patients relative to controls.

	EOS	LOS
NART	↔	↔
WAIS-R	↓	↓
Recognition Memory Test	↓	↓
Extra-dimensional shift ability	↓	↓
Spatial working memory	↓	↓
Tower of London Planning Task	↓	↓

Based on Almeida *et al.* (1995); Elliott *et al.* (1995); Pantelis *et al.*
(1997).

During the past few years traditional neuropsychology has been making room for two different but closely related approaches: (1) the development of cognitive models able to relate neuropsychology to psychopathology, and (2) the use of neuropsychological models in association with neuroimaging techniques. The first is probably better exemplified by the thoughtful work of Frith (1992). In Frith's model (Figure 1), an internal monitor receives information about intended actions, which are then adjusted according to specific goals or plans in order to select the most appropriate response. The model predicts that when an action is initiated internally (i.e. with no environmental stimuli), the monitor is informed about it through a mechanism similar to the corollary discharge. For example, if a subject decides to move his arm to reach out for his cup of tea, the internal monitor will be informed that the action (i.e. movement of the arm) was initiated internally and not as a result of external stimulus. Frith (1992) has argued that if this loop is defective, the subject may initiate an action and not be aware of it. In the example above, the subject may feel that his arm is being moved rather than that he is moving it (delusion of control). In a similar way, one can predict that a defect in the monitoring of inner speech might be experienced as an auditory hallucination. Following this same line of thought, Frith (1992) proposed that many psychotic symptoms can be explained as the result of problematic initiation and monitoring of actions. If this model is correct, one can predict a number of cognitive deficits among these patients, such as perseverative responses in tasks of attention set-shift, increased stimulus response latencies, decreased verbal fluency output, and deficits on tests of planning and working memory. Such an attempt to link the presence of psychotic symptoms to cognitive deficits has already received satisfactory empirical support (Shallice *et al.*, 1991; Frith, 1992).

The work of McGuire and colleagues is a good example of studies that examine the association between psychopathology, neuropsychology, and

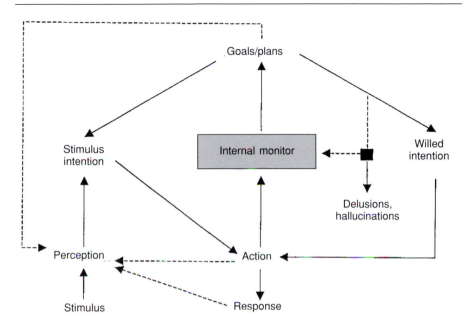

Figure 1. Frith's cognitive model of psychotic symptoms. Dashed lines represent hypothetical connections, and the shaded box represents an interruption or dysfunction to the internal monitor loop. (Based on Frith, 1992 – see text for details.)

neuroimaging. In 1993 they published a paper showing that active auditory hallucinations were associated with increased activity of the cortical areas specializing in language, such as Broca's area (McGuire *et al.*, 1993). Two years later, they tested a cognitive model that linked inner speech with auditory hallucinations (McGuire *et al.*, 1995). They showed that hallucinators were unable to activate the left middle temporal gyrus and rostral supplementary motor area when imagining sentences being spoken to them in another person's voice. These findings suggest that patients who experience auditory hallucinations may fail to activate areas concerned with the monitoring of inner speech.

CONCLUSION

Schizophrenia is associated with intellectual decline. Nonetheless, there is no evidence that patients suffer from a progressive degenerative condition. In addition, there is no indication that the neuropsychology of early and very late onset schizophrenia is different. In fact, there is no such thing as a specific 'neuropsychology of schizophrenia'. The use of extensive cognitive test batteries is unlikely to further contribute to our understanding of the mental processes involved in the emergence of psychotic symptoms. Instead, it seems that a more informative approach may be to investigate the association between discrete psychotic symptoms and specific cognitive models by means of functional neuroimaging. It is still unclear exactly how far this new method of study will take us but certainly it is enabling us to continue to move forwards.

REFERENCES

Almeida, O.P., Howard, R.J., Levy, R., David, A.S., Morris, R.G. and Sahakian, B.J. (1995). Cognitive features of psychotic states arising in late life (late paraphrenia). *Psychol Med* **25**, 685–698.

Arnold, S.E., Trojanowski, J.Q., Gur, R.E., Blackwell, P., Han, L.Y. and Choi, C. (1998). Absence of neurodegeneration and neural injury in the cerebral cortex in a sample of elderly patients with schizophrenia. *Arch Gen Psychiatry* **55**, 225–232.

Braff, D.L., Heaton, R., Kuck, J. *et al.* (1991). The generalized pattern of neuropsychological deficits in outpatients with chronic schizophrenia with heterogeneous Wisconsin Card Sorting Test results. *Arch Gen Psychiatry* **48**, 891–898.

Davidson, M., Harvey, P.D., Powchik, P. *et al.* (1995). Severity of symptoms in chronically institutionalized geriatric schizophrenic patients. *Am J Psychiatry* **152**, 197–207.

Elliott, R., McKenna, P.J., Robbins, T.W. and Sahakian, B.J. (1995). Neuropsychological evidence for frontostriatal dysfunction in schizophrenia. *Psychol Med* **25**, 619–630.

Fleming, K., Goldberg, T.E., Binks, S., Randolph, C., Gold, J.M. and Weinberger, D.R. (1997). Visuospatial working memory in patients with schizophrenia. *Biol Psychiatry* **41**, 43–49.

Frith, C.D. (1992). *The Cognitive Neuropsychology of Schizophrenia*. Lawrence Erlbaum Associates, Hove/Hillsdale.

Frith, C.D., Leary, J., Cahill, C. and Johnstone, E.C. (1991). Disabilities and circumstances of schizophrenic patients – a follow-up study: IV. Performance on psychological tests – demographic and clinical correlates of the results of these tests. *Br J Psychiatry* **159**, (suppl 13), 26–29.

Fujii, D.E.M., Ahmed, I., Jokumsen, M. and Compton, J.M. (1997). The effects of clozapine on cognitive functioning in treatment-resistant schizophrenic patients. *Neuropsychiatry Clin Neurosci* **9**, 240–245.

Gold, J.M., Goldberg, T.E. and Weinberger, D.R. (1992). Prefrontal function and schizophrenic symptoms. *Neuropsychiatry Neuropsychol Behav Neurol* **5**, 253–261.

Goldberg, T.E., Hyde, T.M., Leinman, J.E. and Weinberger, D.R. (1993). Course of schizophrenia: neuropsychological evidence for a static encephalopathy. *Schizophr Bull* **19**, 797–804.

Guy, W. (1988). Abnormal involuntary movement scale (AIMS). *Psychopharmacol Bull* **24**, 781–783.

Hyde, T.M., Nawroz, S., Goldberg, T.E. *et al.* (1994). Is there a cognitive decline in schizophrenia? A cross-sectional study. *Br J Psychiatry* **164**, 494–500.

McGuire, P.K., Shah, G.M. and Murray, R.M. (1993). Increased blood flow in Broca's area during auditory hallucination in schizophrenia. *Lancet* **342**, 703–706.

McGuire, P.K., Silbersweig, D.A., Wright, I. *et al.* (1995). Abnormal monitoring of inner speech: a physiological basis for auditory hallucinations. *Lancet* **346**, 596–600.

Miller, B.L., Lesser, I.M., Boone, K.B., Hill, E., Mehringer, C.M. and Wong, K. (1991). Brain lesions and cognitive function in late-life psychosis. *Br J Psychiatry* **158**, 76–82.

Mockler, D., Riordan, J. and Sharma, T. (1997). Memory and intellectual deficits do not decline with age in schizophrenia. *Schizophr Res* **26**, 1–7.

Morrinson-Stewart, S.L., Williamson, P.C., Corning, W.C., Kutcher, S.P., Snow, W.G. and Merskey, H. (1992). Frontal and non-frontal lobe neuropsychological test performance and clinical symptomatology in schizophrenia. *Psychol Med* **22**, 353–359.

Naguib, M. and Levy, R. (1987). Late paraphrenia: neuropsychological impairment and structural brain abnormalities on computed tomography. *Int J Geriatr Psychiatry* **2**, 83–90.

Nelson, H.E., Pantelis, C., Carruthers, K., Speller, J., Baxendale, S. and Barnes, T.R.E. (1990). Cognitive functioning and symptomatology in chronic schizophrenia. *Psychol Med* **20**, 357–365.

Pantelis, C., Barnes, T.R.E., Nelson, H.E. *et al.* (1997). Frontal-striatal cognitive deficits in patients with chronic schizophrenia. *Brain* **120**, 1823–1843.

Purohit, D.P., Perl, D.P., Haroutunian, V., Powchik, P., Davidson, M. and Davis, K.L. (1998). Alzheimer disease and related neurodegenerative diseases in elderly patients with schizophrenia: a postmortem neuropathologic study of 100 cases. *Arch Gen Psychiatry* **55**, 205–211.

Roth, M., Tym, E., Mountjoy, C.Q. *et al.* (1986). CAMDEX: a standardised instrument for the diagnosis of mental disorder in the elderly with special reference to the early detection of dementia. *Br J Psychiatry* **149**, 698–709.

Sahakian, B.J., Morris, R.G., Evenden, J.L. *et al.* (1988). A comparative study of visuo-spatial learning and memory in Alzheimer-type dementia and Parkinson's disease. *Brain* **111**, 695–718.

Sahgal, A., Galloway, P.H., McKeith, I.G. *et al.* (1992a). Matching to sample deficits in senile dementias of the Alzheimer and Lewy body types. *Arch Neurol* **49**, 1043–1046.

Sahgal, A., Lloyd, S., Wray, C.J. *et al.* (1992b). Does visuospatial memory in senile dementia of Alzheimer type depend on the severity of the disorder? *Int Geriatr Psychiatry* **7**, 427–436.

Shallice, T., Burgees, P.W. and Frith, C.D. (1991). Can the neuropsychological case-study approach be applied to schizophrenia? *Psychol Med* **21**, 661–673.

Spring, B., Lemon, M., Weinstein, L. and Haskell, A. (1989). Distractibility in schizophrenia: state and trait aspects. *Br J Psychiatry* **155**, 63–68.

Stip, E., Lussier, I., Babai, M. and Fabian, J.L. (1996). Seroquel and cognitive improvement in patients with schizophrenia. *Biol Psychiatry* **40**, 434–435.

Tamlyn, A., McKenna, P.J., Mortimer, A.M., Lund, C.E., Hammond, S. and Baddeley, A.D. (1992). Memory impairment in schizophrenia: its extent, affiliations and neuropsychological character. *Psychol Med* **22**, 101–115.

Tombaugh, T.N. and McIntyre, N.J. (1992). The Mini-Mental State Examination: a comprehensive review. *J Am Geriatr Soc* **40**, 922–935.

Waddington, J.L. and Youssef, H.A. (1996). Cognitive dysfunction in chronic schizophrenia followed prospectively over 10 years and its longitudinal relationship to the emergence of tardive dyskinesia. *Psychol Med* **26**, 681–688.

Waddington, J.L., Youssef, H.A., Dolphin, C. and Kinsella, A. (1987). Cognitive dysfunction, negative symptoms and tardive dyskinesia in schizophrenia: their association in relation to topography of involuntary movements and criterion of their abnormality. *Arch Gen Psychiatry* **44**, 907–912.

Weinberger, D.R. (1987). Implications of normal brain development for the pathogenesis of schizophrenia. *Arch Gen Psychiatry* **44**, 660–669.

Late Onset Schizophrenia
Edited by Robert Howard, Peter V. Rabins, David J. Castle
© 1999 Wrightson Biomedical Publishing Ltd

15

Brain Imaging in Late Onset Schizophrenia

GODFREY G. PEARLSON

*Department of Psychiatry, Johns Hopkins Hospital,
Baltimore, Maryland, USA*

INTRODUCTION

Ideally, neuroimaging investigations in late onset schizophrenia patients would help answer the following questions:

1. What is the aetiology and timing of the structural and functional changes in late onset schizophrenia?
2. Can neuroimaging studies identify specific lesions or aetiologies associated with the disorder and determine whether such lesions share a common anatomic localization or represent a single well-defined pathology?
3. Does late onset schizophrenia depend on late-occurring changes unmasking a pre-existing (perhaps genetic) vulnerability?
4. If so, what is the vulnerability and does it consist of a brain lesion of developmental origin, similar to that proposed for early onset cases?
5. Also, is symptomatic onset delayed to the senium because the 'late-occurring changes' referred to above consist of age-related brain alterations?
6. What are these alterations, and can they suffice to cause the emergence of late onset schizophrenia in persons lacking a pre-existing vulnerability?
7. How do the brain changes associated with late onset schizophrenia differ (if at all) from those associated with early onset cases of the disorder?
8. Are the changes associated with late onset schizophrenia diagnostically distinct from those seen in other neuropsychiatric disorders arising in old age?

This chapter reviews the existing neuroimaging literature in an attempt to determine how satisfactorily it provides consistent answers to these questions.

NON-SPECIFIC STRUCTURAL CHANGES

As in schizophrenia with onset in the teens and twenties, various studies have demonstrated increased ventricular-to-brain ratio (VBR) in late onset schizophrenia patients compared with appropriately age- and sex-matched healthy control subjects. The origin of the enlarged ventricles is unknown. It could represent an old, static developmental abnormality or a recent and perhaps progressive one. It could represent generalized tissue abnormality or periventricular changes only. This change is also diagnostically non-specific, being encountered in a wide variety of conditions of diverse aetiologies. Nevertheless, the presence of large ventricles is the best-replicated symptom in LOS.

Computed tomography (CT) studies include those of Rabins *et al.* (1987), Naguib and Levy (1987), Pearlson *et al.* (1987) and Burns *et al.* (1989). Howard *et al.* (1992a,b) found lateral VBR (as well as third ventricular changes) to be no different from that for control subjects but Pearlson *et al.* (1993) found insignificant lateral but significant third ventricular enlargement. Miller *et al.* (1991) found no MRI lateral ventricular differences between patients and control subjects. Overall then, fewer MRI studies than CT show ventricular enlargement in LOS.

Are changes seen in LOS as extensive as those that characterize Alzheimer's disease patients? Rabins *et al.* (1987) found late onset schizophrenia patients to have VBRs greater than those of control subjects but smaller than those of Alzheimer's disease patients with psychotic symptoms. Similarly, Krull *et al.* (1991), assessing VBRs on MRI scans, found values in LOS patients to be intermediate between those of control subjects and Alzheimer's disease patients. Howard *et al.* (1992a) and Almeida *et al.* (1992) found LOS patients *without* Schneiderian first rank symptoms to have ventricular/sulcal enlargement comparable to that of Alzheimer's disease, while LOS patients with first rank symptoms were more similar to elderly controls.

IMAGING STUDIES IN LOS MAY PROVIDE EVIDENCE FOR THE NEURODEVELOPMENTAL HYPOTHESIS OF SCHIZOPHRENIA

Evidence for the neurodevelopmental hypothesis

Due to the non-dominant/non-recessive inheritance pattern of schizophrenia and the evidence noted below, the disorder is frequently hypothesized to require two aetiologic 'hits'. In this proposal, one genetic 'hit' or diathesis is surmised to interact with a second, perhaps environmental, 'hit' in order to produce the conditions necessary for the clinical syndrome to manifest. The second abnormality is presumed to occur most usually in early fetal neurodevelopment, (e.g. maternal pyrexia, or obstetric adversity). Is then late life onset schizophrenia a delay of the same 'two-hit' disorder to old age, or does it represent a different disorder with a separate aetiopathology? Alternatively, is the first or genetic 'hit' identical for both conditions, but the second 'hit' late occurring and perhaps even neurodegenerative in the case of LOS?

Despite the usual onset of 'classic' schizophrenia in early adult life, recent evidence suggests that the disorder develops due to disruptions in fetal brain development that clinically manifest later in life when relevant neural systems reach maturity (Jakob and Beckmann, 1986; Weinberger, 1987; Jones et al., 1992). Non-imaging support for this hypothesis derives from several sources. These include epidemiologic evidence of increased incidence of perinatal insults and obstetrical complications (Kendell et al., 1996; Jones 1997) as well as early behavioural problems (Pilowsky et al., 1993; Weinberger, 1996; Cannon et al., 1997) in the pre-schizophrenic population.

Several MRI studies in young adults with schizophrenia report an excess of gross structural abnormalities in schizophrenia, such as cavum septum pellucidum and callosal agenesis, that clearly reflect abnormal brain development (e.g. Nopoulos et al., 1995, 1997), as do the presence of reversed planum temporale asymmetry and abnormal sulcal–gyral patterns (Kikinis et al., 1994; Bullmore et al., 1995; Barta 1997). Unfortunately, no studies to date have attempted to assess these changes in LOS, so that clear-cut evidence for neurodevelopmental lesions is lacking.

IMAGING STUDIES IN LOS MAY PROVIDE EVIDENCE FOR THE NEURODEGENERATIVE HYPOTHESIS OF SCHIZOPHRENIA

Evidence for the neurodegenerative hypothesis

Staying with the 'two-hit' hypothesis, we proposed above that the second, late-life event in LOS might be age-related or neurodegenerative in character. Is the evidence for this stronger than that for neurodevelopmental problems?

It is possible that the clinical onset of schizophrenia in young adulthood is followed by a continuing, active neurodegenerative process in some patients. Brain imaging, particularly in a longitudinal design, can address this question, but to date studies have yielded conflicting findings. Illowsky et al. (1988), Vita et al. (1988), Kemali et al. (1989), Woods et al. (1990), Jaskiw et al. (1994), Vita et al. (1994), DeLisi et al. (1995) and Mathalon et al. (1997) found evidence for either modest atrophy exceeding that of abnormal ageing or no differences from healthy controls. It is possible that deterioration occurs only in a subgroup of schizophrenic patients, e.g. Nair *et al.* (1997). Elderly, institutionalized early adult life onset schizophrenic patients develop a non-AD dementia (Purohit *et al.*, 1993; Barak *et al.*, 1997). Examination of such individuals using quantitative anatomic measures is important to determine if this occurs commonly in schizophrenia, when the process begins and whether it relates to processes occurring in LOS. To date, no such study has been attempted.

The largest investigation addressing the question of neurodegeneration in early adult life onset schizophrenia is that of DeLisi (1997), who obtained annual MRI scans on 50 young adult schizophrenic patients, followed since first clinical onset, and 20 controls, for 4 or more years. No differences in rate of size change were found for total temporal lobe or hippocampus/amygdala volumes, but schizophrenic patients were characterized by decreased sizes of both hemispheres, right cerebellum, isthmus of the corpus callosum, and left lateral ventricle. This evidence suggests that at least some young people with schizophrenia may manifest neurodegenerative changes.

There is a dearth of similar studies in LOS. Hoffman *et al.* (1991) determined that VBR in patients with schizophrenia aged over 55 years had increased 3 years after an initial scan. In the only direct comparison of elderly early (EOS) and late (LOS) onset schizophrenic patients Corey-Bloom *et al.* (1995) found a more marked increase in ventricular enlargement in the late onset group. More and larger-scale longitudinal studies of LOS are clearly needed to settle these questions, which remain unanswered.

ARE FINDINGS IN LOS DIFFERENT FROM THOSE SEEN IN EARLY ONSET CASES OF SCHIZOPHRENIA?

An essential question to address is whether late onset schizophrenic patients share brain changes with those described previously for 'classic' early onset disease, or, to restate this in slightly different terms, do late and early onset patients have abnormalities in similar brain regions or circuits?

Structural and functional brain imaging abnormalities in early onset schizophrenia include the following: increased ventricular-to-brain ratios (VBRs) on CT or MRI (Johnstone *et al.*, 1976, Weinberger *et al.*, 1979; Pearlson *et al.*, 1987); third ventricular enlargement, (Boronow *et al.*, 1985); cortical atrophy on CT or MRI (Pfefferbaum *et al.*, 1988; Gur *et al.* 1991); both mild generalized loss of cerebral grey matter and local disproportionate grey matter reductions (Pearlson *et al.*, 1997), resting bloodflow abnormalities on SPECT (Gur *et al.*, 1985, Matthew *et al.*, 1988), regional cerebral bloodflow abnormalities during provocative tasks, for example, those of working memory or set-shifting (Berman *et al.*, 1992) and increased dopamine D_2 receptor subtype B_{max} on PET scans (Wong *et al.*, 1986a,b,c; Tune *et al.*, 1994).

Many of these abnormalities are also reported in late onset schizophrenia patients. These include increased VBR on CT or MRI (Naguib and Levy, 1987; Rabins *et al.*, 1987; Howard *et al.*, 1992a, 1994). Several groups (Breitner *et al.*, 1990; Flint *et al.*, 1991; Pearlson *et al.*, 1993) have also described third ventricular enlargement in late onset schizophrenia. Cortical atrophy was described by Howard *et al.* (1992b, 1994) and Pearlson *et al.* (1993) but not by Burns *et al.* (1989). Miller *et al.* (1992) described resting SPECT bloodflow abnormalities in late onset schizophrenia. To date, no bloodflow tasks using provocative cognitive stimuli have been attempted in LOS.

Neuroreceptor PET studies have shown increased B_{max} values for dopamine subtype D_2 receptors by Pearlson *et al.* (1993). That research compared neuroleptic-naive, schizophrenia patients with clinical onset after age 55 to control subjects, using the method described by Wong *et al.* (1986a,b,c) to calculate D_2 receptor B_{max} (receptor density). Because the control subjects were younger, regression values were calculated in the control subjects and a predicted D_2 receptor B_{max} was then computed for the schizophrenic subjects. Standardized residual D_2 receptor B_{max} values for schizophrenic subjects showed significant elevation. This finding is similar to reports of elevated D_2 receptor B_{max} receptors in drug-naive, early onset schizophrenia patients reported using the same method (Wong *et al.*, 1986a), although not by other investigators using a different method (Farde *et al.*, 1987).

Relatively few studies have directly compared late onset schizophrenic patients with elderly early onset schizophrenic patients. Pearlson *et al.* (1993) contrasted 11 late onset patients with 11 early onset individuals, group-matched by age and sex. Groups were compared using the CERAD MRI rating scales for third ventricle and left and right for Sylvian fissure, temporal sulci, temporal horn, lateral ventricles, and cerebral sulci. No significant differences were found between the early and late onset groups, which was interpreted as emphasizing their similarity with regard to brain abnormalities. Below, we discuss that Symonds *et al.* (1997) made a key comparison between age-matched groups of LOS, EOS and control subjects and found no significant differences in ordinal measures of several indices of neurodegenerative measures.

ARE NEUROIMAGING FINDINGS IN LOS DIAGNOSTICALLY SPECIFIC?

The question of the disease-specificity of the brain imaging changes discussed above is important. Pearlson and Petty (1994) noted that many of the reported findings in late onset schizophrenia are non specific in the sense of being unlocalized in the brain. They are also non-specific in that similar brain findings have also been reported for patients suffering from late onset neuropsychiatric disorders, especially depression.

Late onset depression

Late onset depression, like late onset schizophrenia, has a lesser genetic contribution than early onset cases of the same disorder. Late onset depression is also linked to findings of increased ventricular-to-brain ratio on CT or MRI (Pearlson *et al.*, 1987; Rabins *et al.*, 1991) and third ventricular enlargement (Coffey *et al.*, 1989, 1990).

Late-onset depression is also associated convincingly with a higher than expected prevalence of non-specific cerebrovascular changes. This has been shown on MRI and SPECT, (Krishnan *et al.*, 1988; Coffey *et al.*, 1989; Zubenko *et al.*, 1990; Beats *et al.*, 1991; Lesser *et al.*, 1991; Rabins *et al.*, 1991). These findings are discussed in detail in the following section.

The Barta *et al.* (1997) report of reduced entorhinal cortical and superior temporal gyral sizes in late onset schizophrenia is similar to prior reports in early onset schizophrenic patients (e.g. Barta *et al.*, 1990; Pearlson *et al.*, 1997). The 1997 Barta *et al.* study is thus important as it suggests that changes in the temporal lobe reported for early onset schizophrenia but not early onset affective disorder (Pearlson *et al.*, 1997) are also seen in late onset schizophrenia. Rabins *et al.* (unpublished data) compared late onset depressed patients, late onset schizophrenic patients and elderly age- and sex-matched normal controls using the CERAD visual analogue MRI rating scales. This comparison revealed significant differences between normal controls and patients, which differed between the two patient groups. LOS patients differed from normals in having enlargement of the third ventricle and both temporal horns. Depressed patients did not show such abnormalities but differed uniquely from normals in showing enlarged bilateral cerebral sulci, lateral ventricles and Sylvian fissures. Thus, although there are similar non-specific brain changes in the two disorders, there are also distinct differences.

Multi-infarct/vascular dementia

White matter changes, (also known as 'white matter hyperintensities' – 'WMHs' – and 'unidentified bright objects' – 'UBOs') are a visual macroscopic feature derived from the MRI or CT appearance which are commonly noted to occur with increasing age. They likely represent a rather mixed group of histologic findings. Several authors (Awad, 1986a,b; Braffman *et al.*, 1988; Chimowitz, 1992) have found varying combinations of gliosis, myelin thinning, oedema, and perivascular and vascular pathology in post-mortem tissue from brain regions that generated such hyperintense signals on T-2 weighted MRI scans. However, a review of such literature reveals that WMHs do not inevitably correspond with tissue pathology, and that comparable tissue pathology can be found in regions with normal MRI signal. Thus the presence of WMHs may be as much a function of the quantity and/or density, rather than the mere presence or absence, of a group of heterogeneous white matter pathologies.

As noted above, late-life depression is associated convincingly with an excess of such findings. Are similar changes associated with LOS? As discussed earlier in this chapter, late onset schizophrenia may be due to neurodegenerative processes affecting individuals with latent vulnerability to schizophrenia, so that such an association would not be surprising. However, neuroimaging studies using CT or MRI that attempted to link possible degenerative anatomic correlates (atrophy, white matter disease, and strokes) to the disorder have yielded conflicting findings. Several studies report an excess of white matter abnormalities in late onset schizophrenia patients compared with healthy control subjects. These include Miller *et al.* (1986); Miller and Lesser (1988); Breitner *et al.* (1990), Lesser *et al.* (1991, 1992); Flint *et al.* (1991); Miller *et al.* (1991); but not other workers (Howard *et al.*, 1995; Symonds *et al.*, 1997; Rivkin *et al.*, 1999). Although there were suggestions of localized patterns in the earlier positive studies, the changes reported (including periventricular white matter hyperintensities, probable subcortical vascular lesions, and white matter hyperintensities) emphasize that they are neither uniform in nature nor localized to particular brain regions.

Whether such findings occur in association with LOS seems dependent on the choice of cases. The earlier studies, that reported a positive association (e.g. Lesser *et al.*, 1989, 1992; Miller *et al.*, 1992) tended to recruit patients broadly, resulting in inclusion of patients more likely to have microvascular lesions, unsuspected stroke and probable vascular dementia. There is also the suggestion that such cases are perhaps less likely to be clinically typical of LOS. Case series that more carefully screened their population in an attempt to eliminate those most likely to have a diagnosis of organic cerebral disorder (Naguib and Levy, 1987; Krull *et al.*, 1991, Howard *et al.*, 1995) found no excess of white matter hyperintensities.

Several SPECT studies now agree in showing a relative excess in late onset psychosis patients of multiple areas of reduced cerebral blood flow. For example, in a diagnostically mixed group of such patients Lesser *et al.* (1993) showed that approximately 75% had SPECT scan abnormalities of this type. Miller *et al.* (1992) also demonstrated cerebral blood flow abnormalities suggestive of cerebrovascular disease in a proportion of late onset psychosis patients. Further, 83% of the late onset psychosis patients, versus 27% of the control subjects, had one or more small temporal or frontal areas of hypo-perfusion.

Alzheimer's disease

Alzheimer's disease on MRI is characterized by variable amounts of non-specific generalized atrophy, and disproportionate hippocampal and amygdala atrophy (e.g. Pearlson *et al.*, 1992). As noted above, similar ventricular enlargement and cortical atrophy are reported in CT or MRI studies of LOS. A volumetric temporal lobe MRI study by Barta *et al.* (1997) compared elderly patients with Alzheimer's disease to an age- and sex-matched comparison group of late onset schizophrenic patients and to matched normal controls. Patients with Alzheimer's disease showed the expected widespread general and regional cerebral atrophy. Late onset schizophrenic patients showed similar degrees of shrinkage of entorhinal cortex, hippocampus and amygdala to the Alzheimer's disease patients but had significantly more marked volume loss in both superior temporal gyri. This superior temporal gyral finding is similar to prior reports in 'classic' early onset schizophrenic patients, (e.g. Barta *et al.*, 1990). This study suggests that some specific temporal lobe changes reported for 'classic' early onset schizophrenia (e.g. Pearlson *et al.*, 1997) may also be seen in late onset schizophrenia.

CONCLUSIONS

This chapter has attempted to provide a critical review of published papers dealing with neuroimaging in LOS. Emerging data support the concept that early and late onset cases of schizophrenia share common structural and neuroreceptor brain abnormalities.

It remains possible, but unlikely, that both early and late onset forms of schizophrenia represent the same disorder in the sense of sharing the same aetiopathogenesis. In a 'two-hit model' of schizophrenia, for late onset cases, the second 'hit' presumably occurs in late life. Examples of such late-life second 'hits' are the age-associated brain changes (e.g. age-related atrophy affecting a critical structure or pathway, or age-related changes in neurotransmitters or their receptors). For example, elsewhere, we have examined evidence that possible precipitants for late onset schizophrenia include neuronal loss due to normal ageing and vascular or age-related functional changes, especially those affecting females such as postmenopausal oestrogen loss and thus alterations in the relative balance of dopamine D_2 receptors in basal ganglia (Pearlson and Petty, 1994).

A second hypothesis would posit that late onset schizophrenia is an organic phenocopy of the early onset form with only a single 'hit' required. This

Table 1.   Study design differences.

Observation
Wide variability in subject numbers
Variable screening and subsequent exclusion for coarse brain damage, e.g. stroke
Little follow-up to detect incident cases of dementia
No neuropathologic validation
Subject referral bias
Phenomenologic heterogeneity, e.g. delusional disorder versus schizophrenia
Failure to match subjects to controls derived from their community of origin
Variable stringency in patient/control demographic matching
Wide variation in age at onset of disorder, e.g. 45+ versus 65+
Lack of comparison to appropriate psychiatric 'disease control' group
Wide variation in anatomic definitions of regions of interest
Imaging methods semi- or non-quantitative

would presumably consist also of a primary age-associated pathology (e.g. microvascular disease, or early manifestations of a primary dementing illness). The role of late-life brain abnormalities and the relative contributions of neurodevelopmental versus neurodegenerative processes (the latter including microvascular disease) were reviewed here and remain to be elucidated. We concluded on the basis of brain imaging studies that while cerebrovascular pathology may prove an aetiologic factor for a proportion of cases of late onset schizophrenia, the evidence for an association with late onset schizophrenia is less compelling than for late-life depression. Perhaps late onset psychosis as seen by clinicians represents the end result of diverse aetiopathologies, perhaps a mixture of delayed 'classic early onset' and 'organic' secondary cases.

As noted previously (Pearlson and Petty, 1994), different studies of late onset schizophrenia have used widely different inclusion/exclusion factors to select cases. Differences in clinical onset ages and variable stringency in eliminating organic disorders are only two of many prominent examples. These, together with other examples of important differences in study design are listed in Table 1.

Brain imaging can help provide evidence to select among the above competing hypotheses. It is also clear that many late onset schizophrenia patients do not have a specific brain lesion or observable pathologic aetiology to explain their clinical state and that lesions reported in some studies share neither a common localization nor represent a single well-defined pathology.

How can future studies remedy some of the problems of prior investigations? As most studies have been conducted on a relatively small number of intensively studied late onset patients, one need is for new studies to recruit a significantly larger population of late onset schizophrenic patients than have characterized many prior investigations. Another is to compare patients with LOS to a large normative community ageing sample. This will help put brain changes associated with the disorder in the broader context of normal male versus female ageing brains. Another approach is to pool patients and methods across different centres. Neuroimaging studies could be dove-tailed with neuropathologic studies. Longitudinal follow-up is essential to determine whether cognitive or functional decline occurs over a several-year follow-up period. Neuropathologic examination will help elucidate the nature of the underlying pathology, and aid the distinction between developmental and neurodegenerative processes.

Many of the studies of late onset schizophrenia reviewed above included fairly narrowly defined patients, and such case series are less likely to include patients with coarse brain disease. Studies including more broadly defined patients will increase diagnostic heterogeneity and increase the odds of including more 'organic phenocopies', i.e. cases of cerebrovascular and other coarse brain pathology. Inclusion of suitable patient comparison groups (e.g. elderly affective subjects, elderly early onset schizophrenic patients) will help clarify issues related to disease specificity and address the issue of schizophrenia across the lifespan.

Useful information is clearly emerging from neuroimaging studies of LOS, and as study designs improve we can gradually sharpen our questions and refine hypotheses.

REFERENCES

Almeida, O.P., Howard, R., Forstl, H. *et al.* (1992). Should the diagnosis of late paraphrenia be abandoned? *Psychol Med* **22**, 11–14.

American Psychiatric Association (1987). *Diagnostic and Statistical Manual of Mental Disorders, 3rd edn revised*, DSM-IIIR. American Psychiatric Association, Washington, DC.

Awad, I.A., Spetzler, R.F. and Hodak, J.A. (1986a). Incidental subcortical lesions identified on magnetic resonance imaging in the elderly, I: correlation with age and cerebrovascular risk factors. *Stroke* **17**, 1084–1089.

Awad, I.A., Spetzler, R.F. and Hodak, J.A. (1986b). Incidental subcortical lesions identified on magnetic resonance imaging in the elderly, II: postmortem pathological correlations. *Stroke* **17**, 1090–1097.

Barak, Y., Swartz, M. and Davidson, M. (1997). Dementia in elderly schizophrenic patients: reviewing the reviews. *Int Rev Psychiatry* **9**, 459–463.

Barta, P.E., Pearlson, G.D., Powers, R.E., Richards, S.S. and Tune, L.E. (1990). Auditory hallucinations and smaller superior temporal gyral volume in schizophrenia. *Am J Psychiatry* **147**, 1457–1462.

Barta, P.E., Powers, R.E., Aylward, E.H. *et al.* (1997). Quantitative MRI volume changes in late onset schizophrenia and Alzheimer's disease compared to normal controls. *Psychiatry Res* **68**, 65–75.

Beats, B., Levy, R. and Forstl, H. (1991). Ventricular enlargement and caudate hyperdensity in elderly depressives. *Biol Psychiatry* **30**, 452–458.

Berman, K.F., Torrey, E.F., Daniel, D.G. and Weinberger, D.R. (1992). Regional cerebral blood flow in monozygotic twins discordant and concordant for schizophrenia. *Arch Gen Psychiatry* **49**, 927–934.

Boronow, J., Pickar, D. and Ninan, P.T. (1985). Atrophy limited to third ventricle only in chronic schizophrenic patients: report of a controlled series. *Arch Gen Psychiatry* **40**, 266–271.

Braffman, B.H., Zimmerman, R.A., Trojanowski, J.Q., Gonatas, N.K., Hickey, W.F. and Schlaepfer, W.W. (1988). Brain MR: pathologic correlation with gross and histopathology. 2. Hyperintense white-matter foci in the elderly. *Am J Roentgenol* **151**, 559–566.

Breitner, J.C.S., Husain, M.M., Figiel, G.S. *et al.* (1990). Cerebral white matter disease in late-onset paranoid psychosis. *Biol Psychiatry* **28**, 266–274.

Bullmore, E., Brammer, M., Harvey, I., Murray, R. and Ron, M. (1995). Cerebral hemispheric asymmetry revisited: effects of handedness, gender and schizophrenia measured by radius of gyration in magnetic resonance images. *Psychol Med* **25**, 349–363.

Burns, A., Carrick, J., Ames, D. *et al.* (1989). The cerebral cortical appearance in late paraphrenia. *Int J Geriatr Psychiatry* **4**, 31–34.

Cannon, T.D., Bearden, C.E., Hollister, J.M. and Hadley, T. (1997). A prospective cohort study of childhood cognitive deficits as precursors of schizophrenia. *Schizophr Res* **24**, 99–100.

Chimowitz, M.I., Estes, M.L., Fulan, A.J. and Awad, I.A. (1992). Further observations on the pathology of subcortical lesions identified on magnetic resonance imaging. *Arch Neurol* **49**, 747–752.

Coffey, C.E., Figiel, G.S., Djang, W.T. *et al.* (1989). White matter hyperintensity on magnetic resonance imaging: clinical and neuroanatomic correlates in the depressed elderly. *J Neuropsychiatry Clin Neurosci* **1**, 135–144.

Coffey, C.E., Figiel, G.S., Djang, W.T. *et al.* (1990). Subcortical hyperintensity on magnetic resonance imaging: a comparison of normal and depressed elderly subjects. *Am J Psychiatry* **147**, 187–189.

Corey-Bloom, J., Jernigan, T., Archibald, S. Harris, M.J. and Jeste, D.V. (1995). Quantitative magnetic resonance imaging of the brain in late-life schizophrenia. *Am J Psychiatry* **152**, 447–449.

DeLisi, L.E. (1997). Is schizophrenia a lifetime disorder of brain plasticity, growth and aging? *Schizophr Res* **23**, 119–129.

DeLisi, L.E., Tew, W., Xie, S. *et al.* (1995). Prospective follow-up study of brain morphology and cognition in first-episode schizophrenic patients: preliminary findings. *Biol Psychiatry* **38**, 349–360.

Farde, L., Wiesel, F.A., Hall, H., Halldin, C., Stone-Elander, S. and Sedvall, G. (1987). No D_2 receptor increase in PET study of schizophrenia. *Arch Gen Psychiatry* **44**, 671–672.

Flint, A.J., Rifat, S.L. and Eastwood, M.R. (1991). Late-onset paranoia: distinct from paraphrenia? *Int J Geriatr Psychiatry* **6**, 103–109.

Gur, R.E., Bur, R.C., Skolnik, B.E. *et al.* (1985). Brain function in psychiatric disorders, III: regional cerebral blood flow in unmedicated schizophrenics. *Arch Gen Psychiatry* **42**, 329–334.

Gur, R.E., Mozley, P.D., Resnick, S.M. *et al.* (1991). Magnetic resonance imaging in schizophrenia, I: volumetric analysis of brain and cerebrospinal fluid. *Arch Gen Psychiatry* **48**, 407–412.

Hoffman, W.F., Ballard, L., Turner, E.H. and Casey, D.E. (1991). Three-year follow-up of older schizophrenics: extrapyramidal syndromes, psychiatric symptoms, and ventricular brain ratio. *Biol Psychiatry* **30**, 913–926.

Howard, R.J., Forstl, H., Almeida, O. *et al.* (1992a). Computer-assisted CT measurements in late paraphrenics with and without Schneiderian first-rank symptoms: a preliminary report. *Int J Geriatr Psychiatry* **7**, 35–38.

Howard, R.J., Forstl, H., Almeida, O. *et al.* (1992b). First-rank symptoms of Schneider in late paraphrenia: cortical structural correlates. *Br J Psychiatry* **160**, 108–109.

Howard, R.J., Almeida, O., Levy, R., Graves, P. and Graves, M. (1994). Quantitative magnetic resonance imaging volumetry distinguishes delusional disorder from late-onset schizophrenia. *Br J Psychiatry* **165**, 474–480.

Howard, R., Cox, T., Almeida, O. *et al.* (1995). White matter signal hyperintensities in the brains of patients with late paraphrenia and the normal, community-living elderly. *Biol Psychiatry* **38**, 86–91.

Illowsky, B.P., Juliano, D.M., Bigelow, L.B. and Weinberger, D.R. (1988). Stability of CT scan findings in schizophrenia: results of an 8 year follow-up study. *J Neurol Neurosurgery Psychiatry* **51**, 209–213.

Jakob, H. and Beckmann, H. (1986). Prenatal developmental disturbances in the limbic allocortex in schizophrenics. *J Neural Transm* **65**, 303–326.

Jaskiw, G.E., Juliano, D.M., Goldberg, T.E., Hertzman, M., Urow-Hamell, E. and Weinberger, D.R. (1994). Cerebral ventricular enlargement in schizophreniform disorder does not progress. A seven year follow-up study. *Schizophr Res* **14**, 23–28.

Johnstone, E., Crow, T., Frith, C. *et al.* (1976). Cerebral ventricular size and cognitive impairment in chronic schizophrenia. *Lancet* **2**, 924–926.

Jones, P. (1997). The early origins of schizophrenia. *Br Med Bull* **53**, 135–155.

Jones, C.T., Morris, S., Yates, C.M., Moffoot, A., Sharpe, C. and Brock, D.J. (1992). Mutation in codon 713 of the beta amyloid precursor protein gene presenting with schizophrenia. *Nature Genetics* **1**, 306–309.

Kemali, D., Maj, M., Galderisi, S., Milici, N. and Salvati, A. (1989). Ventricle-to-brain ratio in schizophrenia: a controlled follow-up study. *Biol Psychiatry* **26**, 756–759.

Kendell, R.E., Juszczak, E. and Cole, S.K. (1996). Obstetric complications and schizophrenia: a case control study based on standardised obstetric records. *Br J Psychiatry* **168**, 556–561.

Kikinis, R., Shenton, M.E., Gerig, G. *et al.* (1994). Temporal lobe sulco-gyral pattern anomalies in schizophrenia: an *in vivo* MR three-dimensional surface rendering study. *Neurosci Lett* **182**, 7–12.

Krishnan, K.R.R., Goli, V., Ellinwood, E.H. *et al.* (1988). Leukoencephalopathy in patients diagnosed as major depressive. *Biol Psychiatry* **23**, 519–522.

Krull, A.J., Press, G., Dupont, R. *et al.* (1991). Brain imaging in late-onset schizophrenia and related psychoses. *Int J Geriatr Psychiatry* **6**, 651–658.

Lesser, I.M., Miller, B.L., Boone, K.B. *et al.* (1989). Psychosis as the first manifestation of degenerative dementia. *Bull Clin Neurosci* **54**, 59–63.

Lesser, I.M., Miller, B.L., Boone, K.B. *et al.* (1991). Brain injury and cognitive function in late-onset psychotic depression. *J Neuropsychiatry Clin Neurosci* **3**, 33–40.

Lesser, I.M., Jeste, D.V., Boone, K.B. *et al.* (1992). Late-onset psychotic disorder, not otherwise specified: clinical and neuroimaging findings. *Biol Psychiatry* **31**, 419–423.

Lesser, I.M., Miller, B.L., Swartz, J.R. *et al.* (1993). Brain imaging in late-life schizophrenia and related psychoses. *Schizophr Bull* **19**, 773–782.

Mathalon, D.H., Sullivan, E.V., Lim, K.O. and Pfefferbaum, A. (1997). Longitudinal analysis of MRI brain volumes in schizophrenia. *Schizophr Res* **24**, 152.

Matthew, R.J., Wilson, W.H., Tant, S.R. *et al.* (1988). Abnormal resting regional cerebral blood flow patterns and their correlates in schizophrenia. *Arch Gen Psychiatry* **45**, 542–549.

Miller, B.L. and Lesser, I.M. (1988). Late-life psychosis and modern neuroimaging. *Psychiatr Clin North Am* **11**, 33–46.

Miller, B.L., Benson, F.D., Cummings, J.L. *et al.* (1986). Late-life paraphrenia: an organic delusional system. *J Clin Psychiatry* **47**, 204–207.

Miller, B.L., Lesser, I.M., Boone, K.B. *et al.* (1991). Brain lesions and cognitive function in late-life psychosis. *Br J Psychiatry* **158**, 76–82.

Miller, B.L., Lesser, I.M., Mena, I. *et al.* (1992). Regional cerebral blood flow in late-life-onset psychosis. *Neuropsychiatry, Neuropsychol Behav Neurol* **5**, 132–137.

Naguib, M. and Levy, R. (1987). Late paraphrenia: neuropsychological impairment and structural brain abnormalities on computed tomography. *Int J Geriatr Psychiatry* **2**, 83–90.

Nair, T., Christenson, J., Kumar, N., Mayhew, E. and Garver, D. (1997). Progressive ventricular enlargement and neurodegenerative schizophrenia. *Schizophr Res* **24**, 153.

Nopoulos, P.C., Flaum, M., Andreasen, N.C. and Swayze, V.W. (1995). Gray matter heterotopias in schizophrenia. *Psychiatry Res* **61**, 11–14.

Nopoulos, P., Flaum, M. and Andreasen, N.C. (1997). Sex differences in brain morphology in schizophrenia. *Am J Psychiatry* **154**, 1648–1654.

Pearlson, G.D. and Petty, R. (1994). Late life onset schizophrenia. In Cummings, J. and Coffey, C.E. (Eds), *Textbook of Geriatric Neuropsychiatry.* APA Press, Washington, DC.

Pearlson, G.D., Tunc, L.E., Wong, D.F. *et al.* (1993). Quantitative D2 dopamine receptor PET and structural MRI changes in late onset schizophrenia: a preliminary report. *Schizophr Bull* **19**, 783–795.

Pearlson, G.D., Garbacz, D.J., Tompkins R.H. *et al.* (1987). Lateral cerebral ventricular size in late onset schizophrenia. In: Miller, N.E. and Cohen, G.D. (Eds), *Schizophrenia and Aging.* Guilford, New York, pp. 246–248.

Pearlson, G.D., Harris, G.J., Powers, R.E. *et al.* (1992). Quantitative changes in mesial temporal volume, regional cerebral blood flow, and cognition in Alzheimer's disease. *Arch Gen Psychiatry* **49**, 402–408.

Pearlson, G.D., Barta, P.E., Powers, R.E. *et al.* (1997). Ziskind-Somerfeld Research Award 1996. Medial and superior temporal gyral volumes and cerebral asymmetry in schizophrenia versus bipolar disorder. *Biol. Psychiatry* **41**, 1–14.

Pfefferbaum, A., Zipursky, R.B., Lim, K.O. *et al.* (1988). Computed tomographic evidence for generalized sulcal and ventricular enlargement in schizophrenia. *Arch Gen Psychiatry* **45**, 633–640.

Pilowsky, L.S., Kerwin, R.W. and Murray, R.M. (1993). Schizophrenia: a neurodevelopmental perspective. *Neuropsychopharmacology* **9**, 83–91.

Purohit, D.P., Davidson, M., Perl, D.P. *et al.* (1993). Severe cognitive impairment in elderly schizophrenic patients: a clinicopathological study. *Biol Psychiatry* **33**, 255–260.

Rabins, P.V., Pearlson, G.D., Jayaram, G. *et al.* (1987). Elevated VBR in late-onset schizophrenia. *Am J Psychiatry* **144**, 1216–1218.

Rabins, P.V., Pearlson, G.D., Aylward, E.H. *et al.* (1991). Cortical magnetic resonance imaging changes in elderly inpatients with major depression. *Am J Psychiatry* **148**, 617–620.

Rivkin, P., Pearlson, G., Barta, P., Anthony, J., Arria, A.M. (1999). Comparison of white matter hyperintensities in age-matched groups of controls and subjects with late-onset and early-onset schizophrenia. *Intl J Geriatr Psychiatry* (submitted).

Symonds, L.L., Olichney, J.M., Jernigan, T.L., Corey-Bloom, J., Healy, J.F. and Jeste, D.V. (1997). Lack of clinically significant gross structural abnormalities in MRIs of older patients with schizophrenia and related psychoses. *J Neuropsychiatry Clin Neurosci* **9**, 251–258.

Tune, L.E., Wong, D.F., Pearlson, G.D. *et al.* (1994). Dopamine D2 receptor density in schizophrenia patients: a PET study with 11C-*N*-methylspiperone. *Psychiatry Res* **49**, 219–237.

Vita, A., Sacchetti, E., Valvassori, G. and Cazzullo, C.L. (1988). Brain morphology in schizophrenia: a 2- to 5-year CT scan follow-up study. *Acta Psychiatrica Scand* **78**, 618–621.

Vita, A., Giobbio, G.M., Dieci, M. *et al.* (1994). Stability of cerebral ventricular size from the appearance of the first psychotic symptoms to the later diagnosis of schizophrenia. *Biol Psychiatry* **35**, 960–962.

Weinberger, D.R. (1987). Implications of normal brain development for the pathogenesis of schizophrenia. *Arch Gen Psychiatry* **44**, 660–669.

Weinberger, D.R. (1996). On the plausibility of 'the neurodevelopmental hypothesis' of schizophrenia. *Neuropsychopharmacology* **14**, 1S-11S.

Weinberger, D.R., Torrey, E.F., Neophytides, A.N. *et al.* (1979). Lateral cerebral ventricular enlargement in chronic schizophrenia. *Arch Gen Psychiatry* **36**, 735–739.

Wong, D.F., Wagner, H.N. Jr, Tune, L.E. *et al.* (1986a). Positron emission tomography reveals elevated D_2 dopamine receptors in drug-naive schizophrenics. *Science* **234**, 1558–1563.

Wong, D.F., Gjedde, J. and Wagner, H.N. Jr (1986b). Quantification of neuroreceptors in the living human brain, I: irreversible binding of ligands. *J Cerebral Blood Flow Metab* **6**, 137–146.

Wong, D.F., Gjedde, J., Wagner, H.N. Jr *et al.* (1986c). Quantification of neuroreceptors in the living human brain, II: assessment of receptor density and affinity using inhibition studies. *J Cerebral Blood Flow Metab* **6**, 147–153.

Woods, B.T., Yurgelun-Todd, D., Bencs, F.M. *et al.* (1990). Progressive ventricular enlargement in schizophrenia: comparison to bipolar affective disorder and correlation with clinical course. *Biol Psychiatry* **27**, 341–352.

Zubenko, G.S., Sullivan, P., Nelson, J.P. *et al.* (1990). Brain imaging abnormalities in mental disorders of late life. *Arch Neurol* **47**, 1107–1111.

16

Neuroreceptor Studies in Psychotic Disorders in the Elderly: Potential for Understanding Antipsychotic Effects

P. FITZGERALD*‡, SHITIJ KAPUR* AND PHILLIP SEEMAN†

*Department of Psychiatry, and †Departments of Psychiatry and Psychopharmacology, University of Toronto, Ontario, Canada and ‡Department of Psychological Medicine, Monash University, Melbourne, Australia

INTRODUCTION

Imaging modalities are being increasingly applied to the investigation of schizophrenia. These tools measure brain structure (e.g. MRI, CT scanning) or regional brain chemistry (e.g. functional MRI, positron emission tomography (PET), single photon emission computerized tomography (SPECT)). Functional imaging studies may be used to quantify changes in receptor number or to investigate the binding of psychopharmacological agents to receptors in normal and abnormal states. This chapter focuses on the use of imaging studies of neurotransmitter receptors rather than reviewing the entire field of relevant neuroimaging. It illustrates how PET and SPECT imaging may be applied to advance our understanding of psychopharmacological treatment of the elderly.

LESSONS FROM NEURORECEPTOR STUDIES IN YOUNG PATIENTS

Antipsychotic medications have been used in the treatment of schizophrenia and other psychotic disorders for 30 years. While the mechanism of action of these medications is not entirely clear, all of these medications are known to bind to dopamine D_2 receptors. Therefore, it has seemed logical to study the effects of these medications on D_2 receptors in trying to elucidate their mechanism of action.

Table 1.   Doses of typical antipsychotics measured to occupy greater than 60% of D_2 receptors on PET scanning.

Medication	Dose
Haloperidol	2–3 mg/day
Loxapine	15–20 mg/day
Haloperidol decanoate	50 mg/month
Zuclopenthixol acetate (at 31 hours post injection)	12.5 mg

From Nyberg *et al.* (1995a,b); Kapur *et al.* (1996b,c).

PET was first applied to the study of dopamine receptor occupancy in the mid-1980s by Farde and colleagues in Sweden (Farde *et al.*, 1986). The results of studies published by this group over the next 10 years (for example, Farde *et al.*, 1992, 1995; Nordstrom *et al.*, 1993) and a number of studies performed in other centres (Pilowsky et al., 1993; Kapur *et al.*, 1996a) indicate that there is a significant relationship between central dopamine D_2 occupancy and the clinical effects of antipsychotic medication. There are three areas in which a relationship appears to be present. First, occupancy of striatal D_2 receptors appears to predict the development of extrapyramidal side effects (EPSE) fairly accurately. The occurrence of these side effects increases substantially when occupancy increases over 80%. Secondly, occupancy may also predict the development of elevated prolactin, which is associated with a variety of endocrine complications including menstrual cycle disruption and sexual side effects such as anorgasmia. This has not been as intensively studied but there is some evidence that the likelihood of elevation of prolactin increases significantly when D_2 occupancy is greater than 75% (Daskalakis *et al.*, 1998). Finally, a number of studies have attempted to relate D_2 occupancy with effectiveness of antipsychotic medication. When studies have considered classic or 'typical' antipsychotics such as haloperidol, raclopride or sulpiride, relatively consistent results have been found. These studies tend to find that there is a direct relationship between occupancy and clinical response such that occupancy of at least 60–70% of D_2 receptors is required for clinical antipsychotic effect (Farde, 1992; Nordstrom *et al.*, 1993). Importantly, these levels of occupancy are achieved with relatively low doses of medication (Nyberg *et al.*, 1995b; Kapur *et al.*, 1996b; Kapur, 1998) – see Table 1.

Recent research has also provided information about the receptor occupancy of the newer 'atypical' antipsychotics. Both risperidone and olanzapine, two recently developed antipsychotics, are considered atypical due to their relative low potential to produce EPSE. Both of these drugs bind to $5HT_2$ receptors to a greater degree than they bind to D_2 receptors (Farde *et al.*, 1995; Kapur, 1998; Kapur *et al.*, 1998; Nyberg *et al.*, 1998). However, it is also consistently found that the D_2 binding with these medications is greater than 60% when they are clinically effective, in other words in the same range as typical antipsychotics. These medications also increasingly induce EPSE when given in doses that are associated with D_2 occupancy of greater than 80% (greater than 6 mg for risperidone and greater than 20 mg for olanzapine). Additionally, there is some indication that the new atypical antipsychotic sertindole may also block a similar proportion of D_2 receptors when clinically effective (Nyberg et al., 1998).

The picture is different when we consider the prototypical 'atypical' antipsychotic clozapine. Several PET studies of the central binding of clozapine to D_2 receptors have consistently demonstrated binding below that seen with all other systematically studied medications (Farde et al., 1992; Nordstrom et al., 1995; Kapur, 1998) and generally below 60%. Like the other atypicals, clozapine exhibits a high degree of $5HT_2$ binding that occurs even at subtherapeutic doses such as 50 mg in an adult patient (Nordstrom et al., 1995). This is not unusual in the context of the other atypical antipsychotics but the low D_2 binding remains unique and the significance unexplained. There is some indication that the new atypical antipsychotic quetiapine may share this property of unusually low D_2 occupancy at clinically effective doses (Gefvert et al., 1998).

CLINICAL STUDIES OF ANTIPSYCHOTIC TREATMENT IN THE ELDERLY

It is increasingly recognized that the elderly need to be considered as a special subgroup when treated with psychopharmacological agents. However, systematic study of the drug treatment of elderly patients with psychiatric disorders is especially lacking and this situation is particularly problematic in the area of psychotic disorders (Jeste, 1997). There are few systematic studies of antipsychotic treatment considering issues of particular relevance to elderly patients. The data are even more scarce for patients over the age of 75 years.

Despite this, we can make some reasonable statements about antipsychotic therapy in the elderly. First, antipsychotic medications are effective in the management of psychotic symptoms including in patients with late onset psychotic disorders. Efficacy has been demonstrated with both the traditional 'typical' antipsychotics (for example, Honigfeld et al., 1965) as well as with atypical medication such as clozapine and risperidone (see Jeste et al., 1996). Secondly, the elderly appear to require lower doses of antipsychotic medication to achieve equivalent therapeutic responses to those seen in younger patients. This has been demonstrated in a number of studies (for example, Rabins et al., 1984; Craig and Bregman, 1988; Jeste et al., 1988) although there has been criticism of these studies based on the fact that they generally are non-blinded, retrospective or contain small numbers of patients

Table 2.   Age related changes and their relevance for pharmacokinetics in the elderly.

Factor	Age related change
Absorption	No specific changes related to age, may change with the use of concomitant medication (e.g. antacids) or illness
Distribution	Increased for fat soluble drugs secondary to an increase in the fat/muscle ratio
Hepatic drug metabolism	May be a decrease in demethylation or hydroxylation, first pass clearance may fall, no change in cytochrome P450 2D6 activity
Renal excretion	Progressive age related decline
Medication half life	May be increased
Steady state drug levels	May be increased

From Salzman (1982); Rudorfer (1993); Shulman and Ozdemir (1997).

(Jeste *et al.*, 1993). Thirdly, it has been found that the elderly are very sensitive to the development of antipsychotic side effects. Specific problems often occur with orthostatic hypotension, sedation and anticholinergic side effects. In regard to motor side effects there is evidence that the elderly are more at risk for extrapyramidal symptoms and they receive more anticholinergic medication (Avorn *et al.*, 1995). They may, however, suffer fewer acute dystonic reactions (Wilson and MacLennan, 1989). There is a substantially higher incidence of tardive dyskinesia in the elderly treated with antipsychotics (Kane *et al.*, 1988; Saltz *et al.*, 1989) with one prospective study reporting a 26% cumulative incidence over 1 year (Jeste *et al.*, 1993).

It is not clear why older patients require lower doses of medication and are more vulnerable to side effects. One explanation may be pharmacokinetic changes related to age. Certainly there are significant changes in drug distribution, metabolism and clearance, as shown in Table 2.

These changes may partially explain the altered drug effects and there is evidence that neuroleptic blood levels may proportionally increase with age (Forsman and Ohman, 1977; Cohen and Sommer, 1988; Lacro *et al.*, 1996). However, they are probably not sufficient to provide a complete explanation and it is necessary to consider additional factors. The other plausible explanation considers the effect of age related changes on pharmacodynamic effects of psychotropic medication. A number of these changes have been identified in the elderly. These include changes in homeostatic responses to drug effects and changes in receptor and post receptor mechanisms. For example, the effects of a number of benzodiazepine medications have been shown to be altered in the elderly independent of changes in pharmacokinetics (Castleden *et al.*, 1977). Research has also identified changes in adrenergic receptor mechanisms and possibly the cyclic AMP intra-cellular secondary messenger system related to age (Roberts and Tumer, 1988). In relation to the altered effects of antipsychotic medication it is necessary to consider how much this relates to changes in dopamine receptor function as well as the demonstrated fall in receptor number with age.

AGE RELATED DOPAMINE RECEPTOR CHANGES AND THE POTENTIAL FOR RECEPTOR OCCUPANCY STUDIES IN THE ELDERLY

There has been minimal research looking specifically at the receptor binding of antipsychotic medication in elderly subjects with no specific studies published to date conducted in patients in this age group. Additionally, elderly patients have not been included in the general studies performed. Specifically, in all of the PET or SPECT studies of neuroreceptor binding that we have reviewed, there are no patients reported over the age of 50 years and the average age is usually substantially lower (for example 24.2 years in Farde et al., 1992).

There has, however, been some investigation of the effects of normal ageing on the dopamine system. Post-mortem studies have demonstrated a reduction in receptor number with age (Severson et al., 1982, Seeman et al., 1987), although there have been some conflicting findings (DeKeyser et al., 1990), but there has been no evidence of a change in receptor affinity. More recently, several PET and SPECT studies have consistently demonstrated reductions in D_2 receptor number (Wong et al., 1984; Baron et al., 1986; Woda et al., 1992; Antonini et al., 1993; Rinne et al., 1993). The magnitude of this decline varies in the studies between 4 and 8% per decade (Volkow et al., 1996) with the variability of the results attributed to methodological differences between studies and the use of different radiotracers. New data presented by Volkow in the same paper, derived from a study using both the ^{18}F-N-methylspiroperidol ligand and ^{11}C-raclopride indicates that the 'true' figure is probably close to 8%.

Importantly, it is has been demonstrated in several studies that the loss of dopamine receptors begins prior to age 40 and is progressive (McGeer et al., 1977; Volkow et al., 1996). The loss of receptor number appears to have functional correlates in both animals and humans (Roth and Joseph, 1988; Volkow et al., 1998) with the study of Volkow et al. (1998) finding both motor and cognitive test performance decline associated with D_2 loss across several decades of life. This decline is linear with loss of function across all ages studied. The results of these studies imply that despite a significant degree of individual variation, we can expect the majority of elderly individuals to have between one-half and two-thirds of the number of receptors of young

healthy patients, and that the loss of this neuronal function has direct physiological and pharmacological significance.

Do these changes apply to patients with psychosis and more specifically to
elderly patients with disorders such as schizophrenia? There is evidence that
the baseline number of dopamine receptors in schizophrenia is increased in
both young patients and patients with late onset schizophrenia (Wong *et al.*,
1986; Pearlson *et al.*, 1993). These studies have found increases in dopamine
receptors that are bound with spiperone and its derivatives (dopamine D_2,
D_3 and D_4). Similar increases are not found in studies utilizing raclopride
(Farde *et al.*, 1990; Hietala *et al.*, 1994), which only binds to D_2 and D_3 receptors implying that the D_4 receptor may be responsible for the elevation
(Seeman *et al.*, 1993). Despite this relatively higher baseline of D_2-like receptors, the number of receptors in patients with schizophrenia follows the same
pattern of decline over time as that seen in the studies of normal controls
(Wong *et al.*, 1997). Therefore, elderly patients with schizophrenia may, on
average, have more receptors than age-matched normal controls but substantially fewer than younger patients.

At first thought, it appears self evident that this decline in receptor number
will cause the elderly sensitivity to the effects of antipsychotic medication. It
appears logical that as the elderly have fewer receptors, they will be more
easily blocked by medication. However, the situation is more complex.
Receptors are occupied in a *proportional* fashion (Nordstrom *et al.*, 1993;
Kapur *et al.*, 1996b). Therefore, the amount of drug required to occupy 50%
of a person's receptors is, in theory, independent of the total number of
receptors. Thus, despite the loss in D_2 receptors, for an equivalent plasma
level of medication, occupancy in the elderly should be of the same degree
as in the younger individual. Thus, a lower number of receptors does not
automatically imply higher occupancy or greater sensitivity to drug effects.
We propose two distinct alternative hypotheses to explain this sensitivity.

The increased occupancy hypothesis

This hypothesis explains the enhanced sensitivity on the grounds that elderly
patients experience a greater degree of D_2 occupancy for the equivalent
plasma level of antipsychotic medication. In other words, a central mechanism exists such that the relative occupancy of D_2 receptors alters as an
individual ages. Several reasons make it plausible. First, it is possible that the
level of dopamine in the brain falls with age. This would allow a D_2 antagonist a competitive advantage and raise drug occupancy at the receptor.
There is some evidence that changes in dopamine metabolism may not
mirror the reduction in receptor number but currently there is little evidence
to support such a decrease in endogenous dopamine (Eidelberg *et al.*, 1993;
Volkow *et al.*, 1998). Secondly, it is possible that the equilibration of drug

from plasma to CNS increases with age such that a higher CNS concentration, and hence greater occupancy, is achieved for a certain plasma level than in the younger patient. Finally, it is plausible that increased occupancy may result from a change in receptor affinity with ageing. This may be the result of changes in receptor function or be secondary to age related changes in secondary messenger systems. There is some evidence that these systems do alter with age (Roberts and Tumer, 1988).

The decreased capacity hypothesis

This proposes a significantly different explanation for the increased sensitivity of the elderly to antipsychotics. According to this hypothesis, medication sensitivity (therapeutic or to adverse events) is not determined by the percentage of receptors occupied by a drug but by the *absolute number of receptors left unoccupied* that can support signal transduction. In an elderly patient, with fewer overall absolute receptors, the same degree of occupancy will leave fewer absolute receptors left to function normally than in a younger patient.

For example, we can compare a young patient with a baseline of 100 receptors with an elderly patient who has 50 receptors remaining. If both these patients experience 50% occupancy with an antipsychotic, the young patient will have 50 unoccupied receptors remaining whilst the elderly patient has only 25. The neural system in the elderly patient will have less capacity than in the younger patient for signal transduction, possibly providing an explanation for the antipsychotic sensitivity.

CONCLUSION

Receptor imaging studies have contributed substantially to our understanding of the therapy of schizophrenia with antipsychotic medicine in adult patients. These studies have demonstrated and reinforced the role of dopamine blockade in the action of these medications but have raised important questions with regard to the role and mechanism of atypical antipsychotics, especially clozapine. Importantly they have demonstrated a direct relationship between the degree of D_2 occupancy and a number of important clinical effects of these drugs.

The application of these technologies to the study of receptor and drug function in the elderly is lacking and as such reflects the overall state of research in psychopharmacology in this age group. We do clearly know, however, that the elderly are more sensitive to the effects of antipsychotic medication and these drugs are used in substantially lower doses in this age group. Our increasing knowledge of the dynamics of receptor occupancy gives some clues as to the reasons for this sensitivity. Two clear hypotheses are proposed: the elderly may show an increased occupancy or a decreased capacity, or both. We hope that future research will test these hypotheses.

REFERENCES

Antonini, A., Leenders, K. L., Reist, H. et al. (1993). Effect of age on D_2 dopamine receptors in the normal human brain measured by positron emission tomography and ^{11}C-raclopride. Arch Neurol 50, 474–480.

Avorn, J., Bohn, R., Mogun, H. et al. (1995). Neuroleptic drug exposure and treatment of Parkinsonism in the elderly: a case-control study. Am J Med 99, 48–54.

Baron, J., Maziere, B., Loch, C. et al. (1986). Loss of striatal [76Br]bromospiperone binding sites demonstrated by positron emission tomography in progressive supranuclear palsy. J Cerebral Blood Flow Metab 6, 131–136.

Castleden, C., George, C., Marcer, D. et al. (1977). Increased sensitivity to nitrazepam in old age. BMJ 1, 10–12.

Cohen, B. and Sommer, B. (1988). Metabolism of thioridazine in the elderly. J Clin Psychopharmacol 8, 336–339.

Craig, T. and Bregman, Z. (1988). Late-onset schizophrenia-like illness. J Am Geriatr Soc 36, 104–107.

Daskalakis, Z., Christensen, B., Zipursky, R. et al. (1998). Relationship between D_2 occupancy and prolactin levels in first episode psychosis. Biol Psychiatry 43 (suppl), 113S.

DeKeyser, J., Ebinger, G. and Vauquelin, G. (1990). Age-related changes in the human nigrostriatal dopaminergic system. Ann Neurol 27, 157–161.

Eidelberg, D., Takikawa, S., Dhawan, V. et al. (1993). Striatal 18F-striatal uptake: absence of an aging effect. J Cerebral Blood Flow Metab 13, 881–888.

Farde, L., Hall, H., Ehrin, E. et al. (1986). Quantitative analysis of D_2 dopamine receptor binding in the living human brain by PET. Science 231, 258–261.

Farde, L., Wiesel, F., Stone-Elander, S. et al. (1990). D_2 dopamine receptors in neuroleptic-naive schizophrenic patients. Arch Gen Psychiatry 47, 213–219.

Farde, L., Nordstrom, A. L., Wiesel, F. A. et al. (1992). Positron emission tomographic analysis of central D_1 and D_2 dopamine receptor occupancy in patients treated with classical neuroleptics and clozapine: relation to extrapyramidal side effects. Arch Gen Psychiatry 49, 538–544.

Farde, L., Nyberg, S., Oxenstierna, G. et al. (1995). Positron emission tomography studies on D-2 and 5-HT2 receptor binding in risperidone-treated schizophrenic patients. J Clin Psychopharmacol 15, S19–S23.

Forsman, A. and Ohman, R. (1977). Applied pharmacokinetics of haloperidol in man. Current Therapeutic Res 21, 396–411.

Gefvert, O., Bergstrom, M., Langstrom, B. et al. (1998). Time course of central dopamine-D_2 and 5-HT$_2$ receptor blockade and plasma drug concentrations after discontinuation of quetiapine (Seroquel) in patients with schizophrenia. Psychopharmacology 135, 119–126.

Hietala, J., Syvalahti, E., Vuorio, K. et al. (1994). Striatal D_2 dopamine receptor characteristics in neuroleptic-naive schizophrenic patients studied with positron emission tomography. Arch Gen Psychiatry 51, 116–123.

Honigfeld, G., Rosenbaum, M., Blumenthal, I. et al. (1965). Behavioural improvement in the older schizophrenic patient: drug and social therapies. J Am Geriatr Soc 13, 57–71.

Jeste, D.V. (1997). Schizophrenia, antipsychotics and ageing. *Schizophrenia Res* **27**, 103–104.

Jeste, D., Harris, M., Pearlson, J. *et al.* (1988). Late-onset schizophrenia: studying clinical validity. *Psychiatric Clin North Am* **11**, 1–14.

Jeste, D.V., Lacro, J.P., Gilbert, P.L. *et al.* (1993). Treatment of late-life schizophrenia with neuroleptics. *Schizophrenia Bull* **19**, 817–830.

Jeste, D., Eastham, J., Lacro, J. *et al.* (1996). Management of late-life psychosis. *J Clin Psychiatry* **57** (suppl 3), 39S–45S.

Kane, J., Woerner, M. and Lieberman, J. (1988). Tardive dyskinesia: prevalence, incidence, and risk factors. *J Clin Psychopharmacol* **8**, 52S–56S.

Kapur, S. (1998). A new framework for investigating antipsychotic action in humans: lessons from PET imaging. *Molec Psychiatry* **3**, 135–140.

Kapur, S., Remington, G., Jones, C. *et al.* (1996a). Relationship between D_2 receptor occupancy and plasma haloperidol: A PET study. *Eur Neuropsychopharmacol* **6**, 73.

Kapur, S., Remington, G., Jones, C. *et al.* (1996b). High levels of dopamine D_2 receptor occupancy with low dose haloperidol treatment: A PET study. *Am J Psychiatry* **153**, 948–950.

Kapur, S., Zipursky, R., Jones, C. *et al.* (1996c). The D_2 receptor occupancy of loxapine determined using PET. *Neuropsychopharmacology* **15**, 562–566.

Kapur, S., Zipursky, R., Remington, G. *et al.* (1998). The 5-HT$_2$ and D_2 receptor occupancy of olanzapine in schizophrenia: a PET investigation. *Am J Psychiatry* **155**, 921–928.

Lacro, J., Kuczenski, R., Roznoski, M. *et al.* (1996). Serum haloperidol levels in older psychotic patients. *Am J Geriatr Psychiatry* **4**, 229–236.

McGeer, P., McGeer, E. and Suzuki, J. (1977). Ageing and extrapyramidal function. *Arch Neurol* **34**, 33–35.

Nordstrom, A.L., Farde, L., Wiesel, F.A. *et al.* (1993). Central D_2-dopamine receptor occupancy in relation to antiopsychotic drug effects – a double-blind PET study of schizophrenic patients. *Biol Psychiatry* **33**, 227–235.

Nordstrom, A., Farde, L., Nyberg, S. *et al.* (1995). D_1, D_2, and 5-HT$_2$ receptor occupancy in relation to clozapine serum concentration: a PET study of schizophrenic patients. *Am J Psychiatry* **152**, 1444–1449.

Nyberg, S., Farde, L., Bartfai, A. *et al.* (1995a). Central D_2 occupancy and the effects of zuclopenthixol acetate in humans. *Int Clin Psychopharmacol* **10**, 221–227.

Nyberg, S., Farde, L., Halldin, C. *et al.* (1995b). D_2 dopamine receptor occupancy during low-dose treatment with haloperidol decanoate. *Am J Psychiatry* **152**, 173–178.

Nyberg, S., Nilsson, U., Okubo, Y. *et al.* (1998). Implications of brain imaging for the management of schizophrenia. *Int Clin Psychopharmacol* **13** (suppl 3), 15S–20S.

Pearlson, G., Tune, L., Wong, D. *et al.* (1993). Quantitative D_2 dopamine receptor PET and structural MRI changes in late-onset schizophrenia. *Schizophrenia Bull* **19**, 783–795.

Pilowsky, L. S., Costa, D. C., Ell, P. J. *et al.* (1993). Antipsychotic medication, D{-2} dopamine receptor blockade and clinical response: a {+123}I IBZM SPET (single photon emission tomography) study. *Psychol Med* **23**, 791–797.

Rabins, P., Pauker, S. and Thomas, J. (1984). Can schizophrenia begin after age 44? *Compr Psychiatry* **25**, 290–293.

Rinne, J., Hietala, J., Ruotsalainen, U. *et al.* (1993). Decrease in human striatal dopamine D_2 receptor density with age: a PET study with ^{11}C-raclopride. *J Cerebral Blood Flow Metab* **13**, 310–314.

Roberts, J. and Tumer, N. (1988). Pharmacodynamic basis for altered drug action in the elderly. *Common Clinical Challenges Geriatrics* **4**, 127–149.

Roth, G. and Joseph, J. (1988). Peculiarities of the effects of hormones and transmitters during aging: modulation of changes in dopaminergic action. *Gerontology* **34**, 22–28.

Rudorfer, M. V. (1993). Pharmacokinetics of psychotropic drugs in special populations. *J Clin Psychiatry* **54** (suppl), 50S–54S.

Saltz, B., Kane, J., Woerner, M. *et al.* (1989). Prospective study of tardive dyskinesia in the elderly. *Psychopharmacol Bull* **25**, 52–56.

Salzman, C. (1982). A primer of geriatric psychopharmacology. *Am J Psychiatry* **139**, 67–74.

Seeman, P., Bzowe, N., Guan, H. *et al.* (1987). Human brain dopamine receptors in children and adults. *Synapse* **1**, 399–404.

Seeman, P., Guan, H. and Van Tol, H. (1993). Dopamine D_4 receptors elevated in schizophrenia. *Nature* **365**, 441–445.

Severson, J., Marcusson, J., Winblad, B. *et al.* (1982). Age-correlated loss of dopaminergic binding sites in the human basal ganglia. *J Neurochem* **39**, 1623–1631.

Shulman, R. and Ozdemir, V. (1997). Psychotropic medications and cytochrome P450 2D6: pharmacokinetic considerations in the elderly. *Can J Psychiatry* **42** (suppl), 4S–9S.

Volkow, N., Wang, G.-J., Fowler, J. *et al.* (1996). Measuring age-related changes in dopamine D_2 receptors with ^{11}C-raclopride and ^{18}F-N-methylspiroperidol. *Psychiatry Res* **67**, 11–16.

Volkow, N., Gur, R., Wang, G.-J. *et al.* (1998). Association between decline in brain dopamine activity with age and cognitive and motor impairment in healthy individuals. *Am J Psychiatry* **155**, 344–349.

Wilson, J. and MacLennan, W. (1989). Review: drug induced Parkinsonism in elderly patients. *Age Ageing* **18**, 208–210.

Woda, A., Alavi, A., Mozley, D. *et al.* (1992). Effects of age on dopamine receptors as measured with SPECT and IBZM. *J Nucl Med* **33**, 897.

Wong, D., Wagner, H. J., Dannals, R. *et al.* (1984). Effects of age on dopamine and serotonin receptors measured by positron tomography in the living human brain. *Science* **31**, 1393–1396.

Wong, D., Wagner, H. J., Tune, L. *et al.* (1986). Positron emission tomography reveals elevated D_2 dopamine receptors in drug-naive schizophrenics. *Science* **234**, 1558–1563.

Wong, D., Pearlson, G., Tune, L. *et al.* (1997). Quantification of neuroreceptors in the living human brain: IV. Effect of ageing and elevations of D_2-like receptors in schizophrenia and bipolar illness. *J Cerebral Blood Flow Metab* **17**, 331–342.

IV

Treatments

17

Treatment of Late Onset Schizophrenia and Related Disorders

FAUZIA SIMJEE McCLURE and DILIP V. JESTE

Department of Psychiatry, University of California, San Diego, Geriatric Psychiatry Intervention Research Center, San Diego, California, USA

INTRODUCTION

Although onset of schizophrenia after the age of 45 has been a controversial issue, it appears that a sizeable minority of patients present with diagnosable schizophrenia for the first time, after the age of 45. Harris and Jeste (1988) estimated that 23% of hospitalized, acutely-ill patients with schizophrenia reportedly had first onset of their illness after the age of 40. Late onset schizophrenia (LOS) is characterized by paranoid symptomatology (disorganized subtype is very rare), and schizoid or paranoid traits in premorbid personality.

Similarities between LOS and early onset schizophrenia (EOS) include: severity of positive symptoms, chronicity of course, sensory impairment, family history of schizophrenia, early childhood maladjustment, number of minor physical anomalies, increased mortality, overall pattern of neuropsychological impairment, nonspecific magnetic resonance imaging (MRI) abnormalities, and qualitative response to neuroleptics (Jeste *et al.* 1995b, 1998; Lohr *et al.*, 1997). In comparison with EOS patients, LOS patients differ in that they have a high female-to-male ratio, less severe negative symptoms, less severe impairment in learning and abstraction, and a more intact semantic network. In adolescence and early adulthood, LOS patients also have had better premorbid functioning. Additionally, LOS patients may have a larger thalamus on MRI and seem to need lower doses of neuroleptics than age-comparable patients with EOS. In summary, it appears that although there is a similar predisposition and probably similar brain lesions in EOS and LOS patients, LOS patients may have a less severe form and a neurobiologically distinct subtype of the illness (Jeste *et al.*, 1997).

Although management of LOS is an important area of study, there is limited published research addressing treatment of LOS. Moreover, the available studies are often characterized by small sample sizes and are most often case reports or case series rather than well-controlled double-blind trials. In this chapter, the published literature is reviewed and clinical recommendations for the treatment of patients with LOS are offered. Since the number of reports in LOS is limited, studies related to other psychotic disorders (e.g. delusional disorder) in late life are also included. Studies related to these other disorders may be applicable to the population of older patients with LOS. It is hoped that this chapter will help generate interest in research on the treatment of patients with LOS.

NEUROLEPTICS OR ANTIPSYCHOTICS

In general, neuroleptic or antipsychotic medications are the most effective symptomatic treatment for both early and late onset chronic schizophrenia as they both improve the acute symptoms and prevent relapses (Jeste *et al.*, 1993). Alterations in pharmacokinetics and pharmacodynamics, however, complicate pharmacotherapy in older patients; an exaggerated or otherwise altered response to medications may be seen. In comparison with younger patients, geriatric patients show an increased variability of response and an increased sensitivity to medications (Avorn and Gurwitz, 1990; Salzman, 1990).

Antipsychotic medications are broadly divided into conventional or typical neuroleptics and newer or atypical antipsychotics. Conventional neuroleptics block dopamine-D_2 receptors, and newer antipsychotic medications block both dopamine-D_2 and serotonin-$5HT_2$ receptors. Dopamine-D_3 and D_4 receptors have also been identified as important targets for antipsychotic agents (Jackson *et al.*, 1994; Kerwin, 1994).

CONVENTIONAL OR TYPICAL ANTIPSYCHOTICS:
GENERAL CONSIDERATIONS

Beginning with the introduction of the low-potency agent chlorpromazine in 1952, conventional neuroleptics have been available for more than 45 years. Conventional neuroleptic medications include a variety of phenothiazines and butyrophenones. Conventional neuroleptics have proven to be effective for the positive symptoms of schizophrenia but have little impact on the negative symptoms. There is a scarcity of research investigating the effectiveness of these drugs for elderly patients with psychoses.

Side effects are common with conventional neuroleptics. This is of particular concern in elderly patients who are more susceptible to the side effects of drugs. Acute and subacute side effects of neuroleptics include sedation and anticholinergic toxicity (which can lead to urinary retention, constipation, dry mouth, worsening of glaucoma, and confusion) with low-potency neuroleptics such as thioridazine, and extrapyramidal symptoms (or EPS, including Parkinsonism, akathisia, and dystonia) with high-potency neuroleptics such as haloperidol. Although the elderly very rarely develop acute dystonia, they tend to be much more susceptible to other neurological side effects of neuroleptics such as delirium and Parkinsonism (Wilson and MacLennan, 1989). Conventional neuroleptics can also affect cognitive performance, thereby significantly impairing functioning in late life (Wragg and Jeste, 1988; Rosen et al., 1990). A higher incidence of falls (Tinetti et al., 1988) and hip fractures (Ray et al., 1987) has been associated with the use of conventional neuroleptics. A greater susceptibility to the cardiac side effects of neuroleptics has also been found (Soares and Gershon, 1996).

There is a serious risk associated with long-term neuroleptic use. Patients may develop tardive dyskinesia (TD), a movement disorder characterized by involuntary, irregular or repetitive abnormal movements.

In one study (Saltz et al., 1991) of elderly patients, ranging in age from 55 to 99 years, the incidence of TD was 31% after 43 weeks of cumulative neuroleptic treatment. Psychiatric (rather than 'organic') diagnosis and presence of extrapyramidal symptoms early on in treatment were associated with increased vulnerability to TD. Jeste et al. (1999a) reported the cumulative incidence of dyskinetic movements in elderly patients to be 29% following 12 months of typical neuroleptic use. This cumulative annual incidence of TD in older adults is five or six times that reported in younger adults. Higher dosage and longer duration of neuroleptic treatment, possible 'organicity', as well as other factors including alcohol dependence and subtle movement disorder at baseline, were found to increase the risk of TD in the older patient population (Jeste et al., 1995a)

The risk of TD may be reduced or TD may be reversed by discontinuation of conventional neuroleptics. This in itself poses a problem, however; drug withdrawal is usually very difficult in patients with schizophrenia. A recent literature review of 66 studies involving a total of 4,356 patients with schizophrenia or schizo-affective disorder indicated that relapse rates over a mean follow-up period of 9.7 months were 53% when the antipsychotic drugs were withdrawn and 16% when the drugs were maintained (Gilbert et al., 1995). While many of these studies included younger adults with schizophrenia, the rates of relapse following neuroleptic withdrawal seemed to be comparable in those studies which included elderly patients (Jeste et al., 1993).

Thus, it becomes challenging for the clinician to decide whether or not to continue conventional neuroleptic treatment: continued use of the drug is associated with serious side effects while discontinuing the drug can bring about a relapse.

It is more difficult to manage psychosis in elderly patients in comparison with younger patients because the elderly are more sensitive to the side effects of antipsychotic medications. Older patients are also likely to be taking other medications which may increase the likelihood of adverse drug interactions. Hence, it is crucial that neuroleptics be prescribed carefully to this population with attention given to dosing strategies and close observation for possible side effects (Raskind and Risse, 1986; Grossberg and Manepalli, 1995; Jeste *et al*. 1996). Soares and Gershon (1996) point out that misuse of antipsychotics in the elderly is an area of great concern.

STUDIES IN PATIENTS WITH LOS OR RELATED DISORDERS

In a review of studies conducted between 1957 and 1984, which looked at the treatment of LOS, Harris and Jeste (1988) noted that a sizeable proportion of the patients showed an improvement with neuroleptic treatment. Factors such as type of neuroleptic, dosage, blood levels, side effects, and degree of improvement in specific symptoms, however, have not been adequately researched. The numerous limitations of the published literature include small sample sizes, open-label design, absence of validated rating scales for assessing outcome, inconsistent and sometimes unspecified diagnostic criteria, and variable dosage as well as length of treatment. The earlier literature often employs diagnostic terms such as paraphrenia without defining them. A number of reports do not give relevant information about the patient sample or about the pharmacotherapy used. Below we describe selected (and methodologically better) studies of the treatment of LOS and related disorders with conventional neuroleptics that have appeared in the published literature.

Post (1966) reported a complete remission of symptoms in response to at least short-term treatment with trifluoperazine (10–30 mg/day) or thioridazine (50–400 mg/day) in 61% ($N = 43$) of patients and a moderate improvement with these medications in 31% ($N = 22$) of the patients. In a follow-up study consisting of 65 patients who had received treatment with either of the aforementioned medications for a period of 12–41 months, Post (1966) reported that 34% ($N = 22$) of patients remained symptom free. Rabins *et al*. (1984) reported a complete remission of symptoms in 57% ($N = 20$) and moderate improvement in 29% ($N = 10$) of LOS or paraphrenia patients treated with neuroleptics (type of neuroleptic, dosage, and length of treatment were not indicated) and psychosocial therapies. A 2-year follow-up conducted by Rabins *et al*. (1984), with 14 patients over the age of 60, showed that four patients remained completely symptom free. It is not known whether these patients continued with neuroleptics after discharge.

In a study conducted by Pearlson *et al*. (1989), almost half (48.1%, $N = 26$) of LOS patients responded to neuroleptic treatment with complete remission. Complete remission was defined as the absence of hallucinations, delusions, thought disorder, and catatonic behaviour. Partial response was defined by these investigators as either a disappearance of one or more positive symptoms, with persistence of at least one other positive symptom, or a decrease in the frequency of occurrence or in the salience of positive symptoms, resulting in improved overall functioning. Partial response was noted in 27.8% ($N = 15$) patients. Failure to respond to neuroleptic medication, defined as the absence of a change in the presenting positive symptoms, was seen in 24.1% ($N = 13$) patients. Type of neuroleptic, dosage, and length of treatment were not indicated. Presence of thought disorder, which was much rarer in LOS patients, predicted poor response to neuroleptic treatment. For the three groups of patients with complete, partial, and non-response, the percentages of all LOS patients with thought disorder were 11.1% ($N = 6$), 83.3% ($N = 45$), and 5.6% ($N = 3$), respectively ($p < 0.001$). Partial or nonresponse was also predicted by schizoid premorbid personality. For all three groups, the percentages of patients with schizoid premorbid personalities were 35.2% ($N = 19$), 40.7% ($N = 22$), and 24.1% ($N = 13$), respectively ($p < 0.02$). Gender, family history, and first rank symptoms seemed to have no significant impact on treatment outcome.

Wengel *et al.* (1989) treated two women with LOS, who also experienced musical hallucinations, with neuroleptics. In each case, the patients had developed musical hallucinations only after displaying other signs and symptoms of schizophrenia. In one case, trifluoperazine was used, and in the other haloperidol was used in doses up to 40 mg a day. In each of these cases, a decrease in delusions, paranoia, and auditory hallucinations, including musical hallucinations was noted. Musical hallucinations, however, did not disappear completely.

Raskind *et al.* (1979) compared the efficacy of fluphenazine enanthate (5 mg im/2 weeks, for 6 weeks) and oral haloperidol (2 mg tds, for 6 weeks) in 26 patients with late onset paraphrenia. These patients were seen as outpatient psychiatric emergencies who had difficulty with medication compliance. In 11 of 13 patients treated with intramuscular fluphenazine, there was at least a moderate if not marked global clinical improvement in symptoms after 6 weeks. The difference in response between the two groups was not interpreted by the investigators to suggest that fluphenazine was superior to haloperidol as an antipsychotic; rather, the authors concluded that, at least in outpatient populations, poor compliance with oral haloperidol was the most likely reason for the observed superiority of fluphenazine enanthate in their patients. It should be noted, however, that the serum levels of the neuroleptics were not measured.

In order to identify a treatment strategy that was most likely to produce a remission of symptoms, Howard and Levy (1992) investigated the clinical response to treatment in 64 patients with late paraphrenia, all of whom had been prescribed medication for at least 3 months in the preceding year. These authors found that depot antipsychotic medication (either 14.4 mg of flupenthixol decanoate or 9 mg of fluphenazine decanoate every fortnight) was associated with increased treatment compliance, a positive treatment outcome, and a reduced amount of neuroleptic expressed in mg CPZE (chlorpromazine equivalent) daily. Patients receiving oral medications were prescribed, on average, 116 mg CPZE per day while those on depot medication received 90 mg CPZE per day. This difference, however, was not statistically significant ($p = 0.092$).

'Paranoid disorder'

Inconsistent results have been reported in patients with late onset paranoid disorders treated with neuroleptics (and anxiolytics). In a review of the literature, Brink (1979) noted that medications including pipotiazine, sulpiride, lorazepam, clozapine and loxapine effectively reduced paranoid delusions. The literature also suggests good prognosis with these medications for a psychotic paranoid population but poor results for a nonpsychotic paranoid population (Escande, 1983; Szymonowicz, 1983; Panteleeva, 1984; Tuason et al., 1984; Cordingley, et al., 1985; Modell et al., 1985; Soni and Freeman, 1985). Some significant side effects including confusion and catatonic-like features have been reported with these medications. Inconsistent results with psychopharmacological treatment were also noted by Jette and Winnett (1987) in patients with late onset paranoid disorder. Haloperidol had no effect on paranoid delusions; however, in some cases, extreme agitation was temporarily controlled.

Delusional disorder

In older patients, delusional disorder (sometimes referred to as paranoia or paraphrenia) presents a therapeutic challenge. Because of its chronicity, delusional disorder typically does not respond well to antipsychotic medication (Jørgensen and Munk-Jørgensen, 1985; Breitner and Anderson, 1994). To our knowledge, there are no available controlled data on the response of delusional disorder to various pharmacologic interventions. Generally, treatment consists of antipsychotics, as long as they are tolerated, until symptoms improve or remit. It appears that neuroleptics decrease agitation and the intensity of the delusions but do not entirely suppress the delusions (Schneider et al. 1993).

Poor results were reported by Opjordsmoen (1988) in a follow-up study of 23 patients with somatic delusions. Only one-third of the patients showed a favourable outcome, with better prognosis for patients with schizo-affective or mood disorders. Patients with delusional disorder or schizophrenia showed worse outcomes.

Rockwell et al. (1994) studied 10 patients with late onset psychosis with somatic delusions (e.g. a delusional belief that the person has some physical defect, disorder, or disease) with a mean age of 63. These patients were compared with two groups that were similar in age and education (10 normal comparison patients and nine patients with late onset psychosis without somatic delusions). Similar to the aforementioned studies, the delusional patients showed poor compliance with psychiatric treatment recommendations and rarely benefited from short-term psychopharmacologic (mainly neuroleptic) intervention.

Dosage

In four North American clinical centres, the mean daily dose prescribed to LOS patients, whose mean age was 61 years, was 192 mg chlorpromazine equivalents (mg CPZE) compared to 1,437 mg CPZE in a group of young patients with schizophrenia (Jeste and Zisook, 1988).

Jeste *et al.* (1998) found that the mean daily dose of antipsychotics used in patients with LOS was significantly smaller than that prescribed to age-comparable patients with EOS.

In Howard and Levy's (1992) study, the mean dose of prescribed depot was 14.4 mg of flupenthixol decanoate or 9 mg of fluphenazine decanoate every fortnight. Low dosages of neuroleptics in elderly patients have, overall, been found to be both clinically efficacious and better tolerated.

NEW SEROTONIN–DOPAMINE ANTAGONISTS (ATYPICAL ANTIPSYCHOTICS)

The newer antipsychotics have proven to work more effectively than conventional neuroleptics for treating negative symptoms and for treating patients who show treatment-resistance and do not respond to typical neuroleptics. Presently, four new antipsychotic drugs have been approved for use in the United States. These include clozapine, risperidone, olanzapine, and quetiapine. Other newer antipsychotic medications including ziprasidone and zotepine are currently awaiting Food and Drug Administration (FDA) approval.

There are limited data available concerning the use of these newer serotonin–dopamine antagonists in patients with late-life psychoses. In young and middle-aged patients with schizophrenia, these new agents have generally been found to be effective for both positive and negative symptoms of schizophrenia (Kane *et al.*, 1988; Marder and Meibach, 1994; Meltzer and Fibiger, 1996; Small *et al.*, 1997) and show a lower incidence of EPS than conventional neuroleptics.

Although fewer neurologic side effects have been associated with newer antipsychotics, some of these drugs can cause adverse effects such as sedation and postural hypotension.

Clozapine

Clozapine has been available in the United States since the late 1980s (Kane et al., 1988). Well controlled published studies on the use of clozapine in elderly patients, however, are lacking. Results from uncontrolled clinical trials indicate that clozapine is effective in managing treatment-resistant psychotic symptoms as well as severe tardive dyskinesia (Chengappa et al., 1995; Salzman et al., 1995). Clozapine, partly due to its relative inaction on the nigrostriatal dopaminergic system, has a low risk of EPSE. It can, however, cause confusion, postural hypotension, sedation, lethargy, and anticholinergic toxicity (Frankenburg and Kalunian, 1994; Chengappa et al., 1995; Rich et al., 1995; Salzman et al., 1995). In 1% of patients, clozapine causes agranulocytosis, and the risk may increase in elderly patients (Salzman et al., 1995). Evidence suggests that clozapine may improve cognitive functioning in patients with chronic schizophrenia (Hagger et al., 1993). This, however, might not hold true for elderly schizophrenia patients because of its anticholinergic effects (Soares and Gershon, 1996). Overall, clozapine is not a first-line antipsychotic for patients with LOS, and should only be used in patients with treatment-resistant schizophrenia or those with severe TD.

Risperidone

Of the different atypical antipsychotics, risperidone has, to date, been used more widely than the others in elderly patients – with or without schizophrenia. Based on three California open-label studies of risperidone in patients ranging in age from 45 to 100 years at the San Diego VA Healthcare System, Edgemoor Geriatric Hospital in Santee, and the Loma Linda VA Healthcare System in Loma Linda, Jeste et al. (1996) have reported that risperidone is effective as a 'first-line antipsychotic agent'. It produced significant clinical improvement in a majority of older patients with schizophrenia, including those with LOS. When prescribed in appropriately low doses, it was well tolerated in most patients.

Risperidone has also shown potential for improving cognition in older psychotic patients (Jeste et al., 1999a). In an open-label study, risperidone was found to produce a significantly greater improvement in the score on the Mini-Mental State Examination (Folstein et al., 1975) than did haloperidol in a total sample of over 50 patients including some with LOS (Jeste et al., 1998a). In another study, Berman et al. (1995) compared the effects of risperidone and haloperidol on cognition. Twenty patients with stable schizophrenia ranging in age from 57 to 77 received either risperidone or haloperidol. Although initial doses were adjusted as necessary, none of the patients needed to be placed on more than 6 mg of risperidone or 10 mg of haloperidol per day. The Positive and Negative Syndrome Scale (PANSS)

(Kay *et al.*, 1987) as well as several cognitive tests including the Mini-Mental State Examination (MMSE) (Folstein *et al.*, 1975), digit symbol, digit span, trails, word recall, verbal fluency, and an abbreviated Boston Naming Test were administered to each patient at baseline before switching over from their previous antipsychotic medication to the study medication and after at least 2 weeks of receiving a stable dose of the study drug. In comparison with baseline data, patients receiving risperidone ($N = 8$) had significant improvement on the Boston Naming Test ($p = 0.05$) and on the MMSE ($p = 0.05$). However, in those patients who were receiving haloperidol, no significant changes were noted. Also, in the risperidone group ($N = 9$), there was a trend for improvement in negative symptoms ($p = 0.07$) but this was not so with the group receiving haloperidol ($p = 0.16$; $N = 9$).

Very recently, Jeste *et al.* (1998a) compared the 9-month cumulative incidence of TD with risperidone to that with haloperidol in older patients. Sixty-one patients on risperidone were matched with 61 patients from a larger sample of patients who received haloperidol. Patients were matched on age, diagnosis, and length of pre-enrolment neuroleptic intake in order to allow for clinically comparable groups. The median daily dose of each medication was 1 mg. Results suggested that, over this 9-month period, risperidone was associated with a significantly lower cumulative incidence of TD than haloperidol in a high-risk group of older patients. Given the potential seriousness of TD, these data reveal a major advantage for risperidone over haloperidol at least over a 9-month period.

Risperidone should be prescribed in patients with LOS at considerably lower doses than those recommended for younger adults. The initial doses of risperidone should be between 0.25 and 0.5 mg/day, with increases not to exceed 0.5 mg/day. Maximum doses in patients with schizophrenia should remain at 3 mg/day or less. The risk of extrapyramidal symptoms, postural hypotension, and somnolence increases with higher doses.

Olanzapine

In late 1996, olanzapine was approved by the FDA for clinical use, and has been used extensively in younger adults with schizophrenia. The availability of published work in the treatment of elderly patients with olanzapine is limited. In one open-label study (Wolters *et al.*, 1996), 15 Parkinsonian patients, without dementia but with drug-induced psychosis, responded well to olanzapine at doses ranging from 1 mg to 15 mg/day (mean 7 mg/day). Due to drowsiness, one patient discontinued treatment. Side effects of olanzapine include dizziness, sedation, weight gain and some anticholinergic reactions. Jeste *et al.* (1999b) suggest that in elderly patients, the starting dose of olanzapine should be 1–5 mg daily (mean 2.5 mg/day). Maintenance dose is recommended to be between 5 mg and 15 mg per day.

Quetiapine

Quetiapine was brought into clinical practice in 1997. In younger adults with schizophrenia, quetiapine demonstrated significantly better effectiveness and tolerability than haloperidol in a large-scale, double-blind investigation (Arvanitis *et al.*, 1997). Quetiapine has shown very low potential for EPS and little anticholinergic or prolactin-elevating action. Side effects of quetiapine include postural hypotension and drowsiness. In long-term studies of dogs (but not in monkeys or humans), lenticular opacities have been noted. There are some abstracts on the treatment of elderly patients with quetiapine. Jeste *et al.* (1999b) recommend the starting dose of quetiapine in elderly patients to be 12.5–25 mg/day. The optimal target dose is suggested to be between 75 mg and 125 mg per day.

NONPHARMACOLOGICAL TREATMENT

Electro-convulsive therapy (ECT)

Positive results with ECT have been reported by several researchers. Janzarik (1957), for example, studied 50 elderly schizophrenic patients with onset of symptoms after 60 years of age and found that ECT in conjunction with medications such as chlorpromazine resulted in temporary remissions (cited by Post, 1966).

Kay and Roth (1961) reported temporary remissions occurring with the use of ECT or neuroleptics in approximately 25% of their patients. Among patients with late paraphrenia, Frost (1969) reported positive response to ECT in patients who presented with substantial or predominant mood symptoms.

Psychosocial therapies

Although patients with LOS usually require long-term treatment due to the chronic nature of their illness, controlled research studies indicate that psychological interventions can prove to have beneficial outcomes. Social skills training, a widely studied psychological intervention for schizophrenia, as well as cognitive retraining and didactic family counselling have shown positive effects in younger adults. In one study (Rabins *et al.*, 1984), 35 patients with a diagnosis of LOS or paraphrenia were treated with neuroleptics and psychosocial therapies. Upon discharge, 20 patients were symptom free, 10 symptomatic but improved, and five symptomatically unchanged. A 2-year follow-up investigation on 14 patients over the age of 60 revealed that four patients remained symptom free, six patients had relapses with symptom free periods, and three patients experienced chronic symptoms. It is not known how many of these patients over age 60 continued (or were compliant) with neuroleptic treatment upon discharge.

The importance of addressing cognitive and sensory impairments in patients with late onset paranoid disorder, within a group therapy forum, has been stressed by Jette and Winnett (1987). Although correcting such impairments is often difficult and not always possible, patients are encouraged to become aware of how their impairments affect their lives. Jette and Winnett (1987) have described the Hearing Awareness Group which focuses on the effect of hearing loss as well as the process of communication, interpersonal relationships, and the individual's perception of personal worth within the institution. Moreover, these authors note that group psychotherapy can be a complement to individual treatment and can be specially useful in helping participants identify those domains of confusion and misinterpretations of social experience associated with hearing loss. Based on the psychodynamics of late onset paranoid disorder, Jette and Winnett (1987) note that the primary psychosocial intervention with this population may be either individual or group psychotherapy, combined with milieu management. Even though these authors focus on late onset paranoid disorder, the same principles they offer can be applied to LOS patients, many of whom have paranoid delusions.

RESEARCH RECOMMENDATIONS

Future research needs to evaluate the efficacy of psychopharmacological as well as psychological interventions in patients with LOS and other late onset psychoses. We need to determine the relative risk-to-benefit ratios and cost–benefit ratios with different antipsychotics and other forms of treatment for LOS. These studies should include respectable sample sizes based on power analyses with appropriate control groups in order to have more conclusive and generalizable results. Collaborative work with multisite international studies is warranted given the fact that LOS is less common than EOS. Appropriate diagnostic criteria must be applied and reliable rating scales for outcome measures should be employed.

There is also a critical need for investigations of the efficacy of psychosocial interventions since many psychological issues with potential psychopathologic importance arise in later life, including retirement, financial constraints, loneliness, and grief over losses (Sorensen, 1990). Research related to the treatment of LOS will broaden our understanding of the treatment of schizophrenia in general.

CLINICAL RECOMMENDATIONS

The first step in the management of a patient with LOS or other late onset psychosis is a thorough medical work-up to rule out known causes of psychosis such as medical conditions and substance use or abuse. Any treatment should be considered only after obtaining a complete history, psychiatric and physical (including neurological) examination, and necessary laboratory evaluations. Standardized diagnostic criteria such as the DSM-IV (American Psychiatric Association, 1994) along with a definition of age of onset (of prodromal symptoms) should be employed.

Antipsychotics (usually the newer atypical ones) in combination with psychosocial therapies constitute the backbone of management of patients with LOS. A basic principle is to start the patient on low, conservative doses of antipsychotics and increase doses at lower increments than those used for younger patients. Elderly patients are not only more sensitive to adverse effects of medications but also tend to have a slower therapeutic response to antipsychotic medications compared with younger adults.

The British National Formulary recommends that doses of neuroleptics in the elderly should be 25–50% of those given to young adults (Howard, 1996). Indeed, treatment of late onset patients should usually be at even lower doses than those prescribed to age-comparable patients with EOS.

Patients with late onset disease may continue to experience psychotic symptoms despite the great variation in the range of neuroleptic dosages employed. Howard (1996) believes that compliance with treatment is the most important determinant of outcome. Jeste and McClure (1997) note that age-associated cognitive impairment is likely to result in miscompliance rather than simple noncompliance. In other words, elderly patients may not only forget to take their medications, they may take them more frequently, in wrong doses, or at incorrect dosage intervals. In view of physical comorbidity and polypharmacy that are common in the elderly, drug–drug interactions should be watched for carefully. Noteworthy drugs in this category are anticholinergics. Many elderly subjects are on multiple prescribed as well as over-the-counter anticholinergic medications, which may cause urinary retention, constipation, aggravation of glaucoma, confusion, etc. Hence a complete accounting of all the medications that a patient is taking is critical. All unnecessary medications should be discontinued.

The extent of side effects likely to be caused by a neuroleptic, along with concomitant physical illness, a history of the patient's previous therapeutic response to a specific neuroleptic, and other treatments received together, will determine the type of medication that will be best suited for a given patient (Tran-Johnson *et al.*, 1994). The newer atypical antipsychotics are clearly better tolerated and may be more effective than conventional antipsychotics for treating psychotic disorders in the elderly. While the number of studies with these drugs in patients with LOS is limited, it seems that risperidone has so far had more widespread use in the elderly than other atypical agents. Prescribed in suitably low dosages, the atypical agents are generally well tolerated. The optimal length of treatment is not established but varies from one patient to another. If a taper of medication is to be attempted, this should be done very slowly given the risk of relapse. Since there is a certain risk of tardive dyskinesia, periodic assessment of involuntary movements is recommended (Jeste and McClure, 1997).

In treating psychotic disorders in the elderly, supportive psychotherapy, behavioural modification, education of family members and/or caregivers, along with pharmacotherapy should all be considered. Psychosocial treatment is a very important aspect of the management of LOS patients. Establishing a good therapeutic relationship with the patient and providing a supportive atmosphere are vital. The therapist does not agree with the patient's delusional system but should be empathetic and understanding of the patient's distorted thinking.

In order to facilitate overall management of the patient, the clinician should seek the help of the patient's caregivers, family members, friends, neighbours, clergy, or others in the patient's community. Such a network can lead to early detection and treatment of impending relapse and thus avoid unnecessary hospitalizations or legal problems. Social agencies can also be contacted to help the patient obtain appropriate financial, medical, nutritional, or transportation assistance. Conservatorship or guardianship for the patient might also be recommended in order to ensure proper management of the patient's finances.

In summary, appropriately low-dose atypical antipsychotics are recommended for the treatment of LOS, in combination with psychosocial intervention. Such combination therapy is likely to produce the best outcome. A strong and informed support network is also indispensable for the overall well-being of the patient.

ACKNOWLEDGEMENTS

This work was supported, in part, by the National Institute for Mental Health grants MH49671, MH45131, MH43693, MH51459, MH19934, and by the Department of Veterans Affairs.

REFERENCES

American Psychiatric Association (1994). *Diagnostic and Statistical Manual of Mental Disorders, 4th edn* (DSM-IV). American Psychiatric Association, Washington, DC.

Arvanitis, L.A., Miller, B.G. and the Seroquel Trial 13 Study Group (1997). Multiple fixed doses of 'seroquel' (quetiapine) in patients with acute exacerbation of schizophrenia: a comparison with haloperidol and placebo. *Biol Psychiatry* **42**, 233–246.

Avorn, J. and Gurwitz, J. (1990). Principles of pharmacology. In: Cassel, K., Riesenberg, D., Sorenson, L. and Walsh, J. (Eds), *Geriatric Medicine (2nd edn)*. Springer-Verlag, New York, pp. 66–77.

Berman, I., Merson, A., Allen, E., Alexis, C., Sison, C. and Losonczy, M. (1995). Effect of risperidone on cognitive performance in elderly schizophrenic patients: a double-blind comparison with haloperidol. *NCDEU 35th Annual Meeting*, Orlando, Florida, poster no. 93.

Breitner, J.C.S. and Anderson, D.N. (1994). The organic and psychological antecedents of delusional jealousy in old age. *Int J Geriatr Psychiatry* **9**, 703–707.

Brink, T.L. (1979). Hypochondriasis and paranoia: similar delusional systems in an institutionalized geriatric population. *J Nerv Mental Dis* **167**, 224–228.

Chengappa, K.N.R., Baker, R.W., Kreinbrock, S.B. and Adair, D. (1995). Clozapine use in female geriatric patients with psychoses. *J Geriatr Psychiatry Neurol* **8**, 12–15.

Cordingley, G.J., Dean, B.C. and Hallett, C. (1985). A multicentre, double-blind parallel trial of bromazepam (Lexotan) and lorazepam to compare the acute benefit–risk ratio in the treatment of patients with anxiety. *Current Med Res Opin* **9**, 505–510.

Escande, M. (1983). Clinical trial of loxapine succinate applied to the treatment of thirty hospitalized psychotic patients. *Ann Medico-Psychologiques* **141**, 309–322.

Folstein, M.F., Folstein, S.E. and McHugh, P.R. (1975). Mini-Mental State: a practical method for grading the cognitive state of patients for the clinician. *J Psychiatr Res* **12**, 189–198.

Frankenburg, F.R. and Kalunian, D. (1994). Clozapine in the elderly. *J Geriatr Psychiatry Neurol* **7**, 129–132.

Frost, J.B. (1969). Paraphrenia and paranoid schizophrenia. *Psychiatr Clinica* **3**, 129–138.

Gilbert, P.L., Harris, M.J., McAdams, L.A. and Jeste, D.V. (1995). Neuroleptic withdrawal in schizophrenic patients. *Arch Gen Psychiatry* **52**, 173–188.

Grossberg, G.T. and Manepalli, J. (1995). The older patient with psychotic symptoms. *Psychiatric Services* **46**, 55–59.

Hagger, C., Buckley, P., Kenny, J.T. Friedman, L., Ubogy, D. and Meltzer, H.Y. (1993). Improvement in cognitive functions and psychiatric symptoms in treatment-refractory schizophrenic patients receiving clozapine. *Biol Psychiatry* **34**, 702–712.

Harris, M.J. and Jeste, D.V. (1988). Late-onset schizophrenia: an overview. *Schizophr Bull* **14**, 39–55.

Howard, R. (1996). Study on schizophrenia: drug treatment of schizophrenia and delusional disorder in late life. *Int Psychogeriatrics* **8**, 597–608.

Howard, R. and Levy, R. (1992). Which factors affect treatment response in late paraphrenia? *Int J Geriatr Psychiatry* **7**, 667–672.

Jackson, D.M., Ryan, C., Evenden, J. and Mohell, N. (1994). Preclinical findings with new antipsychotic agents: what makes them atypical? *Acta Psychiatr Scand* **380**, 41–48.

Janzarik, W. (1957). Zur problematik schizophrener psychosen in hoheren leben-salter. *Nervenarzt* **28**, 535–542.

Jeste, D.V. and McClure, F.S. (1997). Psychoses: diagnosis and treatment in the elderly. In: Schneider, L. (Ed.), *Updates in Geriatric Psychiatry, New Directions for Mental Health Services*. Jossey-Bass, San Francisco.

Jeste, D.V. and Zisook, S. (1988). Preface to psychosis and depression in the elderly. *Psychiatr Clin North Am* **11**, xiii–xv.

Jeste, D.V., Lacro, J.P., Gilbert, P.L., Kline, J. and Kline, N. (1993). Treatment of late-life schizophrenia with neuroleptics. *Schizophr Bull* **19**, 817–830.

Jeste, D.V., Caligiuri, M.P., Paulsen, J.S. *et al.* (1995a). Risk of tardive dyskinesia in older patients: a prospective longitudinal study of 266 patients. *Arch Gen Psychiatry* **52**, 756–765.

Jeste, D.V., Harris, M.J., Krull, A., Kuck, J., McAdams, L.A. and Heaton, R. (1995b). Clinical and neuropsychological characteristics of patients with late-onset schizophrenia. *Am J Psychiatry* **152**, 722–730.

Jeste, D.V., Eastham, J.H., Lacro, J.P., Gierz, M., Field, M.G. and Harris, M.J. (1996). Management of late-life psychosis. *J Clin Psychiatry* **57** (suppl 3), 39–45.

Jeste, D.V., Lohr, J.B., Eastham, J.H., Rockwell, E. and Caligiuri, M.P. (1998). Adverse effects of long-term use of neuroleptics: human and animal studies. *J Psychiatr Res* **32**, 201–214.

Jeste, D.V., Lacro, J.P., Palmer, B., Rockwell, E., Harris, M.J. and Caligiuri, M.P. (1999a). Incidence of tardive dyskinesia in early stages of neuroleptic treatment for older patients. *Am J Psychiatry* **156**, 309–311.

Jeste, D.V., Rockwell, E., Harris, M.J., Lohr, J.B. and Lacro, J. (1999b). Conventional versus newer antipsychotics in elderly. *Am J Geriatr Psychiatry* **7**, 70–76.

Jette, C.C.B. and Winnett, R.L. (1987). Late-onset paranoid disorder. *Am J Orthopsychiatry* **57**, 485–493.

Jørgensen, P. and Munk-Jørgensen, P. (1985). Paranoid psychosis in the elderly: a follow-up study. *Acta Psychiatr Scand* **72**, 358–363.

Kane, J.M., Honigfeld, G., Singer, J., Meltzer, H. and Clozaril Collaborative Study Group (1988). Clozapine for the treatment resistant schizophrenic: a double-blind comparison with chlorpromazine. *Arch Gen Psychiatry* **45**, 789–796.

Kay, D.W.K. and Roth, M. (1961). Environmental and hereditary factors in the schizophrenias of old age ('late paraphrenia') and their bearing on the general problem of causation in schizophrenia. *J Mental Sci* **107**, 649–686.

Kay, S.R., Fiszbein, A. and Opler, L.A. (1987). The positive and negative syndrome scale (PANSS) for schizophrenia. *Schizophr Bull* **13**, 261–276.

Kerwin, R.W. (1994). The new atypical antipsychotics – a lack of extrapyramidal side-effects and new routes in schizophrenia research. *Br J Psychiatry* **164**, 141–148.

Lohr, J.B., Alder, M., Flynn, K., Harris, M.J. and McAdams, L.A. (1997). Minor physical anomalies in older patients with late-onset schizophrenia, early-onset schizophrenia, depression, and Alzheimer's disease. *Am J Geriatr Psychiatry* **5**, 318–323.

Marder, S.R. and Meibach, R.C. (1994). Risperidone in the treatment of schizophrenia. *Am J Psychiatry* **151**, 825–835.

Meltzer, H.Y. and Fibiger, H.C. (1996). Olanzapine: a new atypical antipsychotic drug. *Neuropsychopharmacology* **14**, 83–85.

Modell, J.G., Lenox, R.H. and Weiner, S. (1985). Inpatient clinical trial of lorazepam for the management of manic agitation. *J Clin Psychopharmacol* **5**, 109–113.

Opjordsmoen, J. (1988). Hypochondriacal psychoses: a long-term follow-up. *Acta Psychiatr Scand* **77**, 587–597.

Panteleeva, G.N. (1984). Clinical efficiency of leponex according to the findings of an international study. *Zh Neuropath Psikhiatr Imeni SS Korsakova* **84**, 393–401.

Pearlson, G.D., Kreger, L., Rabins, R.V. *et al.* (1989). A chart review study of late-onset and early-onset schizophrenia. *Am J Psychiatry* **146**, 1568–1574.

Post, F. (1966). *Persistent Persecutory States of the Elderly*. Pergamon Press, London.

Rabins, P., Pauker, S. and Thomas, J. (1984). Can schizophrenia begin after age 44? *Compr Psychiatry* **25**, 290–293.

Raskind, M.A. and Risse, S.C. (1986). Antipsychotic drugs and the elderly. *J Clin Psychiatry* **47**, 17–22.

Raskind, M., Alvarez, C. and Herlin, S. (1979). Fluphenazine enanthate in the outpatient treatment of late paraphrenia. *J Am Geriatr Soc* **27**, 459–463.

Ray, W.A., Griffin, M.R., Schaffner, W., Baugh, D.K. and Melton, L.J. (1987). Psychotropic drug use and the risk of hip fracture. *N Engl J Med* **316**, 363–369.

Rich, S.S., Friedman, J.H. and Ott, B.R. (1995). Risperidone versus clozapine in the treatment of psychosis in six patients with Parkinson's disease and other akinetic-rigid syndromes. *J Clin Psychiatry* **56**, 556–559.

Rockwell, E., Krull, A.J., Dimsdale, J. and Jeste, D.V. (1994). Late-onset psychosis with somatic delusions. *Psychosomatics* **35**, 66–72.

Rosen, J., Bohon, S. and Gershon, S. (1990). Antipsychotics in the elderly. *Acta Psychiatr Scand* **358** (suppl.), 170–175.

Saltz, B.L., Woerner, M.G., Kane, J.M. *et al.* (1991). Prospective study of tardive dyskinesia incidence in the elderly. *JAMA* **266**, 2402–2406.

Salzman, C. (1990). Principles of psychopharmacology. In: Bienenfeld, D. (Ed.), *Verwoerdt's Clinical Geropsychiatry*. Williams and Wilkins, Baltimore, MD, pp. 235–249.

Salzman, C., Vacarro, B., Lieff, J. and Weiner, A. (1995). Clozapine in older patients with psychosis and behavioral disruption. *Am J Geriatr Psychiatry* **3**, 26–33.

Schneider, L.S., Olin, J.T. and Pawluczyk, S. (1993). A double-blind crossover pilot study of l-deprenyl selegiline combined with cholinesterase inhibitor in Alzheimer's disease. *Am J Psychiatry* **150**, 321–323.

Small, J.G., Hirsch, S.R., Arvanitis, L.A., Miller, B.G., Link, C.G.G. and the Seroquel Study Group (1997). Quetiapine in patients with schizophrenia. *Arch Gen Psychiatry* **54**, 549–557.

Soares, J.C. and Gershon, S. (1996). Prospects for the development of new treatment with a rapid onset of action in affective disorders. *Drugs* **52**, 477–482.

Soni, S.D. and Freeman, H.L. (1985). Early clinical experiences with sulpiride. *Br J Psychiatry* **146**, 673.

Sorensen, L.B. (1990). Rheumatology. In: Cassel, C.K., Riesenberg, D.E., Sorensen, L.B. and Walsh, J.R. (Eds), *Geriatric Medicine (2nd edn)*. Springer-Verlag, New York, pp. 199–211.

Szymonowicz, R. (1983). Dogmatil as long-term therapy in severe psychiatric diseases. *Semaine des hospitaux de Paris* **59**, 1468–1470.

Tinetti, M.E., Speechley, M. and Ginter, S.F. (1988). Risk factors for falls among elderly persons living in the community. *N Engl J Med* **319**, 1701–1707.

Tran-Johnson, T.K., Harris, M.J. and Jeste, D.V. (1994). Pharmacological treatment of schizophrenia and delusional disorders of late life. In: Copeland, J.R.M., Abou-Saleh, M.T. and Blazer, D.G. (Eds), *Principles and Practices of Geriatric Psychiatry*. John Wiley & Sons, New York, pp. 685–692.

Tuason, V.B., Escabar, J.I. and Garvey, M. (1984). Loxapine versus chlorpromazine in paranoid schizophrenia. *J Clin Psychiatry* **45**, 158–163.

Wengel, S.P., Burke, W.J. and Holemon, D. (1989). Musical hallucinations: the sounds of silence? *J Am Geriatr Soc* **37**, 163–166.

Wilson, J.A. and MacLennan, W.J. (1989). Review: drug-induced Parkinsonism in elderly patients. *Age Ageing* **18**, 208–210.

Wolters, E.C., Jansen, E.N.H., Tuynman-Qua, H.G. and Bergmans, P.L.M. (1996). Olanzapine in the treatment of dopaminomimetic psychosis in patients with Parkinson's disease. *Neurology* **47**, 1085–1087.

Wragg, R.E. and Jeste, D.V. (1988). Neuroleptics and alternative treatments: management of behavioral symptoms and psychosis in Alzheimer's disease and related conditions. *Psychiatr Clin North Am* **11**, 195–214.

18

The Place of Non-Biological Treatments

LUIS AGÜERA-ORTIZ* AND BLANCA RENESES-PRIETO†

*Psychiatry Department, University Hospital 12 de Octubre and Department of
Psychiatry, Complutense University, Madrid, and †Regional Ministry of Health and
Social Services, Madrid, Spain.

A DEARTH OF DATA

As stated early by Emil Kraepelin, the field of old age psychosis is probably the darkest subject within psychiatry. The decades that have followed Kraepelin's descriptions of dementia praecox and paraphrenia have seen only partial advances and there have been enormous difficulties in the conceptualization of the different forms of illness and in the clarification of possible aetiologies.

In the present decade, research has been more fruitful and significant advances in the pathophysiology, delimitation of risk factors, clinical presentation, neuropsychology and pharmacological treatment of psychoses presenting in old age have been made. Nevertheless, the psychological aspects of both aetiology and treatment of these late forms of psychosis have received much less attention. This is a problem common to all forms of psychosis but early onset schizophrenia, the brief psychoses, and even delusional disorder, have attracted the interest of the different schools within psychiatry in a more concerted way. Psychoanalysis, psychodynamically oriented therapy (PDT), the cognitive and behavioural therapies (CBT) and the family-systemic therapies have tried to develop forms of treatment deriving from their particular points of view. Their positions, often controversial and not always widely accepted, have helped, however, to advance the practical help and management of younger patients and their families. These benefits have reached the elderly much more scarcely.

THE SOURCES OF INFORMATION

There are several possible sources of information concerning non-drug treatments of psychosis in the elderly, including journals and books, but the subject is not treated extensively in any of them. For example, when a Medline search is performed and the results are restricted to aged patients, the number of hits is surprisingly small, offering no more than a dozen articles of significant interest. Most geriatric psychiatry books include at least one chapter dealing with psychotherapy in old age but they are focused mainly on depression and, to a lesser extent, on anxiety disorders, reflecting the situation found in psychiatric journals (Weiss and Lazarus, 1993).

Another possible source of information can be found in books on psychotherapy. Several authors have made noteworthy contributions to topics related to psychosis but the problem here is the lack of extension of these studies to elderly individuals. Very little has been published in the CBT field, although authors working in PDT have been more productive. A different way of approaching the subject is to consider how much of the information gathered from the psychological management of other diseases can be applied to late life psychoses. From this point of view, depression and dementia are the two most severe illnesses to look at.

Finally, the opinions of clinicians involved in the care of elderly psychotic patients, obtained from surveys, can certainly be a valuable source of information. This chapter presents a comprehensive summary of the information available from all these sources, together with the authors' views and personal experience.

SOME INTRIGUING QUESTIONS AND A CLINICAL PARADOX

Confronted by the problem of late onset psychoses, clinicians are faced with some intriguing questions that have much to do with both aetiology and treatment.

One of the most important questions concerns the age of onset. Why do these patients start exhibiting psychotic psychopathology so late in life? Research from the last few decades has shown some risk factors and the contribution of certain biological states as precipitants for the development of psychosis. They are all addressed in other parts of this book. However, the issue here is to find their psychological or psychosocial counterparts. In fact, the study of the importance of life events or psychosocial correlates for the development of other important mental illnesses is much more developed than that of old age psychosis. Among the available information, it is possible to find, for example, references to the impact of social isolation, which was initially considered one possible cause but can be better viewed now as a consequence of the illness or very probably an interaction of both. The effect of sensory deprivation on the development of paranoid thinking is another factor usually cited. The hypothesis of a possible personality disorder was raised in early investigations, although the relative importance of this has been questioned more recently (Castle and Howard, 1992; Almeida *et al.*, 1995).

All these facts only scratch the surface of the problem. Given the great amount of psychological change and adaptation that any person has to accomplish as part of the ageing process, it is not unwise to presume that emotional agents probably play a determinant role in a supposedly delayed onset of the psychotic illness. This might be an influence exerted by these emotional changes alone or, more probably in conjunction with some of the biological changes necessary but not sufficient for the genesis of the delusional state. Looking at things from this point of view, it is equally important to take into consideration both the causative and the protective factors. In fact, it might well be that the weakening of the latter is more important, in psychological terms, than a possible direct emotional causative effect.

Following this line of thought, one of the most striking findings is the clear preponderance of women in late onset cases. Separation by gender is becoming essential in terms of both the biology and psychopathology of virtually any mental illness. This is especially true in schizophrenia and other related psychoses, where the incidence varies clearly along the age span from early adulthood to old age (see Castle's review in Chapter 12). These sex differences might be explained not only by the effect of age in the different biological processes but also in terms of distinct intrapsychic defence and coping mechanisms.

Another frequent question raised by clinicians is related to treatment effectiveness. Why do some patients tend to respond fairly well to medication while others do not? Is it a simple question of idiosyncratic pharmacological response or of biological constitution, or can we think further in terms of a form of the so-called non-placebo response (Thali, 1988)?

In the diagnosis of the late and very late forms of schizophrenia-like psychoses, a significant depressive disorder has to be excluded. A formal separation of the affective disorders, including the affective psychoses, is necessary. But are these two diseases absolutely separated? Clinical experience shows that patients are far from being free from affective symptoms, mainly in the depressive range. In fact, if patients are followed long enough, it is common to find depressive manifestations ranging from mild depressive symptoms to major depression in at least 50% of cases (Agüera-Ortiz, 1998). The months that follow successful neuroleptic treatment, after the alleviation of delusions and hallucinations, are particularly relevant. Clinicians should pay especially close attention in order to detect newly developed affective symptoms during this period.

Study of the points in common between the late onset psychoses and affective disorders is a field of research that has passed rather unexplored until now. We would like to state clearly our position by affirming that we think that they are basically different disorders. Nevertheless, the information available raises some challenging points that must be taken into account. To cite some of the most obvious, the preponderance of women can point to a certain aetiological relationship with affective disorders which also share this feature. Some authors have also reported a familial aggregation of affective disorders that is more frequent than in matched controls (Howard et al., 1997).

From the perspective of neuroimaging studies, some of the cerebral changes described in late onset cases have been also reported in late onset depression. Probably the clearest findings are the changes in the ventricular-to-brain ratio that have been found in both diseases. The presence of hyper-intensities in subcortical white matter – a typical finding of late-life depression – was reported initially in late onset schizophrenia (Breitner et al., 1990; Lesser et al., 1993) but a more detailed selection of samples, especially excluding patients with clear cerebrovascular disease, has not found an excess of this change with respect to other non-psychotic community dwelling elders (Howard et al., 1995). Some other common factors, from a more psychological perspective, are exposed later in this chapter.

Biological research on the different forms of late onset psychoses has been the mainstream form of investigation, probably in an honest and genuine attempt to find aetiological explanations that may lead to effective treatments. However, a great clinical paradox lies behind this. This paradox refers to the extraordinary problems with which psychiatrists are confronted when they face the patient. These problems are not only of a biological nature but especially they have to do with management needs. By this we mean crucial aspects of illness behaviour such as awareness of illness, the wish to find medical help, difficulties in establishing a therapeutical relationship, compliance with pharmacological treatment and the efficacy of it. What psychiatrists find more often than not is a patient who does not acknowledge his illness, who is not willing to come to the office, and who refuses adamantly any form of medication for a situation that he does not consider a disease at all.

There have been considerable advances in the pharmacological management of psychoses, but the patient must be in a position to accept medication in any of its forms. Clinicians should also have therapeutic alternatives in the case of continued refusal of pharmacological treatment. Additionally, the patient's suffering and the distress experienced by the family must attract the attention of all possible treatment measures. If only for these three reasons, the non-pharmacological management of this kind of patient becomes an absolute necessity.

TREATMENT SHOULD ADDRESS UNDERLYING MECHANISMS

Psychological approaches can take many forms, ranging from the formal psychotherapies to what can be called the psychological management of particular cases. We firmly believe that any approach of this kind must build on a theoretical frame, sufficiently elaborated and sensitive at the same time. However, at the present time, problems related to these ideas are complex and still difficult to understand, and a widely accepted unified theory is lacking. Thus, our opinion, shared also by others (Sadavoy, 1994), is that to take a strong position on the side of only one of the different psychological models available can result in a serious hindrance to the advance of knowledge and to the benefits that patients may obtain.

In fact, the mechanisms underlying very separate forms of therapy such as CBT and PDT can be closer than they may seem, even though the formal application of the therapy techniques is clearly different. Hingley (1997a,b) has recently given support to this assumption. Looking for the most useful parts of the theories that can be applicable to every particular patient can be more useful in the present situation than an excessively rigid psychotherapeutic approach. This position calls for the intervention of open minded therapists, but the kind of situation that we are dealing with is impossible to manage without large doses of flexibility.

Hitherto, several authors have offered interesting insights on the psychological processes of ageing, which can be used as a basis for the management of psychotic patients. The main approaches come from developmental theories, cognitive and behavioural constructs, personality studies and psychodynamic formulations.

Erikson's developmental theory is based on the different stages that any human being has to go through and the tasks that they subsequently must accomplish (Erikson, 1980). The process of ego maturation through the years and the acquisition of different levels of ego identity are central parts of his theory. Passage from one developmental stage to another is achieved only after overcoming the corresponding crisis. Failure to do so results in a state of distress and what he calls identity diffusion. Erikson considered that the successive stages and life crises have a cumulative effect, in that the successful negotiation of the precedent crises helps the person to adapt to the demands of the next stage.

For the last part of life, Erikson described a stage called ego integrity versus despair. By this, he meant the transactions that appear in this very special phase when there is no subsequent one to follow. Lack of a future forces the necessity to look back, and this would be the reason why the practice of reviewing one's life is done more often now than in any other stage. This life review has to make sense, and should leave the individual with a sufficiently satisfying balance between what has been done and what has been lost. Acceptable levels of ego integrity allow the person to benefit from different sources of gratification. These can come from the outside world or the inside world in the form of fruitful relationships with family and friends, a wished-for decrease of the social demands related to retirement, the choice of new and different activities, or the reminiscence of successful elements from the past, for example, in the form of individual achievements or rewarding relationships with others.

Inability to accept changes and losses leads the subject to a conflicting situation where ego integrity is no longer possible and results in a situation of despair. In order to perform this life review, to make reflections about past events, to accept the unstoppable passage of time that subtracts personal capacities and takes the person to the moment of death, the aged person must have the necessary capacity of insight and the personal disposition for it. This is a challenge in which not every person is successful. Failure to achieve this results in various forms of conflictive behaviour well known to old age psychiatrists.

Among other maladjustments, we find different degrees of regression, such as the characteristic attention seeking behaviour exhibited by a considerable number of patients. Another possible situation is the lack of adaptation between the present capacities and the actions actually performed by the old person, for example the abandonment of activities that he or she can still perform, or the intention to continue with tasks that are clearly beyond his or her present capacities. This may also result in attempts to control other people and the environment by trying to exert an authority presently lost. Other alternatives are the frank deterioration of self-image accompanied by depressive thinking, or, in more severe cases, the interpretation of the outer world in a suspicious or unmistakable paranoid way. The detection and management of all these clinical situations and especially of the maladjustment behaviours and the difficulties involved in performing adequate forms of life review are important points that can help in the treatment of the psychotic patient.

Some authors, working from a cognitive perspective, have also postulated a point of view, complementary with this, signalling the importance of ego maturation and the necessary ability to face up to the menaces to self-concept and self-esteem that happen in old age. Externalization of negative affects will be the defensive reaction to protect against the experience of these negative and painful feelings. A pathological attributional style, based excessively on externalization, could be the inadequate response to these menaces and the basis of paranoid ideas (Bentall *et al.*, 1994; Kinderman and Bentall, 1996). This can be easily compared with the projective defence mechanisms postulated by psychodynamic theories.

Hasset (1997) has proposed the integration of some of the above mentioned aspects, taking into account the dimensional approach to personality study, in order to build concepts subject to objective measurement. This is one of the very few attempts to investigate and understand the psychological factors behind the development of old age forms of psychosis. Hasset advances one hypothesis based on possible interactions between the patient's failure to achieve the appropriate ego maturation required in old age, a significant preponderance of certain personality traits like 'openness to experience', the defences generated against threats to the self-concept, and the development of a dysfunctional attributional style based on externalizations. She proposes the measurement of these factors by means of scales already available but not used yet with elderly psychotic populations.

Psychodynamic formulations can also give useful hints to possible aetiological or precipitating factors that could also be subsequently used in the management of patients. Using the concept of personality structure (Bergeret, 1974), it is possible to speak in terms of a psychotic structure that has been compensated by successful defence mechanisms for a long time, maybe exhibiting minor symptoms but not a clear delusional state. Once these defence mechanisms are insufficient to maintain the person within the frame of reality testing, psychosis will appear. In particular, the delusional patient would resort to projection, attributing their own impulses, the origin of conflictive situations, and finally their problems and difficulties, to others. The result is development of acute or chronic persecutory anxiety of different intensity that can lead to varied degrees of suspiciousness and eventually to a delusional state. Boundaries between self and others will thus be softened, and the outside world will be viewed in a threatening way.

Verwoerdt (1987) has proposed an interesting model for paranoid decompensations that can also be viewed as a useful framework for understanding some important aspects of the psychological functioning of the elderly from a psychodynamic perspective. The very clear-cut clinical origin of this conceptualization allows a more general application in the management of the psychotic patient.

Following Verwoerdt's description, the *self* can be divided into a 'bodily self' and a core 'inner self'. Both constitute the unity that enters into relationships and establishes exchanges with the outer world ('external object world'). The *bodily self* acts like a shell that surrounds the *inner self* and acts as a bridge between it and the outer world, containing also the mechanisms of this interaction. Three basic states or stages are possible: depressive, hypochondriacal and psychotic, each involving an increased degree of disturbance based on different levels of regression.

In the depressive stage, interactions with the object world are maintained and are of good enough quality. The hypochondriac stage means a regression and, although the relationships with the outer world are maintained, the emphasis is now within the body. An additional worsening of the situation – and a further state of regression and withdrawal – involves a rupture with external objects that are now considered threatening, and the development of psychotic symptoms. Patients can go along this path in both directions.

We have already stressed the importance that we attach to depressive phenomena in the delusional states of the aged. Depression has been usually related to the experience of loss, a situation that is especially frequent among the elderly. But it is not only losses themselves that are relevant. The concept can be expanded to the difficulties that the ageing person may have to replace lost objects and their loss of aspiration to obtain new objects or gains. These difficulties may result from the painful experiences of multiple or very severe losses that deprive the subject of the necessary mental energy, the fear that they will lose again new attachment objects, or simply verification that there are no more external objects available to them.

Ego strength, in a similar way to Erikson's formulations, has a major importance. The ability to cope with losses and other depressive experiences is crucial to understanding the origin of decompensations. Knowledge about how the person coped with difficulties in earlier years can yield information about the ego strength with which the patient enters old age. Guilt is another usual emotional experience during depressive states. The combination of guilt and an immature ego can be lived, via projective mechanisms, in a persecutory manner in the same way that feelings of envy – a frequent but seldom addressed emotion in late life – can also be transformed and projected outside in the form of persecutory experiences.

The occurrence of important depressogenic life events, or those intrapsychic experiences usually related to depressive emotions in a person with a defective self or personality structure, may not result in the development of clinical depression, if depressive feelings cannot be tolerated or even generated, giving way to more severe forms of psychopathology such as delusional states. Breaking contact with reality may be more tolerable than experiencing important depressive feelings. Depression may become more apparent when delusional symptoms are alleviated with treatment.

The body may act as an interface between the outer and the inner world. Intense regressive trends may result in a loss of interest about people and events, thus increasing attention on the patient's own body. A consequence of this is the development of hypochondriacal symptoms that can precede or follow the emergence of psychotic experiences. We use the term 'hypochondria' and its derivatives in a broad sense, meaning the appearance of somatic symptoms or concerns, not dependent on a physical disease, or excessive in quantity for the severity of the physical disease.

Very isolated and withdrawn patients may experience the outer world as empty or lacking in interest. The only thing that they have left is their own self, that is the body surrounding the world of the mind and representations. As a result, the body becomes the nearest part of the outer world and the one with which the patient establishes relationships. The consequence is that the body then becomes officially ill in the form of an increased risk of developing genuine medical diseases or more frequently in the manner of unexplained physical symptoms. Body functions and physical complaints become the currency in which all psychological transactions are made and the only point of contact and relationship with others.

These symbolic movements of psychic energy from the inner self to the outside through the body or in the opposite direction can be used to detect signs of improvement or worsening of the intrapsychic situation. The development of intense hypochondriacal symptoms may precede a depressive decompensation or under other circumstances, a psychotic state. The emergence of physical complaints in a previously delusional patient can be taken as an indicator of improvement. This can happen not only in elderly psychotics but is also a relatively common experience in younger schizophrenic patients as well.

Accepting the patient's physical concerns and not underestimating them can be a useful tool in the management of the delusional elderly. The patient will be very probably more prone to speak about the state of his body than about the products of his mind and the psychiatrist can use this to establish a therapeutic relationship 'talking the same language' as the patient. In very regressive, disengaged or isolated persons, it can be valuable to facilitate an adequate investment of the body by paying attention to body functions or symptoms or with more elaborated forms of therapy like psychomotor therapy, as explained later.

A very important issue to be reminded of here is the symbolic equivalence that exists between the elderly person's house and his own body. This psychic representation affects not only the psychiatrically ill but is a common experience to old age in general. As the years pass, the place where the old person lives tends to stay unchanged. The physical structure of the house and its contents becomes a relevant part of the world of intrapsychic representations. This is the cause of the general reluctance of aged individuals to make changes in the decoration or structure of their homes. The house and its contents tend to remain unmodified for years, even if this means living in an uncomfortable environment. In fact, the need to perform modifications at home, like small painting jobs or repairs, can be a serious stressor and provoke the development of an overanxious or depressive state. The equivalence of the house to the self body image can explain this psychological functioning particularly characteristic of the aged.

One of the most distinctive symptoms of late onset delusional states is the presence of the so-called partition delusions as described by Howard and others (Howard *et al.*, 1992). Patients experience the menace of, or are attacked by, sounds, gas, odours, rays or other means that pass through walls or ceilings as if they were permeable to these harmful influences. They refer their fear of being poisoned or that they have become ill as being due to these persecutory experiences. In younger people with schizophrenia, delusional menaces are more often centred in their own body. The identification of the elderly with their own house as a symbolic part of their body scheme can help to understand the frequency and relevance of the symptomatology related to the house in this population. Thus, it can be

considered in an equivalent range of emotional experiences to hypochondriasis or any other over-investment of the body.

AN ATTEMPTED INTEGRATION

Models are a useful means of synthesizing and harmonizing findings and
advancing research. In what follows we present a tentative integration of the
above mentioned ideas in an easy to understand manner, always keeping in
mind the risks that accompany the over-simplification of complex problems.

Each individual can be considered to have a particular predisposition to
the development of psychiatric illnesses. This can be understood in terms of
genetics, or of the structural and functional formation of the CNS, but also
in terms of the psychological structuring of the self and personality. These
factors are conformed from the moment of birth or very early in life. Their
expression in the form of an illness depends on other factors generally linked
to environmental influences. The neurodevelopment theories of early onset
schizophrenia are in keeping with this line of thought, in the same way as all
the psychodynamic formulations of a psychotic personality structure. Both
conceptions are by no means incompatible and can be included in a general
vulnerability–stress framework.

Every person reaches adult life and faces elderlyhood with this
background. In our view, these factors continue to exert their action at this
stage of life but are also merged with other influences appearing later. From
the biological point of view, the CNS changes cited at the beginning of this
chapter play an important role. Some of them, like ventricular dilatation,
could be present very early in life, while other signs of atrophy or some of
the vascular changes can be considered to be acquired or of degenerative
origin. Physical illnesses and impairments exert an important action of their
own. From a psychosocial perspective, the main contributing factors are
related to an inadequate process of psychological ageing, the impact of losses
– past and present – incurred, and the emergence of significant personal and
social adversities.

These unfavourable human experiences imply the existence of narcissistic
injuries and menaces to the person's feelings of identity and personal integration. Thus, the path to development of psychological distress and a frank
illness is served. An elaborate and perhaps more mature path to illness is the
development of depressive symptoms. This occurs in more structured personalities that can generate and tolerate the emergence of painful depressive
feelings and are less prone to lose contact with reality. The path to psychotic
illness could be followed by people with a more immature or defective self.
Such individuals make massive use of projective defence mechanisms or
externalization and cannot overtly tolerate depression, at least during the

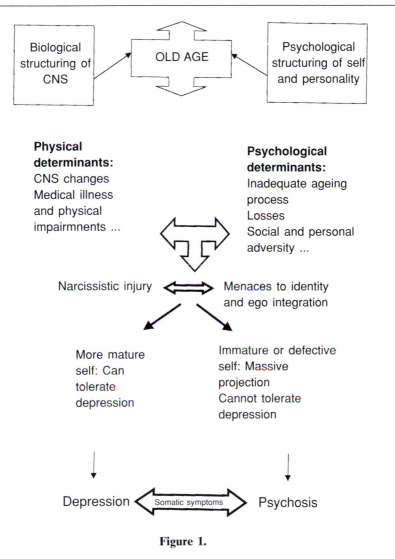

Figure 1.

acute phases. These two different pathways cannot be completely separated and passage from one to the other is possible (Figure 1), as can be seen in the development of psychotic depression or in the emergence of depressive symptoms in psychotic patients when delusions disappear following pharmacological treatment. Somatic symptoms would also extend a bridge between depression and psychosis.

PRACTICAL PSYCHOLOGICAL MANAGEMENT

The psychological approach to the elderly psychotic patient, ranging from formal psychotherapy to the standard office visit, needs the development of some basic skills common to the majority of clinical situations. Since most psychiatric care is nowadays delivered in the community setting in many parts of the world, we will review them from this perspective. Nevertheless, most of the information that follows can also be applicable to the hospitalized patient.

General issues of interview techniques with the aged patient are also appropriate in this clinical situation. In particular, the clinician has to adopt a less abstract or interpretative approach, playing an active rather than a passive role and taking into account possible cognitive difficulties. As with other psychiatric illnesses in aged individuals, assessment of medical conditions and physical factors that can exacerbate psychopathology is a priority. Flexibility is a must, and this includes the length of the interview or session and the interview location (the psychiatrist's own office, other medical facility such as the family physician's office, or the patient's home...). The psychiatrist must also be realistic in terms of the real personal, social and physical limitations of the patient and gain awareness of countertransference movements provoked by the potential for lack of empathy or ageism. It is helpful to delineate explicit, concrete and realistic goals in order to adapt both patient's and doctor's capacities to what can actually be done. In this sense, contextualizing problems is important, as a patient will not present the same difficulties if he or she is living alone, as if he or she is living with other family members or in a nursing home. Provision of formal social resources and support can also be necessary.

Psychopharmacological therapy is the core part of treatment of the delusional elderly. Nevertheless, apart from compulsory treatments, this is practically impossible if it is not made in the context of a wider therapeutic relationship. The phenomena that usually occur during the therapeutic process can be divided into three phases: the initial contacts, the central part of treatment and the termination.

The initial phase

The main goal in this phase is to create a link, a therapeutic alliance based on common trust. It has to be remembered that some patients cannot create solid bonds. This must not discourage the clinician, as the absence of a solid therapeutic alliance does not mean that there is no alliance at all (Verwoerdt, 1987). This alliance is necessary even in the case of a strictly pharmacological treatment, as has been shown for depression (Weiss *et al.*, 1997).

Initial suspiciousness on the part of the patient is enormous but it is important not to forget that he or she is suffering and needs comfort. The clinician must succeed in making the patient accept the need for help, and the kind of help that is offered. It will be necessary from the beginning to accept the patient's hostile behaviour without challenging it directly. The goal is to make the patient change his probable initial view of the doctor or the treatment team from that of a possible enemy to an ally; or in psychological terms, to become what can be called a good figure or good object, one that the patient can count on and that does not cheat or deceive. Only then can a more compliant behaviour be expected and the patient will accept demands to take medications, change behaviours and attitudes, or setting of certain limits. In general terms, the more initial depressive symptomatology the patient has, the easier the alliance becomes, because we will very probably be dealing with a less disturbed patient.

In the building of a trusting relationship, some difficult aspects emerge. Should we always tell the truth – all the truth – to the patient? Should we talk to other people such as family members or neighbours without the knowledge of the patient? In the majority of cases, the answer is the same as in other forms of psychiatric illness, and the patient – especially the suspicious patient – has the right to be aware of what we do. But with the elderly psychotic, it is wise to accept some exceptions, mostly related to the need to obtain and contrast information and to take measures to protect the patient. A good dose of common sense, tact, respect and flexibility is again mandatory.

Another difficulty comes from the necessity of dealing with the delusional thoughts themselves. A well-known and frequent trap for the unwary therapist is to confront the delusions too early. The risk is to get included in the delusional thought or directly lose the patient. Blindly accepting the patient's train of thought does not help either. The advice here is to side-step the delusional line of thinking, neither agreeing nor disagreeing, as is suggested for hypochondriac patients too. Wattis and Martin (1994) proposed the use of dementia-related interviewing techniques in dealing with delusional patients; for example, while not confronting delusions directly, try tactfully to disagree on less sensitive subjects. On the other hand, change the subject if it touches sensitive areas and turn to discuss something more concrete. Also useful is to acknowledge the feelings expressed by the patient but to ignore the content of his reasoning.

A thorough anamnesis and examination can certainly be considered the first form of treatment. Much information is needed, including data on biography, past psychiatric history, physical condition (past and present) and the family and social networks. But it can be very difficult or take a long time to obtain. Data from the patient need usually to be reviewed with information from significant others.

Besides obtaining the usual clinical information, it is important to estimate the patient's degree of regression. This can be expressed in terms of excess of dependence, disability, or hypochondria. Feelings of loneliness must be assessed, since persecutory delusions can also be interpreted as a way of escaping from intense feelings of loneliness, related for example to the death of a spouse or parent. The patient might not accept that he or she feels alone by not telling the whole truth or using statements such as 'I have never needed anybody' or 'Everybody is alone at my age'. The treatment team should make every effort to demonstrate a genuine wish to be near the patient and to help him, showing an honest interest in his state and demonstrating this by creating the occasions to do so or to enquire about his health or well-being. Active interventions, however, must be balanced with the patient's actual need to maintain distances.

Of relevance also is the early assessment of the patient's capacity to tolerate frustration, as frustration will appear sooner or later. Some possible sources of frustration are related to the following facts:

– We are not always going to deal with the same matter that the patient wants us to.
– We will try to turn his fears and concerns into a medical problem and treat it as such.
– We will give more relevance to some of his complaints than to others.
– We will want to prescribe medication and the patient will have to take it.
– This medication will likely have side effects.
– The possibility of admission to hospital is always there and this is a real menace for the patient.

The potential for aggressive behaviour, including the availability of weapons, has to be determined early; information obtained from the family or others is of major importance here. Weapons may be used to harm others and also to commit suicide.

Sensible use of the patient's medical condition or presenting physical complaints can be helpful. Including these or even focusing on them in a substantial part of the initial visits may help to establish a strong relationship. Psychiatry is still a word full of negative connotations and stigma for many aged individuals. Sometimes it helps if the doctor is introduced not as a psychiatrist but as a 'specialist in old age problems'. Even when the patient is aware that he or she is visiting a psychiatrist, the doctor can explain – and demonstrate – that the mental state examination is only a part of the work done in the clinic. Then it is possible for the doctor to address himself most to the physical complaints presented by the patient, while treating both the physical and psychiatric symptoms. Fixing the complaints to the corporal sphere may diminish the occurrence of expansion of delusions, although this does not apply to all patients.

Since bodily concerns, physical symptoms or even hallucinations can be some of the few ways with which the patient makes contact with others, it is necessary to assess the impact of hypochondriacal behaviour in the people surrounding the patient, including their willingness and capacity to accept or tolerate it.

Table 1. Psychological management of the elderly psychotic patient: 'tips and tricks' for the initial contacts.

- Main goal: to create a link, a therapeutic alliance based in common trust
- Many patients cannot create solid therapeutic links, but any degree of attachment is useful
- Initial depressive symptomatology makes the alliance easier
- Management must be oriented to facilitate pharmacological treatment
- Much information is needed, but difficult to obtain: use all available sources
- Assess early:
  the degree of regression (excess dependence, disability, hypochondria)
  the potential for aggressive behaviour, including the use of weapons
  the degree of loneliness
  the capacity to tolerate frustration
- Use medical illness or complaints to help establish the relationship
- The doctor can introduce himself as an 'old age specialist'
- Try to become a 'good object'
- Combat isolation: get in touch, but acknowledge the need for some emotional distance
- Don't ask the patient to do things or set limits before he/she trusts you
- Avoid confronting delusions openly
- Explore fears but respect the needs of dignity and control
- Use reminiscence early

Our advice is to introduce reminiscence in the early phases of contact. Using biographical data, the therapist should extract elements from the history and validate them. Formal reminiscence therapy can be used later but this form of informal support based on past successful elements and the resolution of the needs experienced in difficult times may be of direct help. One must not forget that by the time the patient visits the psychiatrist, the chances are that he has already heard others comment about his mental health or directly claiming that he has gone crazy. This, together with precisely the fact that he is visiting a psychiatrist constitutes a serious attempt to undermine the patient's feelings of dignity and self-control. The use of allusions to successful past situations can counteract these emotions. Sometimes it is the patient who will express this need by saying 'Don't think that I have been like this all my life', then the therapist will only have to follow along this line.

The central phase

The degree of success in the initial contacts will determine in many cases the continuity of treatment. During the central, active treatment phase, one of the main goals continues to be to assure and maintain compliance with both the doctor (and the rest of the therapeutic team) and medication.

Pharmacological therapy is the cornerstone of any kind of care for this kind of patient, and every effort must be made to ensure that they receive it. The possibilities are various, ranging from the patient that promptly accepts medication and has enough family and social support, to the isolated elderly person that refuses it. Whatever the situation, psychological management also continues to be a necessity, especially in the case of those refusing drugs, not only because something has to be done but also for its intrinsic beneficial role.

During this phase, the possibilities for non-biological treatment are diverse, from a formal psychotherapy in the most desirable circumstances to simply continuing to manage the case. We will review next some themes common to the majority of situations.

Once a good quality relationship is established, it is time to investigate the place of significant life events. The possible precipitants of symptoms and their subjective meaning for the patient should be carefully addressed, especially those that could have been experienced as attacks on self-esteem. But any other life events and subjectively important sources of stress should be looked at, even if they do not seem to have a clear association with the delusional disease. These may include quarrelling with neighbours, money affairs, family or domestic differences, and problems with the staff or other people in institutions such as a day centre or a nursing home.

In particular, if the patient has experienced clear losses (be they material or psychological, such as changes in finances, effects of a medical disease, changes in self-image, death of loved ones, etc.) they should be approached and treated as if these losses were the cause of a depressive state, even though the patient does not exhibit clear depressive symptoms. Some of the techniques used for grief therapy are also applicable in these situations. In general, many of the elements used in the psychotherapeutic treatment of depression can be used with these patients (Agüera-Ortiz et al., 1996). In any case, the therapist must be prepared to identify early the presence of depressive signs that can prelude the advent of a full-blown depressive episode, especially when delusional symptoms have disappeared.

The clinician should continue to interest himself in the physical state of the patient, in the functioning of the body systems and the evolution of the diseases that the patient might have. This will be an easy way to keep in touch with the patient and a means to observe his evolution from a different perspective. In fact, once the patient begins to recover contact with reality, an increase of physical complaints is frequently observed. These complaints must be medically explored but in many cases it is not possible to identify an underlying medical condition that explains them. They should then be interpreted as a psychological reinvestment of the body. It is necessary to bear in mind that this reinvestment of the body usually means that an intermediate stage on the way to integration and recovery of mental health has been reached. If the patient continues to recover, physical complaints will be of a transient nature (although they can last months). Otherwise some patients take the route of a corporal over-investment and develop hypochondriacal symptoms sometimes more disturbing than the previous delusional state.

In order to help appropriate forms of body reinvestment, the treatment team should emphasize physical or purely aesthetic aspects. Sensory difficulties should be corrected with the use of spectacles or hearing aids. Activities like visiting the hairdresser, a touch of lipstick or make-up, assuring a proper shave, or renewing clothes, are also simple ways to achieve this and can make a difference.

The development of non-delusional symptoms such as those of depression and more especially those with a physical content helps the patient to 'save face'; that is to say, they provide an acceptable way of exiting the state of severe disturbance that has meant losing contact with reality. They are also a different and more elaborate way of communicating with the environment and in particular with their doctor.

Although a formal reminiscence therapy is not made, the use of reminiscence in this phase is also often very helpful. It is fruitful to support and validate past creative experiences or stages of the patient's life. Delusions can be considered in a way to be the product of a false creativity, not a true creation of the ego. They should be replaced by the patient's authentic personal creations, and this includes not only those that may be present now but also those having happened in the past.

The attitude of the therapist should be one of initially treating symptoms as if all of them were going to be resolved, but paying special attention to those that resist. The reasons why a patient's response to medication is complete in some cases and only partial or non-existent in others are far from clear. It is important to keep in mind that the patient might need some of his pathological productions in order to avoid an even more miserable psychic state, and hence these symptoms tend to be stubbornly resistant to drug treatments. Medication can suppress or soften psychotic symptoms but one needs to place the results in the general context of the often fragile intrapsychic ecology of many patients. A sensible objective can be to respect some specific symptoms that seem to resist medication, because they might have a more important meaning to the patient than is apparent. If the goal is to reach the best equilibrium possible given the actual situation of the patient, the therapist must remember that it is not always beneficial to suppress a symptom without giving a better or at least an acceptable alternative. It would be the equivalent of operating on the deficient vision in a patient with cataracts by removing the crystalline lens without replacing its function with a new lens.

When considering the psychological needs of the affected elderly, one should always try to combat loneliness. The social worker should try to promote contact with peers or engage the patient in social activities, although some patients will resist this very actively. It is wise to suggest activities in which the patient can easily succeed because he or she was previously skilled. An example might be suggesting that the patient resumes playing games like chess, cards or dominoes, sewing or embroidering. This will help him to validate some aspects of his defective self and to turn his mind temporarily aside from paranoid ideation. Members of the treatment team, including the family physician or nurse, can visit from time to time as an additional means of confronting social isolation and to check how things are really going. An unexpected telephone call from the doctor or nurse can improve the sense of not being alone and the feelings of being cared for, not only during the office visits. This has to be done tactfully, since it can also be interpreted by the patient as an attempt to control him or can be interpreted in the context of his delusional world.

Following this line of thought, why not try introducing a pet? The impact of animals in the treatment of mental disorders can be striking, and the so-called 'animal assisted therapy', introduced by Levinson in the early 1970s, is currently attracting increasing attention and research, especially in the fields of dementia and depression (Propsner, 1997; Ridruejo, 1998). Suspicious patients may find more comfort in the company of an animal than that of a person, and the animal's presence can divert the patient's thoughts and perceptions to alternative and more healthy objectives.

Religion may play a role if it is tactfully managed. The positive protective role that religious thoughts may have in psychopathology, especially in the elderly, is well established (Schaie and Willis, 1986). It may be used as a means of reinforcing the fragile self or as an additional way to combat the certainty of delusions or to soften excessively rigid thoughts.

It is of value to remember again the cited equivalence between house and body and to be aware of changes that can be made in the domestic environment. Sometimes the patient has to be helped with services like meals on wheels or introducing modifications in the house, but every change made has to be very carefully planned in terms of the impact that it will cause in the general equilibrium of the patient's life system. Sometimes more serious decisions have to be taken in order to relieve symptoms. This may mean moving the patient temporarily or definitively from the usual place where he lives to another house, with a family member or to an institution.

In general, the therapist should adopt an attitude of demonstrating interest for the patient, avoiding excessive neutrality, and enhancing feelings of confidentiality and trust. Needless to say, all members of the treatment team must be prepared to accept and tolerate resistance to making appointments, changes in them, absences or delays. Sometimes this is related to a lack of awareness of the illness but it may also be interpreted as an intent from the patient to measure the degree of tolerance and trust that the therapist actually has.

Table 2. Psychological management of the elderly psychotic patient: 'tips and tricks' for the central phase of treatment.

- Main goal: to maintain the therapeutic relationship and compliance:
  with doctor and staff
  with medication
- Avoid excessive neutrality: continue enhancing trust
- Tolerate changes in appointments, absences, and delays
- Use psychological approaches, individualizing treatment
- If clear losses, treat as if it was a depression
- Continue showing interest in body and physical illness; be prepared for an increase in physical complaints
- Help physical aspect and physical condition
- Be prepared for the development of depression
- Investigate precipitants of symptoms and their meaning
- Consider the need for some of the symptoms
- Combat loneliness
- Don't forget Body=House; be aware of changes in close environment
- Consider counselling the introduction of a pet
- Continue using reminiscence; support past creative experiences
- Consider the possibility of moving (temporarily or permanently)

Not one of the formal psychotherapies has approached the treatment of the late onset forms of psychosis in enough depth. The clinician has to get by with techniques and ideas used in younger patients or in other forms of old age psychopathology. What follows is a small example of interventions that can be done.

Psychodynamic therapy

From the point of view of psychoanalytic (or psychodynamic in a broader sense) psychotherapy, it is first necessary to review briefly the concept of psychosis. A psychotic process can be understood from this perspective under the following conditions:

- Important difficulties in the perception and relationship with external reality.
- Massive utilization of certain defence mechanisms such as projective identification, disavowal, splitting of the object and splitting of the ego.
- Difficulties in establishing personal boundaries.
- Difficulties in establishing bonds with objects and frequent attacks to the bonds.
- Confusion between the word presentations of and thing presentations of things, with difficulties in establishing links between them, resulting in problems for symbolization.

From a psychoanalytical perspective, the treatment of psychosis has always been controversial. Freud maintained an ambivalent position to the problem. He maintained that it was impossible for the psychotic patient to establish the transferential relationship essential to any analytical cure. Nevertheless, many authors after Freud have tried to demonstrate the opposite. Some have defended the possibility of an orthodox psychoanalytical treatment while others have developed therapeutic modalities different to the type cure, that can be summarized under the heading of applied psychoanalysis (individual analytically inspired psychotherapy face to face, group psychotherapy, psychoanalytic psychodrama, etc.). A question should be raised, following Hochman (1986), on whether the term 'psychoanalysis of psychosis' is a correct formulation or if it can only be maintained thanks to an abusive conceptualization, which includes for example the extension of the diagnosis of psychosis to the borderline states or narcissistic personalities, or consideration of the notion of transference in a lax sense, that is, all the different forms of relationship between the therapist and patient.

Being strict in concepts, terms and formulations, it seems difficult to accept the indication for a standard psychoanalytical treatment for the psychotic disorders in general, and more especially in the case of aged persons. This position is not contrary in any way to the acknowledgement of the potential utility of the treatments that are an adaptation or application of psychoanalysis.

Both adult and elderly psychotic patients have great difficulties in integrating outside reality, perceiving it clearly and separating it from their intrapsychic reality. As previously stated, there are also important defects of symbolization. These circumstances make it absolutely necessary that any form of treatment takes into account the reality. Thus, it will not be possible to perform forms of psychoanalytical psychotherapy within a rigid setting, and a generalized use of elements such as free association or interpretation (even if the patient is seen face to face and the number of sessions is reduced), unless the therapist accepts serious risks of an important psychic regression with dangerous consequences.

It is also essential to remember that this, or any other, form of psychotherapy cannot be done without the necessary integration of the other types of treatment, such as pharmacology or rehabilitation, which are other ways to help establish contact with reality. Medication and psychotherapy should, in many cases and ideally, be provided by the same clinician or at least by a well integrated team. Empathy is of major importance in the treatment of any psychotic patient. Words must not be isolated from acts. The psychotic patient needs both, so both must be offered in an integrated manner. In a number of instances, the psychodynamic approaches to therapy can be better provided in an institutional setting rather than in the usual individual person to person sessions. Such a setting is not necessarily hospitalization as an inpatient. Institutions like day-hospitals or their equivalents can also offer adequate support for treatment. Thus different forms of psychodynamically inspired institutional treatment developed for younger patients can be of much value (Hochman, 1986). Institutional therapy can provide the patient with proofs of the cited empathy because he can have frequent opportunities to experience it, not only through verbal contact but also through acts and facts. Acts are much less frequently encountered in the standard person-to-person therapy.

One of the main objectives of psychodynamic interventions should be to help the patient reconcile himself with his own mental activity, favouring the symbolization processes as much as possible.

Cognitive behavioural therapies

There are a growing number of studies on the role of this form of therapy, mostly related to early onset schizophrenia. One of the most interesting is the London–East Anglia study on therapy with pharmacological treatment resistant patients (Kuipers et al., 1997; Garety et al., 1997). The authors of this well controlled research report an improvement rate of up to 50% in this difficult population. The main predictor of success found was the degree of flexibility about delusions (the possibility that they are not true). Another finding that can be attractive for our field of interest is that impairment in cognitive functions as measured by the investigators did not interfere with treatment outcome. A proportion of the elderly psychotic population do not respond to pharmacological treatment and exhibit minor cognitive impairments. Even though one cannot extrapolate the findings directly to our patients, the research merits an extension to advanced age.

Other techniques used with psychotic patients include the modification of delusional beliefs and control over hallucinations (Fowler et al., 1995), and the reinforcement of coping strategies to overcome both symptoms and the situations that induce or exacerbate them (Garety et al., 1994).

A different potentially applicable field of research is compliance therapy (Kemp and David, 1996; Kemp et al., 1996). Compliance with medication is a major concern in both young and old patients. The form of therapy described by Kemp and colleagues claims a threefold improvement in compliance with pharmacological treatment. Of interest also for the elderly population is that cognitive function was not found to show a relationship to measures of insight or to the degree of compliance itself.

Reminiscence therapy

Therapies based on reminiscence or life review are based on the observations of certain authors, especially Butler (Butler, 1963; Butler and Lewis,

1977), about the process of reactivation of memories experienced by the ageing individual faced with the perception of the reality of death. It is a procedure that provides a more global and complete meaning to what has happened in life until then. Reminiscence is characterized by the return and expression of memories of past events, especially the most significant, both positive and painful.

Reminiscence happens spontaneously during any form of therapy, particularly with the elderly. It can be enhanced by the use of facilitating elements like old photographs, objects, music, old papers, the invitation to talk about past events, or anything that has a definite meaning to the patient.

The possibilities of working with the past and memories vary depending on the patient and the severity of the illness, but should be tried relatively early in most cases and used whenever possible. Coleman (1986) reported that the patients who benefit most from the therapeutic use of reminiscence are those who produce memories spontaneously but in a painful form because of a dissatisfaction with the past, and those who suppress reminiscence because of a dissatisfaction with the present. It is evident that a significant number of psychotic elderly belong to one of these two categories.

Psychomotor therapy

Psychomotor therapy is a complex and elaborate form of therapy developed from the creative genius and impulse of the Spanish psychiatrist Julián de Ajuriaguerra in the 1950s. A simplified definition of its technique is the use of the body and its movement to touch affects. Although it makes use of talk, words are not always necessary and they are substituted by other forms of relationship like movement or relaxation. This is one of the main advantages because it makes it possible to work with patients who are reluctant to make verbal contact, who refuse to talk about emotionally meaningful topics, or when simply words interfere or are insufficient for the diagnostic or therapeutic processes (Agüera-Ortiz, 1993).

Psychomotor therapy makes use of concepts related to the body scheme, the subjective experience of time and space, muscular tone and the different positions between relaxation and movement. Two phases can be differentiated:

Examination. Psychomotor examination techniques can provide very useful information on the patient's body functioning, his adaptive capacities, the balance between an organic or emotional dominance of his process, and the level of concordance and relationship between conflicts expressed (or hidden) verbally and body functioning related to those emotions. The examination has diagnostic value in itself, and can be followed (or not) by therapy.

Therapy. Therapy can be applied individually or in a group. The methods comprise among others, active techniques such as soft exercises resembling gymnastics, working with gait and equilibrium, coordination, the use of voice and shouting, dance, and playing therapeutic games. The passive techniques include the passive mobilization of limbs, the therapeutic use of massage and touch, working with breathing, and especially different relaxation techniques.

Psychomotor therapy was originally developed for child psychiatry but currently it is being used with neurological and psychiatrically diseased elderly patients. Despite the fact that it is not very well known, particularly in Anglo-Saxon countries, it is a very successful form of therapeutic approach, with a history of more than 40 years, that can be used with patients with different ranges of severity. In the hands of a competent therapist it is possible to create a safe, less paranoid atmosphere where patients can feel safe and experience pleasant feelings, both in the corporal and the psychic sphere. It helps with readaptation to the environment and can lessen the rigid armour that paranoid patients build around themselves.

Again, experience with older psychotic patients is not very wide. Nevertheless, it has already proved beneficial, in the same way as with other very disturbed patients such as severe depressives, overanxious regressives or the demented. Working with delusional or post-delusional persons needs a tactful, skilful therapist, because even the more naive intervention like a soft relaxation technique may result in a worsening or reappearance of delusions or hallucinations. Psychomotor therapy can be used safely and effectively in an ambulatory setting. It is also a suitable alternative for inpatients, in particular the more severely disturbed.

The field for research with these or other models is open. Adaptations of the techniques and procedures successfully used with other kinds of patients are lacking despite the necessity of them. For example, a field surprisingly scarcely explored is the adaptation of the great range of psychosocial and rehabilitation therapies already used in younger people with schizophrenia to patients with late onset. Another promising field of interest is the analysis of coping strategies and the subsequent interventions aimed at reorienting and ameliorating the activities to face psychotic phenomena (Abelskov, pers. comm.).

Therapy termination

The majority of primary psychotic diseases tend to be chronic in nature and the late onset forms are not an exception. Maintenance of pharmacological treatment for months or years is necessary more often than not in order to achieve a reasonable remission of symptoms and prevent relapses. Some kind of psychotherapeutic intervention should always be part of the treatment, at least during the time that medication is necessary.

As patients get better, they tend to need a less frequent follow-up or can even be discharged. As with other types of severe mental illness, it is often advisable to consider what can be called an 'open discharge'. This means that, even in cases of an excellent resolution of symptoms, some kind of contact and follow-up should be maintained. This can be assured by distancing the frequency of appointments to one or two per year, or asking the patient and the family to call from time to time, even if it is obvious that everything is going right. The patient will feel better if he knows that the team, the clinic or the institution will be available in case of need. Certain patients may wish to stop coming to the clinic when their symptoms are relieved but the psychiatrist should insist in keeping up at least the kind of loose relationship that will facilitate the prevention of relapses. On the other hand, those patients with more depressive symptomatology can experience the termination of the active therapeutic intervention as some kind of abandonment. These patients need to make some sort of contact or to count on the possibility that they can do so. The clinician should realize this and act accordingly. For most patients, a long-term commitment should be the rule.

Persistence in therapy and drop-out is an issue in all kinds of elderly patients. Mosher-Ashley (1994) reported the results of a large sample of aged subjects who had received psychotherapy for various diagnoses in a community mental health centre. Total completion of the psychotherapy plan as judged by the therapist was achieved by only a small proportion of the sample (less than 12%) but about 60% completed at least ten sessions. Persistence in therapy was found to be related to nursing home residence, the presence of religious beliefs and receiving therapy at home. It is interesting to note from this study that the continuity of psychotherapy was not related to the source of referral (self-referral or other), age or gender. Especially relevant to our field of interest is the finding that the presence of suspiciousness was not significantly related to early termination or drop-out, the opposite to what is usually expected.

THE ROLE OF THE FAMILY AND OTHERS

Contrary to what is commonly said or written, late onset schizophrenia patients often do have families and are in contact with them in various ways. Patients are often included in social networks where the family is the essential nucleus (Semple et al., 1997). Consequently, family members can play a crucial role in the patient's treatment plan. Table 3 shows a schematic way of classifying the possible role of family members, depending on their existence and availability, understanding availability not only as physical proximity but also as willingness to collaborate.

Table 3. Potential roles of the family in helping with the management of the psychotic elderly patient.

Family		Lives with patient	
		Yes	No
Available	Yes	++	+/–
	No	+/–	–/–

+ or – signs express more or less favourable situations.

In fact, family members may be reluctant to intervene in the management of the patient. Especially if the situation is long-standing, the persons involved may be full of resentment and have changed their attitudes from co-operative to frankly hostile. It must be taken into account that certain family members may be sick themselves. Depression is not uncommon and psychosis is more frequent than expected, especially in the case of a child living at home with a psychotic parent.

The family can help the patient and we can help the patient's family. The treatment team needs the support and assistance of the family in order to obtain information and to ensure the continuity of visits to the clinic and treatment compliance. As psychotic conditions tend to be chronic in nature, the family can be confronted with the patient's disruptive behaviour for years. Delusions are not the only symptoms that are difficult for close family members to tolerate. Hypochondriacal and other bodily symptoms can also be a significant source of distress. In the beginning the patient may receive positive support from the family or significant others. Nevertheless, if the situation continues unresolved, they may no longer be able to tolerate the situation. This can create more anger and paranoid feelings on the part of the patient. A true family crisis can be precipitated, and the various family members will probably be playing different roles, not all of them sufficiently adaptive. Sometimes a team approach is more convenient because contacts with family members may be better handled by different members of the team.

It is necessary to inform the family about the nature of the symptoms, and that it is impossible to suppress them by logical argument. Alternatives should be given on how to deal with delusions, for example by tactfully showing evidence against them. To show a supposedly stolen object can be helpful for the patient if it is done in a way that reassures him and diminishes the focus on the delusion, but not if it is done in a way that is interpreted as an accusation that he is not telling the truth. The prognosis of the illness and the importance of medication has to be sufficiently explained.

As is usually recommended in the case of families with a demented person, it is necessary to identify the main care-giver. We should assess the possible excess of stress and signs of mental illness in this person, and look not only for signs of depression – which will be the most frequent case – but also of psychosis. The inclusion of different family members in the evaluation and treatment processes is often advisable. The need to contact other people and include them in the treatment plan can be extended to neighbours or other people related to the patient.

The general practitioner often plays an important role in the management of the patient, sometimes the only role. In this case, the psychiatrist will have to inform the GP about the peculiarities of the illness and explain the symptoms and behaviours that can be expected from this kind of patient. The various alternative treatments should be discussed and decisions taken collaboratively. Creating an effective liaison through frequent consultations will improve the likelihood of the patient being treated successfully.

CONCLUSION

Psychotic illnesses are severe psychiatric disorders at any age. They are usually difficult to treat and the outcome is not always as good as the psychiatrist may wish. Ignorance on crucial aspects of aetiology and psychopathology often limits the possibilities of treatment. But this ignorance should not lead to an oversimplification of the problems or to a therapeutic nihilism. Psychotherapeutic treatments have not been extensively used to date and the efficacy of the different forms needs to be further investigated. But complex problems need multiple and imaginative approaches.

The elderly psychotic patient should not be excluded from receiving psychological help. He may benefit from adaptations of different psychotherapeutic measures. This can include the more classic techniques such as psychodynamic and cognitive behavioural therapies or the newer forms of treatment specially designed for the aged, for example reminiscence or psychomotor therapy. Psychotherapeutic work may influence the psychological precipitants of the psychotic crisis and alleviate the symptoms. It can also help in the early detection and management of non-psychotic symptoms that can secondarily appear during treatment, such as the emergence of depressive symptoms or hypochondriacal concerns. In fact, both examination and management of symptoms can be more easily performed if they are considered within the framework of a three-dimensional axis constituted by psychosis, depression and hypochondria. More research is also needed to clarify the role of the non-psychotic psychopathology in the general picture of the illness.

Any form of psychotherapeutic action with elderly patients suffering a psychotic illness should aim at least to:

– Help the patient gain insight about the illness and how to cope with symptoms.

- Make a reassessment of the past, reliving strengths and achievements.
- Reinforce and reinvest the patient's emptied and suffering self.

Clinicians should never forget that they are treating not only the delusions or hallucinations but also the person who has created them. This person has lived a long life and has a history of emotions and experiences that almost always offers chances to make a psychological approach possible and a truly comprehensive treatment a reality.

REFERENCES

Agüera-Ortiz, L. (1993). La práctica de la Terapia Psicomotriz en Psicogeriatría. *Psiquiatría Pública* **5**, 95–108.

Agüera-Ortiz, L. (1998). Results of a Survey on the Late Onset Forms of Psychosis (unpublished report). Psychiatry Department, Complutense University Madrid, Spain.

Agüera-Ortiz, L., Reneses-Prieto, B. and Calcedo-Barba, A. (1996). Qué papel juegan las psicoterapias en el tratamiento de la depresión en el anciano? In: Calcedo Barba, A. (Ed.), *La depresión en el anciano. Doce custiones fundamentales*. Fundación Archivos de Neurobiologia, Madrid, pp. 225–252.

Almeida, O.P., Howard, R.J., Levy, R. and David, A.S. (1995). Psychotic states arising in late life (late paraphrenia). The role of risk factors. *Br J Psychiatry* **166**, 215–228.

Bentall, R.P., Kinderman, P. and Kaney, S. (1994). The self, attributional processes and abnormal beliefs: towards a model of persecutory delusions. *Behav Res Therapy* **32**, 331–341.

Bergeret, J. (1974). *La personalité normale et pathologique*. Dunod, Paris.

Breitner, J.C., Husain, M.M., Figiel, G.S., Krishnan, K.R. and Boyko, O.B. (1990). Cerebral white matter disease in late-onset paranoid psychosis. *Biol Psychiatry* **28**, 266–274.

Butler, R.N. (1963). The life review: an interpretation of reminiscence in the aged. *Psychiatry* **26**, 65–70.

Butler, R.N. and Lewis, M.I. (1977). *Aging and Mental Health (2nd edn)*. Mosby, St Louis.

Castle, D. and Howard, R. (1992). What do we know about the aetiology of late-onset schizophrenia? *Eur Psychiatry* **7**, 99–108.

Coleman, P. (1986). Issues in the therapeutic use of reminiscence in the elderly. In: Hanley, I. and Gilhooly, M. (Eds), *Psychological Therapies for the Elderly*. Croom Helm, Beckenham, pp. 41–64.

Erikson, E. (1980). *Identity and the Life Cycle*. Norton, New York.

Fowler, D., Garety, P. and Kuipers, E. (1995). *Cognitive Behaviour Therapy for Psychosis: Theory and Practice*. Wiley, Chichester.

Garety, P., Kuipers, E., Fowler, D., Chamberlain, F. and Dunn, G. (1994). Cognitive-behavioural therapy for drug resistant psychosis. *Br J Med Psychol* **67**, 259–271.

Garety, P., Fowler, D., Kuipers, E. *et al.* (1997). London–East Anglia randomised controlled trial of cognitive-behavioural therapy for psychosis—III: predictors of outcome. *Br J Psychiatry* **171**, 319–327.

Hassett, A.M. (1997). The case for a psychological perspective on late-onset psychosis. *Austr NZ J Psychiatry* **3**, 68–75.

Hochmann, J. (1986). Réalité partagée et traitement des psychoses. *Rév française de psychanalyse* **50** Novémbre-Décembre, 1643–1662.

Howard, R., Castle, D. and O'Brien, J. (1992). Permeable walls, floors, ceilings and doors. Partition delusions in late paraphrenia. *Int J Geriatr Psychiatry* **7**, 719–724.

Howard, R., Cox, T., Almeida, O. *et al.* (1995). White matter signal hyperintensities in the brains of patients with late paraphrenia and the normal, community-living elderly. *Biol Psychiatry* **38**, 86–91.

Howard, R.J., Graham, C., Sham, P. *et al.* (1997). A controlled family study of late-onset non-affective psychosis (late paraphrenia). *Br J Psychiatry* **170**, 511–514.

Hingley, S.M. (1997a). Psychodynamic perspectives on psychosis and psychotherapy I: Theory. *Br J Med Psychol* **70**, 301–312.

Hingley, S.M. (1997b). Psychodynamic perspectives on psychosis and psychotherapy II: Practice. *Br J Med Psychol* **70**, 313–324.

Kemp, R. and David, A. (1996). Psychological predictors of insight and compliance in psychotic patients. *Br J Psychiatry* **169**, 444–450.

Kemp, R., Hayward, P., Applewhaite, G., Everitt, B. and David, A. (1996). Compliance therapy in psychotic patients: randomised controlled trial. *Br Med J* **312**, 345–349.

Kinderman, P. and Bentall, R.P. (1996). Self-discrepancies and persecutory delusions: evidence for a model of paranoid ideation. *J Abnormal Psychol* **105**, 106–113.

Kuipers, E., Garety, P., Fowler, D. *et al.* (1997). London–East Anglia randomised controlled trial of cognitive-behavioural therapy for psychosis. I: Effects of the treatment phase. *Br J Psychiatry* **171**, 319–327.

Lesser, I.M., Miller, B.L., Swartz, J.R., Boone, K.B., Mehringer, C.M. and Mena, I. (1993). Brain imaging in late-life schizophrenia and related psychoses. *Schizophr Bull* **19**, 773–782.

Mosher-Ashley, P.M. (1994). Therapy termination and persistence patterns of elderly patients in a community mental health center. *Gerontologist* **34**, 180–189.

Propsner, N. (1997). Pets helping to heal the elderly. *New Jersey Medicine* September, 32.

Ridruejo, P. (1998). Terapia asistida por animales en psicogeriatría. *Proc VII Meeting Spanish Psychogeriatric Society*. Aran, Madrid.

Sadavoy, J. (1994). Integrated psychotherapy for the elderly. *Can J Psychiatry* **39** (suppl. 1), S19–S26.

Schaie, K.W. and Willis, S. (1986). *Adult Development and Aging*. Little, Brown & Co., Boston, MA.

Semple, S.J., Patterson, T.L., Shaw, W.S. *et al.* (1997). The social networks of older schizophrenia patients. *Int Psychogeriatrics* **9**, 81–94.

Thali, A. (1988). Des amanithes phalloïdes et autres poisons – psychodynamique de l'effet non-placebo. *Rééducation* **3** June, 34–42.

Verwoerdt, A. (1987). Psychodynamics of paranoid phenomena in the aged. In: Sadavoy, J. and Leszcz, M. (Eds), *Treating the Elderly with Psychotherapy. The Scope for Change in Later Life*. International Universities Press, Madison, CT, pp. 67–93.

Wattis, J. and Martin, C. (1994). *Practical Psychiatry of Old Age*. Chapman & Hall, London, pp. 165–166.

Weiss, L.J. and Lazarus, L.W. (1993). Psychosocial treatment of the geropsychiatric patient. *Int J Geriatr Psychiatry* **8**, 95–100.

Weiss, M., Gaston, L., Propst, A., Wisebord, S. and Zicherman, V. (1997). The role of the alliance in the pharmacologic treatment of depression. *J Clin Psychiatry* **58**, 196–204.

V

Consensus Statement

19

Consensus Statement of the International Late Onset Schizophrenia Group†

ROBERT HOWARD, PETER V. RABINS, MARY V. SEEMAN,
DILIP V. JESTE
and the Members of the International Late Onset Schizophrenia Group*

SUMMARY

Schizophrenia, whether of early or late onset, from childhood to old age, is fundamentally heterogeneous and presumably consists of a group of related illnesses. We believe that there is sufficient evidence to justify recognition of late onset (onset after the age of 40 years) schizophrenia and a very late onset (onset after 60) schizophrenia-like psychosis.

THE CASE FOR HETEROGENEITY WITH INCREASED ONSET AGE

Schizophrenia-like psychoses can arise at any time in the life cycle between childhood and old age. The expression of such psychotic symptoms shows greatest variation when onset age is at both extremes of life. Variations in epidemiology, symptomatology, pathophysiology, and treatment response with age at onset can help to provide important clues to causative risk factors.

---

†A longer version of this Consensus Statement is in press with the *American Journal of Psychiatry*. This prepublication abstract is published with permission of the American Psychiatric Association.

---

*Kirsten Abelskov, Osvaldo P. Almeida, Nancy C. Andreasen, David J. Castle, Jean-Pierre Clément, Shitij Kapur, David W.K. Kay, Sudhir Khandelwal, Luis Agüera-Ortiz, Godfrey D. Pearlson, Anita Riecher-Rössler, Phillip Seeman, Noriyoshi Takei.

Epidemiology

Female sex is associated with later age at onset. Incidence curves for males and females are different and some preliminary data suggest three adult peaks corresponding to early adult life, middle age and old age (Van Os *et al.*, 1995; Sham *et al.*, 1996). Very late onset cases may arise in the context of sensory impairment and social isolation (Kay and Roth, 1961)

Symptomatology

Early and late onset cases are more similar than different in terms of symptoms (Pearlson *et al.*, 1989; Howard *et al.*, 1993; Jeste *et al.*, 1997). The only study of a large representative sample found almost no differences up to age 60 (Hafner *et al.*, 1998), but in clinical samples, extreme old age is associated with a low prevalence of formal thought disorder and affective blunting and higher prevalence of visual hallucinations (Rabins *et al.*, 1984; Pearlson *et al.*, 1989; Almeida *et al.*, 1995a).

Pathophysiology

Regardless of onset age, schizophrenia is associated with a generalized cognitive impairment relative to age-matched unaffected subjects (Almeida *et al.*, 1995b; Jeste *et al.*, 1995). No difference in type or severity of cognitive deficits has been found between early versus late onset cases. Later onset of schizophrenia is, however, associated with somewhat milder cognitive deficits, especially in the areas of learning and abstraction/cognitive flexibility (Jeste *et al.*, 1997). Brain imaging findings are essentially similar regardless of onset age (Pearlson *et al.*, 1993; Howard *et al.*, 1994; Corey-Bloom *et al.*, 1995). In the old age onset group no excess of focal structural abnormalities have been reported (Howard *et al.*, 1995a; Symonds *et al.*, 1997).

Aetiology

Familial aggregation of schizophrenia is more common in earlier than in later onset cases (Howard *et al.*, 1997). Some studies suggest familial loading for affective disorders in later onset schizophrenia cases. The prevalence of a family history of Alzheimer's disease, vascular dementia, dementia with Lewy bodies or ApoE genotype is not increased in later onset cases (Howard *et al.*, 1995b).

AGE AT ONSET CUT-OFF POINTS

Categorization by specific age of onset ranges is relatively arbitrary. There was general agreement that cut-offs have clinical utility and act to stimulate research effort. Epidemiological evidence is strongest for a cut-off at age 60 to define the very late onset group. Some clinical studies support another cut-off at age 40, although some epidemiological evidence suggests that this age point may be too high for the middle group.

NOMENCLATURE

Consensus was reached that cases arising between age 40 and 60 should generally be called late onset schizophrenia. Cases with onset after the age of 60 should usually be called very late onset schizophrenia-like psychosis.

ASSESSMENT AND TREATMENT

Regardless of age of onset, psychiatric and medical examinations and available investigative procedures should be performed to exclude identifiable aetiologies. The presence of sensory impairments and social isolation should be sought and appropriate remedial action taken. The place of non-pharmacological treatments has not been adequately investigated.

Drug treatment should be commenced at very low doses and increases in dose should be made slowly. Use of low dose depot medication may be successful in ensuring compliance. The atypical antipsychotic agents are clearly advantageous in the treatment of late onset cases, because of the reduced likelihood that they will cause extrapyramidal symptoms or tardive dyskinesias.

REFERENCES

Almeida, O., Howard, R., Levy, R. and David, A.S. (1995a). Psychotic states arising in late life (late paraphrenia): Psychopathology and nosology. *Br J Psychiatry* **166**, 205–214.

Almeida, O., Howard, R., Levy, R., David, A.S., Morris, R.G. and Sahakian, B.J. (1995b). Cognitive features of psychotic states arising in late life (late paraphrenia). *Psychol Med* **25**, 685–698.

Corey-Bloom, J., Jernigan, T., Archibald, S., Harris, M.J. and Jeste, D.V. (1995). Quantitative magnetic resonance imaging in late-life schizophrenia. *Am J Psychiatry* **152**, 447–449.

Hafner, H., Hambrecht, M., Loffler, W., Munk-Jørgensen, P. and Riecher-Rössler, A. (1998). Is schizophrenia a disorder of all ages? A comparison of first episodes and early course across the life cycle. *Psychol Med* **28**, 351–365.

Howard, R.J., Almeida, O.P., Graves, P. and Graves, M. (1994). Quantitative magnetic resonance imaging volumetry distinguishes delusional disorder from late-onset schizophrenia. *Br J Psychiatry* **165**, 474–480.

Howard, R., Castle, D., Wessely, S. and Murray, R.M. (1993). A comparative study of 470 cases of early- and late-onset schizophrenia. *Br J Psychiatry* **163**, 352–357.

Howard, R., Cox, T., Almeida, O., Mullen, R., Graves, P., Reveley, A. and Levy, R. (1995a). White matter abnormalities in the brains of patients with late paraphrenia and the normal community living elderly. *Biol Psychiatry* **38**, 86–91.

Howard, R., Dennehey, J., Lovestone, S., Birkett, J., Sham, P., Powell, J., Castle, D., Murray, R. and Levy, R. (1995b). Apolipoprotein E genotype and late paraphrenia. *Int J Geriatr Psychiatry* **10**, 147–150.

Howard, R., Graham, C., Sham, P., Dennehey, J., Castle, D.J., Levy, R. and Murray, R. (1997). A controlled family study of late-onset non-affective psychosis (late paraphrenia). *Br J Psychiatry* **170**, 511–514.

Jeste, D.V., Harris, M.J., Krull, A., Kuck, J., McAdams, L.A. and Heaton, R. (1995). Clinical and neuropsychological characteristics of patients with late-onset schizophrenia. *Am J Psychiatry* **152**, 722–730.

Jeste, D.V., Symonds, L.L., Harris, M.J., Paulsen, J.S., Palmer, B.W. and Heaton, R.K. (1997). Nondementia nonpraecox dementia praecox? Late-onset schizophrenia. *Am J Geriatr Psychiatry* **5**, 302–317.

Kay, D. and Roth, M. (1961). Environmental and hereditary factors in the schizophrenias of old age ("late paraphrenia"). *J Ment Sci* **107**, 649–686.

Pearlson, G.D., Kreger, L., Rabins, P.V., Chase, G.A., Cohen, B., Wirth, J.B., Schlaepfer, T.B. and Tune, L.E. (1989). A chart review study of late-onset and early-onset schizophrenia. *Am J Psychiatry* **146**, 1568–1574.

Pearlson, G.D., Tune, L.E., Wong, D.F., Aylward, E.H., Barta, P.E., Powers, R.E., Tien, A.Y., Chase, G.A., Harris, G.J. and Rabins, P.V. (1993). Quantitative D_2 receptor PET and structural MRI changes in late-onset schizophrenia. *Schizophr Bull* **19**, 783–795.

Rabins, P.V., Pauker, S. and Thomas, J. (1984). Can schizophrenia begin after age 44? *Compr Psychiatry* **25**, 290–294.

Sham, P., Castle, D., Wessely, S., Farmer, A.E. and Murray, R.M. (1996). Further exploration of a latent class typology of schizophrenia. *Schizophr Res* **20**, 105–115.

Symonds, L.L., Olichney, J.M., Jernigan, T.L., Corey-Bloom, J., Healy, J.F. and Jeste, D.V. (1997). Lack of clinically significant gross structural abnormalities in MRIs of older patients with schizophrenia and related psychoses. *J Neuropsychiatry Clin Neurosci* **9**, 251–258.

Van Os, J., Howard, R., Takei, N. and Murray, R.M. (1995). Increasing age is a risk factor for psychosis in the elderly. *Soc Psychiatry Psychiatr Epidem* **30**, 161–164.

Index